MEDICAL TESTS

Cathey Pinckney
and
Edward R. Pinckney, M.D.

Facts On File, Inc.

MEDICAL TESTS

This is an abridged version of *The Encyclopedia of Medical Tests*, Revised and Updated Edition, published by Facts On File, Inc., in 1982.

The nature of medical testing is that it is constantly evolving and subject to interpretation. Therefore, while the authors of this book have made their best efforts to ensure the accuracy and completeness of the material presented, the reader is advised that no claim can be made that all relevant information concerning the medical tests described in this book is included here. Additionally, the reader is advised that this book is not a manual for self-diagnosis or self-treatment, and is further advised to consult with his or her physician in search of answers or treatment for any medical problems.

Printed in the United States of America

MEDICAL TESTS

Contents

Introduction

"Is there any test that will tell me if I have cancer?"

Some medical tests can hint that cancer might be present; there are a few tests that might even help locate where a cancer might be lurking. But there is no test, at this time, that can guarantee a definite answer for everyone.

"Can a doctor predict whether I will have a heart attack?"

It is not possible to predict future heart disease in healthy people. There are, however, medical tests that can offer early warnings sufficient to prompt preventive measures.

"I think my son is taking drugs; is there any way to be sure?"

There are simple tests a doctor can perform in his office that can expose the use of narcotics. But not all dangerous drugs are readily detected; LSD, for example, is almost impossible to spot.

"Can I find out whether my baby will be born all right?"

While there are several different ways of discerning congenital abnormalities and potentially tragic metabolic disturbances in an unborn baby, not all inherited disabilities can be detected at present. In addition, neither a positive nor a negative test is always accurate.

"My memory seems to be going; is it possible to determine whether something is wrong and do something about it?"

There are ways to test for most kinds of memory defects. Some tests can reveal the specific cause of a loss of memory, which, when determined, may be quickly reversible.

"We just came back from a trip abroad and have been sick ever since. Could we have picked up a strange bug?"

It is not difficult to uncover the germ—or, more likely, the parasite—that is causing repeated bouts of fever, stomach and intestinal problems and even joint aches. The tests take a great deal of patience and uninhibited participation by those who are afflicted. And some forms of hepatitis from exotic countries still cannot be unmasked.

"I can't get pregnant; isn't there some way to prove it's not my fault?"

It is possible to determine, through a series of tests, whether a man is sterile, or so deficient in the production of normal sperm as to be functionally sterile. It is sometimes possible to learn exactly why a woman cannot conceive.

"It seems that medical tests are not always precise. How much can I rely upon a test result?"

Very few medical tests are infallible; most are subject to endless sorts of error; while occasional tests are disease-specific (that is, positive or abnormal results strongly suggest the presence of a specific disease), most can show positive results in the presence of a wide variety of conditions; most tests can also show negative (normal) results even when a specific illness is known to be present. Never depend on the results of one test. Whenever a test you have taken shows a positive or abnormal test value, be sure to have that test repeated two or three times, preferably at different laboratories or in a different doctor's office.

"If that's the case, how can I ever trust any medical test? More importantly, how can I be sure I have all the information necessary to understand a test's results?"

You can never be sure that the result of any single medical test, or even of a single battery of medical tests, is reliable. A test should never be regarded as anything more than a means of confirming other clinical observations: your symptoms, the physical signs you exhibit, your family's medical history and your doctor's observations. If a test result corresponds with everything else, fine; if it does not, you must neither forego proper therapy nor undergo potentially dangerous treatments on the basis of the test alone. Once you are aware that most medical tests are not absolutely reliable, you are well on your way to understanding test results as your doctor does. Your doctor also has an obligation to tell you everything you need to know about any test before you undergo it.

"But what if my doctor won't discuss the details of medical tests with me?"

You have the moral right—and ultimately, the legal right—to be told all medical facts about yourself, including medical test results and their meanings. In Colorado, Hawaii, Illinois, Indiana, Minnesota, Oregon, Virginia and Wisconsin, state laws require doctors and hospitals to allow patients to review and/or obtain copies of their medical records. Ohio courts have ruled that patients have a property right to their records, because the records can help determine the course of future treatments. In California, doctors are supposed to give patients copies of their records, although they may keep the originals from their patients' eyes. Florida law requires physicians, but not hospitals, to show patients their records; in Connecticut, Louisiana and Massachusetts hospitals must show patients the information on their charts, but doctors are not required to do so. Oklahoma law permits a patient to see physical health records, but records concerning mental illness may be restricted if a psychiatrist so demands. Anyone who was once a patient in a hospital or other medical facility operated by the United States government may review all original health records or obtain copies of them. If direct requests fail, you can always obtain a subpoena (court order) forcing the doctor or hospital to provide you with your records; these are almost always granted, unless your doctor can prove to the judge that the information would harm you more than it would help. States change their laws concerning access to medical records periodically, so find out what your state's laws provide so that you can use them in your own behalf.

And you can use this book. When you are told that you should have a specific medical test, or several different tests, you can look each test up and find why it is usually performed; what it is supposed to reveal; whether it is performed on your blood, your urine, some other secretion or excretion or directly on your body; normal and abnormal values and what they might signify; and a reasonable assessment of the test's accuracy. You will also be made aware of any risk factors involved and the degree of pain or discomfort that might be endured by the average person. In several instances you may be surprised to learn that some of your normal daily activities, some of the foods you eat and some of the medicines you take could have an adverse effect on the test's results, producing a false value. Your doctor, or whoever performs a test on you, should inquire about anything that might interfere with testing—but this is not always done, and the consequences could be disastrous for you.

It may seem at times that medical tests can result in miracles. To the parents whose newborn baby is tested for phenylketonuria (PKU), found to have the enzyme deficiency and put on a diet in time to prevent mental retardation, the test is a miracle. And imagine the feelings of a family whose father collapses with what seems to be a heart attack when, within an hour, medical tests prove that he does not suffer from a heart problem at all and that he will recover completely by the next day.

Yet medical tests may also have other, wholly non-miraculous results. Take the case of one 45-year-old automobile dealer. He had experienced slight chest pains off and on for several years, but his doctor had never been able to make a precise diagnosis; his electrocardiogram results were always normal. Finally, the man was referred to a specialist who performed a vectorcardiogram, a variation on the standard electrocardiogram in which subjective rather than objective interpretation of test results plays an important role. The heart specialist thought he detected evidence of a previous heart attack (also known as a myocardial infarction or coronary thrombosis) and told the patient that he had to move immediately from his two-story home to a one-story home so that he would not have to climb stairs; that he could never physically exert himself again; that he had to abandon his ethnic diet for one abhorrent to his taste and incompatible with his way of life; that he had to give up his job because of the constant emotional involvement it required; and, finally, that he had to forego any and all excitement if he wanted simply to stay alive. All this on the basis of one medical test and one doctor's blind belief in that test. The man followed the doctor's recommendations for two miserable years.

Now for the good news. On an impulse, the invalid auto dealer sought out a new doctor. The tests, including the vectorcardiogram, were repeated by a different specialist, and no evidence of any heart disease was found. A third physician was called upon; he confirmed the absence of any disability. The patient was then told that he could return to his former life-style without fear. He has since lived happily for 10 years. With the help of his new doctor, he sued the doctor who had caused him to alter his lifestyle so severely. In court, the doctor could not offer any tangible proof (other than his subjective interpretation of the vectorcardiogram) that heart muscle pathology was, indeed, present; the patient collected a tidy sum to help compensate for the years of misery he had endured.

Never, under any circumstances, rely upon the good or bad results of a single medical test. Any medical test report that could change your life must be repeated at least twice—and in different settings, such as another laboratory or another doctor's office—before it can be considered a valid part of your medical record. What is more, it is a rare medical test whose results cannot be confirmed, supported or substantiated by several other, entirely different medical tests. Equally important, should a test seem to indicate the absence of disease whose presence you or your doctor strongly suspects, that test, too, must be duplicated and triplicated by others before its results are accepted.

If you think this warning is superfluous, you should know that when medical laboratories were tested for accuracy in government surveys, more than one out of every seven test results were found to be either in error or totally unreliable—and that means that the results of at least four million tests every day are inaccurate. Defective testing reagents (chemicals) cause many of these erroneous test results. The Food and Drug Administration reports weekly that test chemicals found to be out of date, contaminated or mislabeled have been seized or recalled.

When thousands of sphygmomanometers (blood pressure measuring devices) were evaluated, one out of every four was found to give wrong readings—mostly on the high side. Similar surveys showed that thousands of electrocardiograph machines were improperly calibrated, and that numerous X-ray machines, often operated by inadequately trained technicians, produced ineffective or faulty X-ray pictures. Again, do not become overly concerned about an initial test that seems to indicate the presence of a medical problem; have the test verified and keep in mind that the odds are more with you than against you.

In the event a laboratory or other test proves erroneous you have strong legal recourse, since the courts have held that a mistake in medical testing is negligence on the part of the testing facility or doctor. This applies to both medical tests that falsely indicate the presence of a disease and to tests that fail to recognize signs of an existing or impending affliction.

When you undergo any medical test, you have the right to expect absolute accuracy. You also have the right to know and understand just what each medical test is supposed to detect; how well it should perform; what extraneous information it might show; what, if any, dangers or possible complications it might involve; and, most of all, just what its results mean to you.

Your rights in medical testing. First and foremost, whenever you have a medical test—whether it requires the use of some machine such as an X-ray, electrocardiograph, spirometer (a device for measuring lung function) or audiometer (an instrument for evaluating hearing thresholds), or the microscopic or chemical examination of one or more of your secretions, excretions, blood or other body fluids—you have the right to assume that every phase of the test will be performed correctly by trained people using properly maintained, precisely calibrated equipment. This amounts to an implied warranty offered to you by the doctor who orders the test and who ultimately interprets the results, as well as the testing facility and the manufacturer of any equipment, chemicals or other products involved in the test. Any error, no matter how slight, is not to be tolerated and should be compensated for, usually by some monetary award.

Just imagine being told you have a high blood sugar, and the subsequent grief that could cause, all because a laboratory technician left the tourniquet on your arm too long just prior to drawing a blood sample; the abnormal concentration of blood in your lower arm would cause almost all evaluations of your blood chemistry to be erroneously high. Or imagine your doctor failing to diagnose diabetes because the laboratory technician left your blood sample standing around for a few hours before analyzing it; as a result, your blood-sugar level would be mistakenly reported as low and your metabolic disease might then progress to dangerous and even irreversible levels.

Almost every clinical laboratory will repeat any medical test, without charge, should you or your doctor feel the test result does not complement your complaints or symptoms or your doctor's suspicions. Although this may help weed out a technical or human error, it is often better to have the test repeated at a totally different facility.

Another of your rights is that you be informed just how precise a test can be, assuming all technical criteria have been met and human error has been eliminated. For even when a test is performed correctly, its results are not necessarily conclusive proof of the existence or nonexistence of a medical problem. Virtually every medical test can be evaluated by three parameters: sensitivity, specificity and predictive value or relative accuracy.

Sensitivity reflects the ability of a medical test to show a positive (abnormal) value where the disease being tested for is actually present. If a test used to detect a specific disease confirmed the correct diagnosis in every case, it would have a 100 percent sensitivity index. If a test showed positive results in only 70 percent of those who had the disease, it would have a 70 percent sensitivity. Unfortunately, few tests have a 100 percent sensitivity rating. The vast majority of medical tests do not always reveal the presence of the disease they are intended to detect. One example is the stress electrocardiogram, which is administered while the patient walks or runs on a treadmill, climbs a few steps or exercises vigorously. The test is designed to show potential heart damage as well as to reveal previously undetected minimal heart damage; patients with the latter condition are considered more susceptible to future heart attacks. Experience has shown, however, that a stress electrocardiogram fails to show potential abnormalities or identify existing heart disease in more than half of all patients who undergo the test.

Just as sensitivity indicates how well a test will confirm a disease diagnosis where the disease is present, a test's *specificity* reveals to what degree that test will falsely imply the presence of a disease in a healthy person or fail to detect the disease in a sick person. Ideally, a test for a particular disease should never show a positive result in anyone who does not have that disease. If a test shows a false result in 25 percent of those who take it, it has a 75 percent sensitivity. A negative result from a test with such moderate sensitivity would not necessarily mean that the presence of the disease could be ruled out. But no test has 100 percent specificity and in too many instances a healthy person has received a test result implying sickness. Once again, the stress electrocardiogram provides a good example; of the people who have taken this test, more than half of those with no known heart disease have gotten results that falsely indicated existing pathology.

As with all medical tests, even sensitivity and specificity are relative. They may vary with the quality controls in different laboratories as well as with the doctor's or laboratory's criteria for normal values.

The third parameter for measuring a test's precision is *predictive value,* or relative accuracy. Predictive value is determined by a mathematical formula that weighs the ratio of true positives (how often the test is right) against false positives (how often the test is wrong) and arrives at an overall figure which indicates the probability of the existence of a disease should a medical test show a positive result for that disease.

Before you submit to any medical test your doctor should make you aware of the sensitivity, specificity and predictive value of that test.

Obviously, there is much more to sensitivity, specificity and predictive value. For instance, these parameters may be affected by the incidence of the particular disease for which a patient is being tested. When a disease is very prevalent, a great many people may show a positive test result without having any symptoms; in contrast, when a disease is rare, a positive test may have much greater significance. Your doctor should take such factors into account when explaining a test's value in your particular case. He might also simply summarize sensitivity, specificity and predictive value by describing the test's *marginal benefit* to you; that is, just how much more knowledge about you and the suspected diagnosis will the doctor have after the test is performed?

The variation in the accuracy and significance of medical tests can be shown by comparing the stress electrocardiogram test to one of the newer tests for diagnosing syphilis. Because the stress electrocardiogram fails to detect heart problems in a great many patients (poor sensitivity) and falsely indicates heart problems in many other people (poor specificity), it is considered to have a very low predictive value, or a relatively low accuracy rating. In contrast, most of today's direct tests for syphilis have a predictive value close to 100 percent; that is, they almost always show a positive result for someone who has the disease (excellent sensitivity) and rarely show a positive result for someone who does not have the disease (excellent specificity). Of incidental interest, many of the older, now out-of-date tests for syphilis, while detecting most cases of the disease (good sensitivity), also showed a positive result for people who had cold sores, jaundice, infectious mononucleosis, bronchitis, pneumonia, childhood diseases (mumps, measles, chicken pox) and some forms of arthritis, and even for women experiencing a normal pregnancy (very poor specificity). Consequently, the older tests, such as the Wassermann, Kline, Kahn, and VDRL, had a low accuracy rating.

Bearing all this in mind, do not be surprised if your doctor insists that you undergo a not-too-accurate stress electrocardiogram test. He probably has spent anywhere from $5,000 to $25,000 for his stress electrocardiogram equipment (treadmill, monitoring machines and related instruments), and at anywhere from a $100 to $300 charge for each stress test, he must do at least one test a week for a year in order to recoup his initial investment and allow the gadget to start making its expected profit.

Before you submit to any medical test, your doctor should make you aware of the commonly accepted accuracy and significance of that test as well as his own interpretation of the test's true value. Only when you know how accurate a test is, as well as your chances of coming up with a false result, can you judge the relative worth of that test for you—and your money.

Why many medical tests are performed. Medical tests are sometimes ordered for reasons over which you have little or no control. On occasion, a test may be demanded by a school, by an employer, by some governmental agency (such as a health department) or by a hospital, whose "routine" admission requirements often wastefully duplicate previous tests, primarily for profit. Most often, however, such tests are for the protection and benefit of the community, health facility or business and not primarily for your personal welfare.

A great many tests are, in reality, nothing more than "fishing" expeditions. True, often a patient has so many vague complaints that a doctor will order a battery of tests, hoping that at least one will lead to a more circumscribed diagnosis. Younger doctors are trained to practice medicine in this manner, substituting the findings of medical tests for the observations of experience. It used to be that doctors questioned and examined their patients far more carefully and applied testing to confirm their suspicions; today, the tests usually come first and it is the test results, more than the patient's complaints, that guide the doctor's ultimate application of therapy.

Defensive medicine. At this point it is important to bring up the matter of "defensive medicine." The ever growing threat of malpractice suits has forced most physicians to erect a pseudo-legal barrier of protection against the slightest possibility of being sued by a patient. And the foundation for this protective shield is the medical test.

Doctors openly admit they are ordering more tests than ever. A recent American Medical Association survey showed that more than three out of four physicians admitted they ordered X-rays, electrocardiograms and a multitude of other medical tests far beyond the requirements of sound medical practice for the sole purpose of having a better defense in the event of a subsequent malpractice suit. It is difficult, at times, to relate many tests a patient undergoes to his or her complaints; it is even more difficult to justify such tests in terms of the ultimate diagnosis. But still they are ordered and performed.

Physicians have learned that a jury will not consider an honest scientific impression based solely on education and experience as sufficient evidence that they acted in good faith. In malpractice trials, according to later admissions by jury members, far more weight is given to a laboratory test which is performed by a machine and which has an ultimate written value that can be seen than to a diagnosis based primarily on a doctor's learned ability. *Failure* to order a certain test—no matter how removed that test might be from the patient's symptoms or how indeterminate for arriving at a diagnosis—is a key element in numerous suits alleging physician negligence. Diagnostic error resulting from inadequate medical testing is the basis of half of all medical malpractice claims against general practitioners and internal medicine specialists.

A physician practicing in the state of Washington examined a patient who had stomach problems. As part of his medical testing, he performed a chest X-ray, a standard electrocardiograph and even some of the enzyme tests. The same tests were repeated two weeks later, and although the enzyme tests were slightly abnormal, the patient had no complaints relative to his heart. Eight years later, after the patient had died of heart disease, the patient's wife sued the doctor for not having given her husband a stress electrocardiogram. The court found the doctor guilty of not having performed the additional diagnostic test and said it was his duty to disclose to the patient every test available to help diagnose all theoretically possible non-life-threatening causes of stomach pain. Thus, the doctor was found guilty of malpractice for not performing a medical test with an accuracy rating of less than 50 percent.

Because of defensive medicine, a patient with a common cold has a 90 percent chance of having his blood tested for 20 or more different substances. A study in New York state law showed that a patient complaining of a sprained ankle will have *both* ankles, legs and feet X-rayed (primarily to show any difference between the two ankles, legs or feet) along with nearly a dozen chemical tests that could indicate bone pathology, a bone metabolism defect (such as gout), rheumatic disease, anemia and even chronic alcoholism. This is true even in cases where the doctor is 99 percent sure it is nothing more than a sprain. More than any other reason, including the increased ability to diagnose disease, the existing legal process is responsible for the growth of medical testing.

On being a participatory patient. One way you can participate in test evaluation is to ask your doctor what the reason is for the test.

By fully understanding the need for a test and its purpose and knowing your past medical history and, especially, that of your family, you may come up with the answer to some obscure medical problem. You could even avoid a great deal of supplementary, possibly painful and irrelevant testing. For instance, if diabetes runs in your family, there is a better-than-average chance the condition will afflict you; consequently, you should inform your doctor of such a potentially inherited trait so that he can first concentrate on the obvious rather than spread his testing far and wide for the cause of your symptoms. Since many forms of anemia, heart and kidney problems, eye and ear difficulties and even skin disorders are genetic in origin, information on your family's illnesses could be particularly relevant to your medical problem.

Another reason for you to know why your doctor is ordering one or more tests for you is to prevent duplication of testing. It is not unusual for one doctor to follow the same line of reasoning as another doctor, based on your complaints, and repeat tests that you have already had. Your symptoms, for example, may make a doctor think the problem is related to your kidneys; if you tell your doctor you have had kidney tests repeatedly without any abnormal findings, you might avoid possible complications resulting from needless testing. Unless your doctor can justify repeating tests that were done in the past, you should not subject yourself to such a waste of time and money and an unnecessary hazard.

The obvious concern arises, "But what if my doctor won't tell me why he is ordering a test and what if he says that I wouldn't understand the results anyway?"

Nonsense! It is not difficult for a patient to understand that a doctor is looking for some sort of problem, a thyroid condition for example, and that the tests ordered are to determine the specific nature of the problem. (Of course, if you feel cold when others around you are warm, or if you always seem to be hot in a cool environment, you are already more than halfway to your diagnosis.) Furthermore, how complicated can a thyroid problem be? To be sure, there are always a very few people who have some rare and exotic type of illness, but the vast majority of thyroid gland dysfunctions are common, easily diagnosed and even more easily treated.

Again, assuming you learn that your doctor is searching for a suspected thyroid condition, you should find out just what other information the tests might, rightly or wrongly, reveal. It is all too common for a particular test to hint at another, totally different condition that may or may not exist. Unfortunately, thousands of people are treated needlessly for essentially fictitious diseases simply on the basis of some random test finding totally unrelated to the original search. It is even sadder than much of this seeming misfeasance is due more to the patient's ignorance of or lack of interest in his condition than to incompetence or greed on the part of the doctor. By becoming a participatory patient you will assure yourself of the best possible care.

"That's fine," you say, "but what if my doctor still won't tell me anything?" You have a legal right to know what your doctor has decided about your condition, and how he came to his decisions. Do not be put off by the idea that the jargon is similar to a foreign language or that the terms will be too difficult to understand. In almost all instances the information a doctor writes in a patient's chart is in plain English, and a medical dictionary can be consulted for any terms that are not explained. The information is about your physical well-being and may have a direct bearing on your life. You must make the decision to use it in your best interests.

When your doctor orders you to undergo any medical tests, one of the best examples of patient participation is to ask: "What will you do if the test value is abnormal? What will you do if the test value is normal?" If the doctor gives the same answer to both questions, you should then ask, "Why do the test?"

Risks vs. benefits. Every medical test carries some degree of risk that must always be weighed against the expected benefits. Your doctor is legally required to warn you about all possible risks before you undergo any test. Only then can you make an informed decision about whether the possible information to be derived from the test is worth the possible dangers that might accompany the procedure. The doctrine of "informed consent" protects you from being forced to make a decision without first being offered all relevant information in plain English.

Unfortunately, the law also assumes that your submission to a medical test—especially the simpler ones, such as blood examination—implies your consent. In many courts the very fact that you willingly let your blood be taken, or exposed your body to an electrocardiogram or X-ray, or allowed your doctor or a technician to look inside of you with some sort of observation device has been considered sufficient evidence that you had the opportunity to question your doctor or the technician about all prospective dangers and either did so or deliberately avoided doing so. In such cases it can be very difficult to prove that potential risk factors were purposely hidden from you. Therefore, never assume a medical test is relatively harmless until you feel you have had that test procedure explained to your satisfaction.

Invasive vs. non-invasive tests. When considering risk factors, a distinction must be made between invasive and non-invasive tests. Any test that involves penetration of the body is, literally, an invasive test. An invasive test normally poses a much greater risk than a test that does not penetrate the skin or an orifice of the body. The use of plethysmograph to detect thrombosis of the leg is non-invasive; the injection of dyes or nuclear radioactive substances into the leg is not only invasive, but carries a greater degree of risk without always offering a greater significance for diagnosis. While some doctors feel that the simple sticking of a needle into the arm to draw blood should not be considered invasive, in truth it is, as is the insertion of a sigmoidoscope, a bronchoscope or a catheter. Recent research has revealed that the use of an invasive test itself is sufficient to produce a false abnormal test result where no abnormality exists, and where an equally productive non-invasive test would show a normal result.

Whenever an invasive procedure is ordered, ask if there is a non-invasive test that would be just as efficient.

Consequences and alternatives. Of course, there is another aspect to the risk factor of testing: knowing and understanding just what the consequences may be both in having the test and, equally important, in *not* having the test. Forgoing a proposed medical test might be much more dangerous than any possible risk associated with the test. If you are told to have a Pap test to look for early signs of cancer and you hesitate, you may hesitate for too long and your cancer, assuming it exists, may grow to an incurable stage. For years a woman refused her doctor's advice to have a Pap test. When she died of cancer, her family sued the doctor, claiming the physician had failed to impress her sufficiently about the dangers of not having the test. A doctor is required to disclose all information relevant to a meaningful decision by the patient, generally including the nature of the proposed medical test or procedure, its purpose, the risks involved *and* the alternatives to it. Only in this way can the patient's decision not to have the test be considered an "informed refusal."

Alternatives may include different but related tests. The use of an echocardiogram in place of angiography is a good example. An echocardiogram entails no invasion of the body (no needles, no catheter, no dyes, no radioactive chemicals) and, consequently, no pain or discomfort. Angiography, however, is a prolonged, painful procedure that poses dangers. Many cardiologists feel that an echocardiogram can provide sufficient data for a diagnosis in the vast majority of cases where the two tests could be used.

And there are a great many alternatives to various radiographic tests that are potentially far less harmful. Computerized tomography (CT or CAT scanning) is a painless, non-invasive technique that provides a more efficient means for studying the brain than pneumoencephalography, an X-ray test in which air is injected through the spinal cord into the brain. CAT scanning may also eliminate the need for a myelogram, a potentially dangerous procedure in which dye is injected into the spinal canal to study the vertebrae and their spacing; if some of the dye remains in the canal, leg paralysis can result. Plethysmography, the application of a blood pressure cuff around the leg attached to recording instruments, can often reveal a thrombosis (blood clot) as efficiently and with far less risk than the injection of a dye into the supposedly clogged vein to make it stand out on an X-ray (the dye itself can cause thrombosis).

In attempting to detect developing physical defects, as opposed to inherited metabolic disorders, the use of a sonogram (a picture produced by soundwaves) may offer as much information about a fetus as an amniocentesis test, which has inherent dangers for both mother and child. Ultrasound testing can replace many other potentially harmful tests used for diagnosing liver, gallbladder, kidney and other gland problems. It can also differentiate cysts, clots, abscesses and other masses from solid growths, thereby eliminating the need for a great deal of unnecessary exploratory surgery. In addition, many new tests utilizing radioimmunoassay techniques (which examine blood samples for minute chemical imbalances) can be substituted for some risky and uncomfortable poking and digging around in your body in the search for cancers.

But unless you are made aware of the alternatives, you cannot make an informed decision about whether or not to undergo a test or battery of tests. While one doctor may well prefer and even insist on a more hazardous test approach, you are entitled to know the reasons for his choice and just why he considers the alternatives inappropriate.

Your final, ultimate right in medical testing is to be made aware of any existing test that might make a difference in your way of life. After a 38-year-old woman gave birth to a child with a congenital defect, she sued her doctor for not informing her that there was a practical test (amniocentesis) which could have warned of the possibility of a birth defect. The court not only awarded the woman a cash settlement but forced the doctor to pay the cost of her daughter's medical care for life. In another, somewhat similar case, a woman who was not tested for rubella (German measles) when she became pregnant gave birth to a defective child; she sued her doctor, who was then required to make financial restitution for not informing the woman that the rubella test existed and should be perfomed on all pregnant women.

While knowledge of existing medical tests is not the responsibility of the patient, you should be aware of all available tests relevant to any medical problem or condition you may have.

Should any test, whether performed as a screening panel or as an individual test in the privacy of your doctor's office, indicate a reportable disease, your doctor *must* notify the proper government authorities. In addition to infectious diseases, such as tuberculosis, typhoid and sexually transmitted diseases (venereal diseases), diabetes, epilepsy, heart ailments, senility, alcoholism and any other affliction that could affect your ability to drive a car must also be reported.

Costs. The vast majority of patients do not pay for medical testing directly but have it paid for through health insurance plans. Although most people do not care about the cost of testing, they are wrong in assuming that someone else is paying for it. Employers' payments for workers' health care are reflected in the cost of merchandise; so, indirectly, you are still paying for the increasing cost of medical tests. Surprisingly, the cost of medical testing, both direct and indirect, runs close to $140 billion a year, or nearly half the total cost of all medical care. While hospital bills seem to be the greatest single health cost item, medical testing accounts for the largest portion of a hospital bill—even larger than the separate costs for a patient's room, nursing care, use of operating rooms and maintenance. At the same time, medical tests provide the greatest source of income for hospitals, which is why many hospitals demand that every patient undergo a battery of tests upon admission—even though they may have been performed the day before in a doctor's office or a laboratory. Duplicate testing generally has more financial than diagnostic value.

In general, commercial laboratories charge the lowest fees for medical tests, and hospitals charge the highest fees; the cost of tests performed in doctors' offices usually falls somewhere in between. Hospitals justify their relatively high fees by claiming that the profits from testing make up for financial losses in other areas. There are no controls or regulations governing the cost of medical tests, although some insurance companies and certain govermental agencies may limit the amount of money they will pay for a particular test. Geographical location and the affluence of the community where it is performed also affect the cost of a test; an electrocardiograph in a small midwestern town will average $25 while an identical test in Beverly Hills, Calif. runs from $50 to $150.

Although there are no firm figures for the cost of specific medical testing, studies indicate that assuming the usual growth in the number of medical tests, the cost of laboratory tests now totals almost $30 billion; radiology and related testing techniques amount to $20 billion, $1 billion of which goes for coronary angiography alone; electrocardiography, endoscopy, biopsy, eye, ear and other instrumental tests add up to $40 billion; and the additional expense of hospitalization solely for testing purposes is $50 billion.

And yet these figures are not half as surprising as some other observations made by other researchers who attempted to assess the value of medical tests. One study showed that in spite of the expense of medical testing, only five percent of all laboratory tests actually resulted in altered patient care or had any impact on a patient's diagnosis or treatment. Another study revealed that the majority of doctors never even looked at the reported results of medical tests after they were recorded on hospital charts.

Doctors are constantly being reminded of the profit to be made from medical testing by salesmen at medical meetings and by articles in medical journals. One recent advertisement for an electrocardiograph machine in a major scientific publication was headlined: "Buy the EK-8 now and receive enough ECG supplies to reward you with $3,000 potential income." The ad went on to say that if a doctor purchased the machine, the company would then furnish, free, enough supplies to produce 150 electrocardiograms, which, at a minimum fee of $20 per ECG, would cover the entire cost of the machine. A doctor performing no more than five electrocardiograms a day would have his money back in 30 days and well over $20,000 profit before the year was over. (Most physicians and hospitals charge far more than $20 for an electrocardiogram; in 1981, in a similar advertisement aimed at doctors, the minimum fee was raised to $25.)

Lest you think that doctors must invest a great deal of time and money learning how to read and interpret electrocardiograms, there are many services that read ECGs for doctors and charge from $1 to $2 per reading, depending on the volume of business. Some even transmit the ECG and its analysis over the telephone while it is being performed.

It has become extremely profitable for a physician to perform most blood and urine tests in his own office. Machines that perform dozens of routine examinations, at a minimum cost to the patient of $5 per test, are now available to doctors for less than $1,000. A doctor who performs tests in his office can charge a health insurance plan or governmental health program or agency several hundred dollars for the same number of tests a clinical laboratory, using automated equipment, will perform for a fraction of the cost. He can also perform 10 different urine tests by simply dipping a 25¢ strip of chemically-coated plastic into his patient's urine specimen and charge $5 or more for each test.

There are commercial clinical laboratories that charge doctors $6.50 to carry out up to 27 different chemical analyses of a patient's blood; some will even perform 42 tests for $14.50. Incidentally, the quality of work performed by a laboratory in a doctor's office is not always under direct supervision, evaluation, inspection or control by government or professional agencies, as is the case with most commercial laboratories, which must demonstrate their competence regularly.

An article in a recent medical journal described how any physician could easily triple his income by performing most medical tests in his office. It was estimated that such testing would add at least $60,000 in net income to a doctor's earnings.

Thus, medical testing has far more of an economic than scientific impact on a patient's care. At the same time, doctors admit that the present fee system for medical care far better rewards physicians who rely on medical tests and testing apparatus than those who use cognitive skills—a doctor's reasoning and judgment based on training and experience. As one doctor put it: "Why not gastroscope [perform an examination of the walls of the esophagus, the stomach and, at times, the first part of the small intestine] every patient at five hundred dollars for fifteen minutes' work, when an hour's time devoted to listening to and examining a patient will only bring in eighty-five dollars at best?" Backing up this philosophy, a study by the Congressional Office of Technology Assessment, called "The Cost-Effectiveness of Upper Gastrointestinal Endoscopy," concluded: "Current financial incentives undoubtedly encourage physicians to perform many more endoscopies than are clinically justified at this time. Steps should be taken to discourage the unnecessary use of this procedure and to lessen the financial incentive by lowering reimbursement to doctors who perform such tests."

It is easy to see why X-rays and other tests that require expensive instruments or machines are much more in vogue than in necessary service.

Of course, there is the other side of the coin. As one internist put it: "Try and limit a patient's testing to one or two evaluations; he'll go right out and find another doctor who will perform an endless barrage of tests. It seems as if you can never test a patient enough—and relevance is never considered by either party."

While health insurance plans and government-sponsored medical care programs actually reward doctors in proportion to their use of medical tests, and while fear of malpractice has forced an increase in testing, the patient's faith in medical tests is an equally important factor in their increasing use. Patients mistakenly believe that having as many tests as possible ensures better medical care.

In most instances, if you are a member of a health insurance plan and your doctor is also part of that plan, the total cost of medical testing is paid to the doctor, with no extra charge to you. If, however, your doctor is not a member of your insurance plan and has not agreed to accept the insurance fee as total payment, you may have to make up the difference. Depending on the number of tests performed, this could amount to hundreds of dollars. Before you undergo a test, check with your doctor to see if there will be any additional costs to you.

Where tests are performed. Most medical tests are performed in a doctor's office, at a commercial laboratory or in a hospital. A sample for a blood test can be obtained anywhere—even at home—and then analyzed at any one of the three usual places. Almost all tests that involve X-rays, including those that use dyes or radionuclear substances as well as computerized tomography, can be performed in a doctor's office, although the latter is most often carried out in a radiologist's office or a hospital. Heart function examinations, including exercise testing, usually take place in a physician's office. A few tests, such as cardiac catheterization as part of angiography, and some endoscopy procedures, are more likely to be performed in a hospital setting; doctors prefer to have a patient check into the hospital the night before a test so as to control his or her activities and environment prior to testing. Some physicians like to keep their patients in the hospital an extra day after certain complicated or extensive examinations, such as angiography, or dilatation and curettage. Where a test is done may depend as much on who the referring doctor feels is the best qualified to perform the test and interpret the results as where the equipment is located. There are no hard and fast rules about where a test should be performed; the doctor's convenience, not the patient's, may well be the deciding factor.

Patient-related causes of inaccurate test results. The more tests that you undergo, the greater the possibility that some hint of a non-existent disease process will arise. While test results may make it appear that you have incipient diabetes, heart or kidney trouble, a hormone deficiency, a hidden infection or even cancer, the cause may well be something you ate, drank or did the night or day before. Although you really have no control over the ineffective chemicals, inefficient machines and other sources of error in a laboratory, you can reduce the possibility of a faulty test result caused by your own activities.

Here is a list of things that can affect the results of medical tests.

Medications. Aspirin, laxatives, cold pills, cough preparations, sleeping aids, vitamins, nose drops, pain relievers and, especially, stomach antacids can markedly alter a test value. Prescription drugs have an even greater influence on medical testing. In 1972 the American Association of Clinical Chemists published a list of over 9,000 different adverse effects on laboratory tests caused by drugs alone and the list has been growing ever since.

Birth control pills (oral contraceptives), which many women do not regard as a medicine, can greatly alter the value of more than 60 medical tests, including 15 of those most frequently performed. Alcohol, too, can affect test values; a very small amount will distort blood pressure testing, lipid tests (such as for cholesterol and triglycerides), the prothrombin time test and any form of diabetes testing (glucose, insulin, etc.).

Before you undergo any test, inform your doctor and/or laboratory performing the test about every medication you are taking; the doctor can then decide whether to have the medication discontinued prior to the test or taken into account when the test results are evaluated.

Diet. A great many food substances can alter test results. For example, iodine from table salt, fish, hot dogs or other foods can totally disrupt the outcome of certain thyroid function tests. Foods containing large amounts of vitamin K (green leafy vegetables or fish) may cause abnormal values in prothrombin time tests; some of the chemicals in commercial French-fried potatoes will adversely affect prothrombin time for a week. Drinking milk before a calcium or phosphorus test will lead to inaccurate results. Coffee can cause a false positive uric acid test. Even water can affect test results; there are times when water should be avoided prior to testing, just as there are times when a specified amount must be consumed. Consumption of bone meal tablets as a food supplement can cause cancer-like abnormalities on X-rays.

Routine activities. A patient's daily routine, including his sleeping habits, can have a direct effect on certain tests, especially hormone evaluations. If a patient works all night and sleeps during the day, the physician should be informed of this. Physical activity or lack of it can influence the results of a great many tests. For example, a renin test will have different results depending on whether a patient has been lying down or standing up just before blood is taken. Excessive exercise, including running, can produce what seems to be abnormal values even though there is no disease process.

Work-related factors, such as indirect contact with certain chemicals on the job, can alter many test results. The amount of noise in a work location and even the lighting conditions can change the body's hormone production, which in turn can distort certain test results.

Attitude. If a patient experiences stress or anxiety a few days before a test or at the time the test is performed, the altered mental attitude can produce an abnormal test value. A patient who is kept waiting a long time for a test appointment may have a false abnormal result, especially if waiting causes him or her to miss another important appointment. The test values for a blood sample from a male patient can be altered by the fact that the sample was taken by an attractive female technician.

Physical factors. Sex, age, height, weight and body surface area must be taken into account when interpreting the results of a medical test. It is perfectly normal for a woman to have a sedimentation rate twice as high as that of man. Most pulmonary function tests and some hormone tests are dependent on size and physical build. Test results may even vary because of changes in the weather. Some families have genetic traits that produce abnormal test values even though no true disease condition is present. More than 100 million people have an inherited glucose-6 phosphate dehydrogenase enzyme deficiency (rare in central European Caucasians), which causes a hemolytic type of anemia (destruction of red blood cells) in reaction to certain drugs and false abnormal test values in testing for certain other types of anemia.

If the test you want to know about is not in the book... The medical tests listed in this book are those in regular, if not always frequent, use. Some tests are utilized only by specialists; other tests are almost routine with a visit to the doctor. Although new medical tests are introduced to doctors every day, most of these are experimental and will never gain professional acceptance. Such tests, often without any proven scientific value, are most frequently performed in hospital settings where research and teaching predominate. Other tests may become outmoded, either because newer, more specific, easier, less complicated or less expensive substitutes come along, or simply because the tests never really proved their worth in spite of their common use.

But most old, outmoded tests do not die; they rarely—regardless of their cost or value—even fade away. While a majority of doctors now consider the basal metabolic rate (BMR) test to be one of the least accurate means of measuring thyroid function, it is still used relatively frequently. This may be because many antiquated but profitable BMR measuring machines are still around, or because some doctors feel more comfortable employing this once-standard test as a confirmation of nuclear age techniques. Should your doctor order this test for you, the chances are quite slim that your health insurance company will pay for it. Nor will most insurance companies reimburse you or your doctor for a cephalin flocculation test to help diagnose liver disease, yet many laboratories still receive requests for, and perform, this particular test.

As a matter of fact, in 1981 dozens of different tests were declared outmoded, unnecessary, unreliable and even useless by various professional medical organizations, health insurance programs such as Blue Cross and Blue Shield and even the Food and Drug Administration. And yet, in spite of this ostensibly cost-saving measure, most doctors say they will still order almost all of the "outmoded" tests solely to protect themselves from malpractice suits. And, backing up the doctor's attitudes, a spokesman for the American Bar Association's Commission on Professional Liability has stated: "If the doctor doesn't request some test that he should have, there *is* a potential for liability." Furthermore, he said that if a patient were subsequently to come down with a condition completely unrelated to what the doctor was treating the patient for, if the condition might have been detected with the help of a medical test—no matter how outmoded or obscure—the patient's lawyers might well use this "oversight" to justify awarding money to the patient. Again, no matter how obsolete or ineffective a doctor or an insurance company may consider a given test, if a lawyer can convince a jury that the test in question *might* have been of some value, the doctor could be found negligent.

You should know which medical tests have been classified as outmoded, whether by medical associations, insurance companies or government agencies. When such tests are ordered for you, most likely you will have to pay for them yourself, unless your doctor can convince a medical review board of the absolute necessity of that test under your specific circumstances.

But the fact that one state insurance company may consider a medical test outmoded does not necessarily mean that reimbursement will be refused in another state. Each insurance plan sets up its own rules, and only your doctor knows which medical tests are covered.

Outmoded or unproved tests, at present, include:

- Amylase isoenzymes that detect the different forms of amylase to help distinguish between pancreas disease and alcoholism
- Angiography using motion picture film or when employed to obtain quantitative measurements of the heart's chambers
- Ballistocardiography to help diagnose heart disease
- Basal metabolism rate to help diagnose thyroid function

- Capillary fragility or coagulometer to help differentiate blood clotting diseases
- Cephalin flocculation as a measure of liver disease
- Chromium poisoning tests
- Congo red to confirm amyloid disease
- Drug abuse screening for narcotics, barbiturates, caffeine or nicotine when performed on body tissues
- Drug monitoring for certain drugs, such as guanase, iodine or digitalis, in the urine
- Endoscopy when contrast dye is employed to outline the bronchial tubes for X-rays or for nuclear scanning of the lung
- Feces examination for calcium or starch to help diagnose malnutrition disorders
- Gastric analysis for pepsin (a stomach enzyme that aids in digestion) or as part of the diagnex blue test to evaluate stomach acid
- Hair analysis
- Icteric index as a measure of liver disease
- Impotence testing employing ultrasound or the penile tumescence monitor
- Leucine aminopeptidase in the urine to help distinguish liver disease from bile duct problems
- Non-protein nitrogen as a measure of kidney function
- Pesticide poisoning tests
- Phonocardiogram to help detect heart disease
- Pneumoencephalography (radiography of the brain using air as the contrast medium)
- Pregnancy tests employing rabbits, frogs or rats
- Protein-bound iodine as a measure of thyroid function
- Pulmonary function tests when used primarily for screening, a sometimes routine procedure for hospital patients
- Red blood cell indices, which are simply mathematical calculations based on other blood tests, such as hemoglobin, hematocrit and red blood cell size
- Skin reaction testing for brucellosis, cat-scratch fever, certain fungus diseases, certain sexually transmitted diseases (Frei), psittacosis and trichinosis
- Streptococcal agglutination testing
- Syphilis testing employing the treponema pallidum immobilization technique
- Thymol turbidity as a measure of liver disease

In contrast to the tests now considered outmoded, two tests that were once so classified have now been restored to the good graces of health insurance payment; they are:

- Culture and sensitivity studies to indicate the exact cause of an infection and also show which drugs will likely be most effective in fighting the organism responsible for the disease
- Lead screening to help detect lead poisoning

With each passing year more and more medical tests will undoubtedly be labeled as superfluous—or possibly unprofitable—but do not be surprised if you are ordered to undergo an antiquated test; be even less surprised when it turns out that you must pay for the test directly in spite of your health insurance coverage.

Again, the tests listed in this book are in actual use regardless of any controversy over their value. Where possible, their significance and value are stated. To many physicians, the value of certain tests is relative; one doctor may swear by a particular test that another doctor abhors. Yet it is the ultimate diagnosis that counts and every doctor is entitled to utilize the procedures that he feels will result in successful diagnosis and treatment. Tests in themselves cannot and do not make diagnoses; they assist, amplify and confirm a doctor's thought processes—nothing more.

Two caveats. If, after reading this introduction, you are still not sure of the need to participate actively in your medical testing, remember that in several recent studies anywhere from 25 to 50 percent of abnormal test results reported to doctors were *not* followed up by those doctors. Surprisingly, some doctors simply ignored test reports that indicated the possibility of pathology—even when the tests were ordered by the doctors themselves and were not required as part of a hospital admission program. If you go through the trouble of having a test performed, you should see to it that the results of that test are not simply made known but fully explained to you. It is your body and your life.

Finally, it must be stressed that this book is not a manual for self-diagnosis. Although some tests may be indicative of specific disease processes, no test or battery of tests can be considered conclusive in determining the cause, presence or absence of illness. Even when an abnormal test value is consistent, it alone may not be considered diagnostic. A medical test must always be interpreted in the context of the patient's symptoms and the doctor's other findings. A test in itself is relatively meaningless; it is only one of many guides to a patient's health.

How To Use This Book

Finding a test. Tests are listed in alphabetical order under the name most commonly used by doctors. Where a test is known by other names or terms, the most customary alternative references are listed in the index. For example, the most common name for a thyroid function test is T_4. Some doctors use the term thyroxin and others may order a hyperthyroid test. Yet all these terms refer to the same test. In addition, there are more than a half dozen other thyroid tests, all of which assess the functioning of the thyroid gland. If a test is not listed, it is probably not in common use. The tests selected for inclusion in the book were drawn from a survey of those tests regularly, even if infrequently, performed at several hospitals, many different commercial laboratories and in the offices of 50 physicians representing all the various specialities in medical practice.

If there are different but closely related tests that might reveal similar information, such tests are noted. Tests that appear in **boldface type** are described separately under their own names.

When performed. Medical tests are performed primarily to confirm a doctor's diagnosis. Because so many medical tests do not have a specific purpose, the same test may be performed to help diagnose many different diseases. Physicians also order medical tests when their suspicions do not coincide with a patient's symptoms or complaints. In such cases it is not unusual for a doctor to order a battery of different tests with the hope that one or more test results will raise a red flag and help narrow the focus toward a precise diagnosis.

Normal values. The normal values cited for a test are those commonly accepted by the medical profession. Where laboratory test results are reported in numerical form, a patient need not understand the exact meaning of the measurement associated with that numerical value (mg per 100 ml, mMol, mEq), but he or she should be able to note whether the reported value of a test lies within or outside the normal values for that test. In almost all instances normal values reflect the test results found in 95 percent of supposedly healthy people. In the case of laboratory test results, normal values may vary from laboratory to laboratory, primarily because of different technical procedures employed; a normal value obtained by one laboratory may well be considered abnormal by a different laboratory. In the case of non-laboratory tests, such as X-rays, electrocardiograms, reflex tests or nuclear scanning observations, a doctor usually draws his own conclusions on the basis of training, knowledge and experience with a large measure of subjective evaluation. Thus, all normal values should be considered primarily as reference points, and are sometimes called "reference range." Some medical tests have such a wide range of values within normal limits that it takes a significant deviation from the normal to indicate the possible presence of a medical problem.

Certain doctors, however, define reference range, or limits of normal values, much more narrowly than the majority of their colleagues. This, of course, leads to a far higher index of disease suspicion. It is therefore important to know each doctor's concept of normal values and whether it differs from commonly accepted standards.

A test result that is within normal limits does not guarantee that the disease being tested for is not present. Sometimes a shift in test values, even within the limits considered normal, can be as much an indicator of illness as an abnormal value. It is the clinical interpretation of a test value by a doctor, taking into account all other related facts, that ultimately determines whether a test result is normal or abnormal.

Abnormal values. Depending on the type of test, abnormal values are either expressed in numerical terms or described. Since in numerous medical tests an abnormal value could be caused by any of a hundred different diseases, only the most common conditions reflected by an abnormal value are listed.

It must be reiterated that a single abnormal test value does not necessarily signify the presence of a disease. Because of the likelihood of error in medical testing any test with an abnormal result must be repeated, preferably by a different physician or laboratory. When a reported abnormal test value is critical, most doctors will insist on a third evaluation before attributing significance to the results. Consideration must also be given to those daily activities of a patient that may directly affect medical test results and cause false abnormal values (diet, drugs, smoking, etc.).

Risk factors. Almost every medical procedure, be it a test or a treatment, involves some risk. The hazard posed by sticking a needle into a vein, while negligible, does exist. General risk factors for blood testing, the insertion of catheters and needles, the use of contrast substances (dyes), the application of X-rays and radioactive substances and the employment of electrical instruments, which comprise the vast majority of tests, are listed here and simply noted in each appropriate test. Where a specific medical test involves greater risk factors, the dangers are described under the test heading.

General risk factors.

Blood testing. Blood is normally taken from a vein in the antecubital area (inside the arm, in front of the elbow, where the arm bends); samples are also drawn from arteries or veins in the groin area, the neck, the back of the hand, the finger tip, the ear lobe and from the heel. In the case of infants, blood is commonly obtained from veins along the side of the head.

Although the dangers related to the insertion of a small needle through the skin are relatively minimal, there are a few possible complications. The most notable hazard is called hematoma, which usually occurs when the needle goes through the vein to the opposite side of the intended vein puncture site or when the technician makes several unsuccessful attempts to find the vein. Blood then extravasates (leaks) into the surrounding areas, swelling the adjacent tissue and usually turning the skin black and blue. A hematoma is rarely dangerous and usually disappears within a few weeks. More often than not this occurs in a patient who has been taking large amounts of aspirin or a drug prescribed to keep the blood from clotting; it may also occur in a patient who has high blood pressure. Although the reported incidence is extremely rare, there is the remote possibility that a severe hematoma could cause destruction of any tissues affected. Another extremely rare risk is the breakage of the needle within the body; although this problem is not necessarily serious, a subsequent surgical procedure might be required to locate and remove the needle. When needles and glass syringes are cleaned and reused, as opposed to utilizing disposable ones, there is always the risk of infection, especially hepatitis, depending on the the effectiveness of resterilization.

Catheter and needle insertion. A catheter is a thin rubber or plastic tube that is inserted into the body, most commonly in the arm, groin area or neck, to pass through to a specific location (guided by X-rays) in order to deliver test materials to a precise spot (heart chambers, arteries of the heart, kidneys or particular areas of the brain). At times, depending on the area to be tested, a rigid metal needle is used in place of a catheter.

Although the dangers are almost as remote as using a needle to obtain blood for testing, they do exist. Needles are usually used to guide a catheter into the body. Catheters sometimes break off in the body, necessitating surgery to effect their removal. The risk of infection from catheters increases proportionately with the amount of time they remain in the body, which is almost always a prolonged period.

Needles and/or catheters are also inserted into the bladder to obtain sterile urine samples; into joint spaces, where the risk of bone infection is not uncommon, even when meticulous antiseptic techniques are observed; and into the ducts of various body glands, such as the salivary glands, to obtain test material. Whenever ducts are probed, in addition to the risk of infection and catheter breakage, there is always the scant but real possibility of tearing or rupturing the duct, causing a condition that usually requires surgery and is difficult to repair.

Contrast substance (dye) use. Many tests involving organs of the body depend on the use of a contrast dye, either swallowed, inserted by catheter or enema or injected into the blood stream. The dye, no matter what its chemical name, is resistant to X-rays and thus markedly enhances an organ's image on an X-ray picture. When swallowed, the dye, usually a barium mixture, fills the gastrointestinal tract from the esophagus through the stomach to the intestines, outlining each portion of the bowel much more than if the intestines contained nothing but food or air. The failure of the dye to outline a portion of the organ being studied usually indicates a "filling defect," or abnormal area. Different chemical dyes are used to study different organs of the body.

New evidence indicates that some contrast dyes, especially those used in angiography, may cause damage to chromosomes; this is in addition to that caused by prolonged X-ray exposure. The subsequent offspring of young people on whom the contrast substance is used could consequently be affected. Otherwise, the risk attending the use of any contrast dye is primarily one of allergy, although other adverse reactions have been reported. In general, one out of every 58 patients receiving a contrast dye as part of a testing procedure has some sort of detrimental response. For every 10,000 to 40,000 times a test using a contrast dye is performed, a patient dies as a direct result of the test. The risk factors increase dramatically with patients who have any sort of allergy, and those with known allergies must be pre-tested meticulously for the slightest sensitivity to contrast dye prior to undergoing such a test.

X-ray and radioactive substance application. The application of X-rays and radioactive chemicals to the body is not innocuous no matter how minimal their use or how common the procedures. X-ray dosage can be cumulative and not show any evidence of damage until many years later. Some of the risks of excessive X-ray exposure include hair loss, skin changes that may lead to cancerous lesions and even organ changes.

Some other, lesser or more remote risk factors include loss of elasticity from the skin (this makes the skin look much older than it is, particularly the facial area) and possible deleterious effects on the reproductive organs. Whenever X-rays are taken, even such small pictures as dental X-rays, a lead shield should be placed over the lower abdomen to protect the ovaries or testicles.

Electrical instrument use. Any time a testing machine utilizes electricity, there is always the risk, although minute, of electric shock and even electrocution. While such instruments are usually kept in proper working order, there have been enough instances of faulty equipment or operator carelessness to warrant mention of this hazard. In addition, it is also dangerous to use electrical instruments in the vicinity of explosive gases or chemicals, such as anesthetic gases, including even ether.

Failure of electrical equipment presents another risk factor. In many tests, such as computer tomography or nuclear scanning, television cameras or cathode ray tubes are used to visualize internal organs. In several different X-ray examinations involving contrast dyes, television is used to watch the dye disbursement. It is not unusual for a television screen to go dead or for some highly integrated electrical circuit to fail at the precise moment it is needed. While the electrical mishap is not directly harmful, it may necessitate a prolonged delay of the testing procedure, which, in the case of a catheter inside the heart, a dye inside the knee or injected radioactive material, can be dangerous. Electrical failures may thus force repeat testing, indirectly doubling or tripling any of the test's original inherent risk factors.

General pain/discomfort factors. In describing the amount of pain or discomfort a person might feel in undergoing various tests, it is difficult to be specific. Every individual perceives and tolerates pain differently. The quantity and quality of pain is so subjective that it is impossible to say one kind of pain is minimal while another is excruciating. The prick of a needle in the arm and the subsequent drawing of blood may be a negligible annoyance for one person and agony for another. Only you can really know the extent to which you feel and react to pain and other forms of discomfort. There are patients who feel tormented when forced to lie motionless on a hard table, as is often required for many different X-ray examinations, nuclear scanning procedures and ultrasound observations and even for an electrocardiogram and an electroencephalogram.

For some people embarrassment can be far more uncomfortable than pain. Having to urinate on command may be quite a trial. The necessary exposure and probing of the body can also cause distress. More than a few people are mortified when they have to furnish a stool specimen for a feces examination; yet even that experience may not be as bad as having to undergo a semi-public enema or other rectal survey. And, in spite of the so-called new sexual freedom, there are still many women who feel embarrassed when they have a gynecologic examination, just as there are many men who become unsettled when tested for impotence, fertility or sexually transmitted diseases. For a patient who is claustrophobic, pulmonary function tests conducted in small sealed chambers can be insufferable.

Fear or anxious anticipation of a test procedure or test result is fairly common. The time required for a test, including waiting time, can cause apprehension. For example, a glucose tolerance test requires at least five hours, during which time blood and urine samples are collected every hour, or even every half-hour. Almost all X-ray tests that utilize dyes require you to lie still for one to two hours after the tests are completed so that you can be treated immediately for any allergic reaction. Any test that involves physical activity should be explained so that you will not be shocked when you find you have to exert yourself, for example, walking uphill on a treadmill for several minutes.

You also should be alerted to all consequent physical reactions to tests. After certain eye examinations, the drops in your eyes may blur your vision for hours—even to the point where it would be dangerous to drive a car. If skin tests are to be performed you may want to wear long-sleeved clothing to avoid feeling self-conscious about the many conspicuous red blotches on your arms after leaving the doctor's office. All potential invasions of body areas in the course of an examination should be explained to you ahead of time. Other conceivable vexations such as repeated feces collection should never come as a surprise. Thus, the more you know about the details of any test, the less anxiety you may experience.

Blood testing. Most people rate needle puncture as a momentary, slight pain. The amount of discomfort, of course, depends to a large extent on the technician (usually called a phlebotomist) who draws the blood—be it from the arm, finger tip or elsewhere. For a number of people the apprehension of the needle coming toward them is more distressing than the actual pain of the insertion. Some people (usually children) automatically scream throughout the process. An experienced technician who can locate the best vein and insert the needle into the vein without hesitation will automatically reduce the level of perceptible pain. If, however, you find needle puncture particularly painful, there are ways to alleviate the pain. A local anesthetic (a cream, ointment, liquid or even a freezing spray) can be applied to the test area a moment or two beforehand. Injections of nerve-end numbing drugs under the skin are sometimes used, but many people feel the burning from the drug insertion is as painful as the needle itself. In most instances, a smaller-size needle is less traumatic; the large needles so commonly used are primarily for the technician's convenience to hasten the procedure. Disposable-type needles are always much sharper and therefore less irritating than needles that are resterilized and reused—most often without being resharpened.

Catheter and needle insertion. Many tests require the insertion of a catheter into a blood vessel, body organ or body cavity. Needles are sometimes used to insert dyes and other radio-opaque substances and radioactive chemicals. They are also employed to obtain body tissue or fluid specimens for study.

In essence, a catheter is nothing more than a flexible needle and is used accordingly, especially to direct a diagnostic substance to a particular part of the body, such as the kidneys or heart. If repeated sampling must be performed, it is not unusual to insert a catheter and leave it in place until the test is completed; it is much more comfortable than a rigid needle. In almost all instances the area where a needle or catheter is inserted is anesthetized first, leaving the skin or organ surface numb. Catheters are also inserted into body orifices, such as the urethra (where urine exits from the body) to collect a sterile urine specimen or to allow dye to fill an organ, e.g., the bladder. Most people consider such procedures quite uncomfortable but not unbearable. Unfortunately, it is difficult to apply completely effective anesthesia to such passageways.

Most other tests may well cause discomfort, but should any

test have an inherent ability to cause pain, a doctor or technician can usually alleviate the pain by one or more methods.

Where performed. The cost of a test may depend more on where that test is done than on the simplicity or difficulty of performing it. More than 90 percent of all tests can be and are performed in a doctor's office, assuming the office has the necessary laboratory facilities, instruments or equipment such as an operating room, an X-ray machine or an electrocardiograph. In the case of blood tests, some doctors, or their assistants, draw the patient's blood and then send it to a commercial laboratory. Other test specimens, such as urine, feces, biopsies, material for culture, etc., may also be obtained in a doctor's office and then sent out for evaluation. Where special or unique equipment is required, patients may be referred to a hospital or teaching center. Should a test require careful observation afterward, it is almost always performed in a hospital. There are times when a doctor will send a patient to a hospital for a test more as a matter of the doctor's—as opposed to the patient's—convenience. On the other hand, in some cases health insurance companies will reimburse the doctor or the patient for the cost of the test only if it is performed in a hospital, regardless of the necessity for hospitalization.

Accuracy and significance. The interpretation of the accuracy and significance of any medical test is relative. The conclusions arrived at came from a review of the current medical literature and a consensus of physicians who most often utilize the tests. Even though some tests may seem indicative of specific disease processes, no test or even a battery of tests can be considered absolutely conclusive in determining the cause, presence or absence of illness. The significance of any medical test must always be interpreted within the context of a patient's medical history and symptoms and the doctor's observations from physical examination of the patient. A medical test in and by itself is relatively meaningless; it is only one of many clues to a patient's condition. Doctors do not always agree on the accuracy or the significance of a test. Many doctors swear by a test that their colleagues deem virtually worthless. Much of a test's significance depends on how a physician applies the result of that test to his patient's condition.

As but one example of the relativity of a test's accuracy and significance, in the same issue of a medical journal one doctor reported that the accuracy of the occult blood test for colon cancer was 92 percent—more than twice as accurate as a direct sigmoidoscopy examination—while another doctor wrote about how most medical articles cite the same test as yielding almost 60 percent false-negative reactions—where the pathology was not detected by the test.

The American College of Physicians, a group of specialists whose members are primarily internists, cardiologists and experts in metabolic and endocrine diseases, has been studying the relative value of medical tests for many years. Its finding thus far is: "Unfortunately, there exists no unambiguous method for evaluating medical technology, and the many studies lead to confusing conclusions." In other words, at the present time there are no absolute standards for the accuracy and significance of medical tests.

A

ACID PHOSPHATASE

Acid phosphatase is an enzyme found primarily in the prostate gland. The male hormone testosterone causes the prostate to secrete acid phosphatase into the bloodstream. Blood is taken from an arm vein for serum examination. Urine and prostatic secretion are occasionally tested. Direct aspiration of the prostate by needle is also used to test for prostate disease.

When performed: If there is a suspected abnormality of the prostate gland; to help identify metastasizing carcinomas (spreading cancers).

In suspected rape the vaginal fluid may be tested for prostatic acid phosphatase to prove sexual intercourse took place. Many rapists have abnormal sex gland functioning and do not produce sperm; a woman who has been raped may not show a positive sperm test but will usually show a positive acid phosphatase test. In addition, sperm usually disappear after a day or two, but the acid phosphatase remains for at least 72 hours. (Sperm have, however, been found up to seven days after intercourse. See **Semen.**)

Normal values: Several different methods are used to measure acid phosphatase; the values vary with the method used. The most common values are 0 to 2.0 Bodansky units; 0 to 0.65 Bessey-Lowry units; 0 to 5.0 King-Armstrong units; and 1 to 1.9 IU per liter.

Abnormal values: Acid phosphatase is elevated with metastatic carcinoma (spreading cancer) of the prostate and the spread of some other cancers (a normal acid phosphatase is not an assurance of no cancer), Paget's disease (thickening and softening of the bones), and a form of bone cancer called multiple myeloma. The King-Armstrong method can detect moderate rises in cases of pneumonia and hepatitis, as well as with certain cancers. The Bodansky method is more specific for prostatic cancer. Prostatic examination or massage will also elevate serum acid phosphatase levels, as will the taking of the drug clofibrate (Atromid-S).

The newer radioimmunoassay technique to detect prostatic acid phosphatase (RIA-PAP) is more sensitive and should make it possible to obtain an earlier diagnosis of prostate cancer.

Risk factors: Negligible (see general risk factors for blood testing).

Pain/discomfort: Minimal (see general pain/discomfort factors for blood testing).

Accuracy and significance: This test is considered the best laboratory test for detecting prostate disease in its early stages. Radioimmunoassay testing is considered 90 percent accurate. A negative RIA-PAP test is considered about 85 percent accurate in indicating the absence of prostate cancer. A positive test can be caused by conditions other than prostate cancer (anemia, severe infections, hormone diseases that affect bones, thrombophlebitis, heart attack, diabetes, kidney disease and other forms of cancer). Most doctors regard a rectal examination as the most accurate test for prostate cancer.

AGGLUTINATION

Agglutination means the clumping or gathering together of cells (usually red blood cells) into a mass; normally each cell exists separately. This phenomenon can easily be seen under the microscope; in many instances it can also be viewed with the naked eye when the lumps settle into the bottom of a test tube or clump together on a glass slide.

Agglutination occurs as a reaction against various diseases, primarily infections. Whenever the body is exposed to bacteria, viruses, fungus, or a toxin that contains antigens (the agents that cause disease), it reacts by producing antibodies. These antibodies then attempt to fight off the specific organism that has invaded the body. Antibodies found in a patient's blood indicate that the patient has already been exposed to a particular infection. The exposure may have occurred many years previously or it may be of very recent origin.

The principle behind agglutination testing is always the same: to see if antigens of a known condition have already caused a defensive (antibody) reaction against that condition. If antibodies are present and clump with the known antigen, the test is called positive. Some antigens combine with antibodies only in cold temperatures, some need warm temperatures, some clump better when exposed to latex particles, and some show clumping best when sheep red blood cells previously exposed to the disease are used. Sometimes the cells flocculate, or fall like snowflakes, clumping at the bottom of the tube.

A single positive agglutination test is not usually sufficient to make a diagnosis. To determine if the disease is recent enough to be the cause of a patient's symptoms, two or three agglutination tests are performed within a few weeks. The serum is diluted first with equal parts of an innocuous solution and then progressively down to one part serum to well over a thousand parts of diluent (e.g., 1:1,064). The result is reported by titer (the highest titer represents the weakest solution in which agglutination occurs). A noticeable rise in titer with each test usually indicates an active disease with more and more antibodies being formed daily. Blood is taken from a vein and the serum is tested. Thus sometimes the test is called "serology."

A related test, **Complement Fixation,** is also used to diagnose mysterious infections. The two tests may be given together. At times the same disease will give a positive reaction to the agglutination test as well as the complement fixation test. At other times a particular disease will respond only to one of them.

Coombs' test for agglutination (there is a Direct Coombs' and an Indirect Coombs') is used primarily in blood conditions. A positive Direct Coombs' usually signifies erythroblastosis fetalis (the Rh anemia of newborns) and hemolytic anemia (where a person's own antibodies destroy his red blood cells). The Indirect Coombs' is used to detect Rh blood-type factors. Unfortunately, a great many drugs, including penicillin, cause a positive Direct Coombs'.

There are a number of new adaptations of agglutination and **Complement Fixation** tests. The fluorescent antibody study (FA) is one such adaptation. It is a technique which treats a specific disease antigen with a fluorescent dye that attaches itself to a patient's antibodies—if they are present in the patient's blood—thereby signifying the presence of the disease. This test also provides quantitative results that indicate the progress of the disease. Some doctors designate the particular procedure to be used, and refer to a direct fluorescent antibody test (DFA) and an indirect fluorescent antibody test (IFA).

Another recent adaptation is the enzyme-linked immunosorbent assay (ELISA); it too is used to detect antibodies to bacteria, parasites, some viruses, and certain antigens. Although the methods are similar to those used in radioimmunoassay (see **Nuclear Scanning**), this procedure employs an enzyme rather than radioactive chemicals to bind the antibodies. Far more rapid results are possible with these two adaptations (some report results the same day) than with standard agglutination techniques.

When performed: The test is used most often when there is a persistent fever, such as occurs with an infection that cannot be diagnosed. Specific infections for which different forms of agglutination tests are conducted include:

Amebiasis
American trypanosomiasis
(a form of sleeping sickness)
Brucellosis
(undulant fever, usually resulting from association with cows, sheep, or goats and their unpasteurized milk)
Cryptococcosis
(a fungus-caused meningitis)
German measles or **Rubella**
(an agglutination test is required by law in some states at the time of marriage or pregnancy to determine if a woman has had the disease, and to immunize her if not); see **Rubella.**
Histoplasmosis
(a fungus-caused lung infection)
Infectious **mononucleosis**
Legionnaires' disease
(pneumonia)
Melioidosis
(a generalized infection common in drug addicts)
Q-fever
(a rickettsial pneumonia; rickettsia are a form of bacteria)
Rat-bite fever
Schistosomiasis
(swimmer's itch)
Streptococcal infections
Tapeworms
Toxoplasmosis
Trichinosis
(primarily from eating raw, infected pork)
Tularemia
(rabbit-handling fever)
Typhoid fever
Typhus
Virus conditions

Agglutination tests are also performed to help diagnose rheumatoid arthritis; to ascertain the specific cause of certain allergic reactions, such as to cow's milk; to diagnose certain anemias caused by the Rh factor; to determine a person's blood type, such as A, B, AB, O, or Rh; and even to ascertain pregnancy.

By noting which type of blood a person's serum agglutinates, the physician can determine that person's blood type and therefore the type of blood that would be safe for transfusion if ever needed.

Whether a mother will react to the Rh factor during pregnancy is also determined in the same way. By mixing a woman's urine that contains the hormone increased during pregnancy with the antiserum for that hormone and observing for agglutination, the physician can ascertain if the woman is pregnant.

Normal values: While agglutination reactions to disease should not be present, an old, forgotten infection can cause a positive test. Usually, though, the titer is quite low, averaging less than a 1:64 dilution. Unless this titer suddenly rises (is present in much greater dilutions) within a few days, it is not considered evidence of any active disease. When it comes to blood typing, there are no normal values.

Abnormal values: If the titer of a patient against a specific disease rises within a few days to a week, it can reasonably be concluded that the patient is manufacturing a great many antibodies against that disease and therefore is harboring the organism that causes the disease. Sometimes agglutination tests are performed against a number of different infectious diseases; the one that shows the highest, increasing titer usually indicates the diagnosis. A titer over 1:64 is needed to be of definitive value.

Well over half of all people with rheumatoid arthritis show a positive agglutination test to latex particles (the reason is not known), but then so do some people with systemic lupus erythematosus and chronic infections. A few drugs such as methyldopa (for high blood pressure) and some pain relievers can cause a false positive test; in contrast, excessive use of certain antibiotics can mask a positive agglutination test, making it appear negative.

Risk factors: Negligible (see general risk factors for blood testing).

Pain/discomfort: Minimal (see general pain/discomfort factors for blood testing).

Accuracy and significance: Most agglutination tests, and particularly those using IFA, DFA, and ELISA are considered 90 percent accurate. There are a few exceptions, however. The test for Legionnaires' disease has approximately an 80 percent accuracy while the test for trichinosis has only about a 60 percent accuracy. A negative test is not regarded as conclusive evidence of the disease's absence.

ALBUMIN/GLOBULIN (A/G Ratio)

Albumin and globulins are the main total plasma proteins in the blood. These proteins aid in maintaining the osmotic pressure of the blood (keeping a balance between the percentage of chemicals and plasma), provide nutritive substance for tissues, and carry essential substances such as hormones, vitamins, drugs, and enzymes throughout the body. There are four different globulins; the largest in number are the gamma globulins, which carry the immune bodies to help fight disease. The average person produces about 15 g of plasma proteins a day. Blood is taken from a vein and the plasma or serum is tested. The results are stated as a ratio of the amount of albumin to the amount of all the globulins.

The different forms of the primary plasma proteins are also detected through electrophoresis (a technique rather than a test). This method of applying an electrical charge to the proteins and observing their migration on paper gives an indication of the amounts of albumin and the globulins. Although the patterns that result may indicate the presence of disease, they are not considered specific.

Albumin and globulin are also measured in other body fluids; the presence of albumin (protein) in the urine is an indicator of kidney disease. However, people with a condition known as orthostatic albuminuria automatically excrete albumin in the urine when they are on their feet for long periods of time. It signifies no disease.

When performed: If there are problems of food absorption; to distinguish starvation from other diseases; in various liver and kidney diseases; when there is a question of infections, especially when there seems to be no resistance to infection; when cancer is suspected.

Normal values: The total proteins (primarily the sum of the albumin and the globulins) average 7 g per 100 ml. Usually there is almost twice as much albumin, 4.5 g per 100 ml, as there are globulins, 2.5 g per 100 ml; and when the amount of albumin is divided by the amount of globulins, the normal A/G ratio averages two to one (2:1). Ratios from 1.5:1 to 2.5:1 are within normal limits. No protein should be detected in the urine.

Abnormal values: With diseases that affect the blood proteins, the amount of albumin is usually decreased and the globulins increased, thereby reversing the usual A/G ratio. In liver conditions especially, the amount of albumin decreases because of that organ's inability to manufacture it; gamma globulins increase, since they are made outside the liver. In kidney problems both the serum albumin and gamma globulins decrease, but the alpha and beta globulins increase. In starvation, because little or no protein is eaten, all the blood proteins are decreased. The same decrease in the proteins is found when food cannot be absorbed because of various diseases.

Alpha antitrypsin (AAT), an antienzyme globulin, is decreased in inherited liver disease in children and lung disease in adults. Another globulin, **Alpha Fetoprotein** (AFP), usually disappears from the blood after birth but is sometimes found in adults with liver and other cancers.

Risk factors: Negligible (see general risk factors for blood testing).

Pain/discomfort: Minimal (see general pain/discomfort factors for blood testing).

Accuracy and significance: The majority of doctors consider the presence of albumin in the urine to be the most accurate indicator of kidney disease. There is one exception. Some physically active people, such as athletes, may show small amounts of albumin in the urine; however, after lying down for several hours, they should have no albumin in the urine. In general, albumin/globulin tests do not specify a particular disease, and they should be viewed as confirmation of other diagnoses.

ALCOHOL

Testing for the body's ethyl alcohol content—whether in the blood, the breath, or the urine—is most commonly related to the legal question of driving while drunk. Police and highway officers often measure alcohol concentration in the breath, which reflects blood levels. After alcohol is consumed, it reaches a peak in the blood in about half an hour's time. It takes about three hours to eliminate each ounce of alcohol ingested. Thus a blood alcohol test is fairly reliable for many hours after the last drink. The blood alcohol test is also an important diagnostic tool when an unconscious person is brought to an emergency facility.

Blood, breath, or urine may be tested. Blood is taken from a vein. Breath is usually collected in a bag or balloon, or it may be exhaled directly into a measuring instrument. In the urine test, the individual must first empty the bladder and then wait a minimum of 20 minutes before the test sample is taken so that the specimen accurately reflects the amount of body alcohol at the time of testing.

When performed: The test is performed not only to determine if alcohol has been consumed but, of greater importance, to determine the degree of alcoholic intoxication so as to apply proper treatment. It can also help determine the cause of coma and is used to discriminate antihistamine or tranquilizer overdosage from alcohol toxicity.

Normal values: Normally there is no measurable amount of alcohol in the body. When less than 0.05% of the blood (50 mg per 100 ml) is composed of alcohol, it is usually not considered intoxication in the legal sense.

Abnormal values: Three ounces of an average (86-proof) liquor will usually produce symptoms of intoxication and cause a blood alcohol level of over 0.05%, which in many states is sufficient to cause prosecution as "under the influence." Other states have laws that stipulate more than 0.10% as evidence of intoxication; a few states insist on alcohol levels of 0.15% before issuing a citation. Ten ounces of liquor will usually produce stupor or coma and will cause blood alcohol levels to measure 0.4%. Twelve ounces at one time has caused death. Urine levels are always about 50% higher than corresponding blood levels. Breath values parallel blood values.

Abnormally high test values will result if, just prior to inserting the needle to take blood, the technician wipes the skin with alcohol, or if the individual belches while breathing into a bag or measuring device. The use of alcohol-containing mouthwashes prior to a breathing test can also cause higher values.

Risk factors: Negligible (see general risk factors for blood testing).

Pain/discomfort: Minimal (see general pain/discomfort factors for blood testing).

Accuracy and significance: If performed properly, the test is considered very reliable. Any evidence that the specimen has been improperly collected, handled, transported or evaluated in the laboratory usually disqualifies the test result for legal purposes. Urine tests are not as accurate as blood tests; breath tests, when properly performed, are considered as accurate as blood tests. While a false positive test result is rare for blood alcohol, a true positive test occurs in only about half of all people afflicted with alcoholism.

ALCOHOLISM

The **Alcohol** test (whether from blood, breath, or urine) is a measure of the amount of alcohol in a person at the time the test is taken. It does not in any way indicate whether the patient is a chronic user of alcohol. There are, however, tests that can reveal whether a person is a heavy drinker, or even an alcoholic, in spite of that person's denial. One such test is the measurement of enzymes, either gamma glutamyl transferase (GGT) or gamma glutamyl transpeptidase (GGTP). Others include the folic acid test (see **Folates**), **Uric Acid** test, measurement of **Zinc** levels in the blood or urine, measurement of **Sweat,** and measurement of certain amino acids in the blood such as alpha-amino-n-butyric acid and glutamate dehydrogenase (GDH) that indicate liver damage.

Outside the realm of biochemistry, there is the Self-Administered Alcoholism Screening Test (SAAST). Originally known as the Michigan Alcoholism Screening Test, and subsequently modified and improved upon by the Mayo Clinic, the test consists of 35 questions; the answer to each is designated as "alcoholic" or "non-alcoholic." The questions are quite direct; two examples are: "Have you ever lost friendships because of your drinking?" and "Has your wife, husband, or other family member ever gone to anyone for help about your drinking?" When the test was compared with drunken driving arrest records and enyzme measurements, it was found to be about 95 percent accurate.

When performed: Whenever alcoholism is suspected or when patients are admitted to hospitals in coma or undiagnosed unconscious conditions; to aid in uncovering patients who might become alcoholics; to aid in the treatment of patients who show symptoms of alcoholism but who deny drinking; to follow the progress of a patient's therapy.

Normal values: Normal values range from 30 to 45 units per liter (men usually have higher amounts) for GGT; less than 25 units per liter for GGTP. Amino acids have varying normal values.

Abnormal values: GGT will rise to 500 to 1,000 units per liter depending on how heavily the person has been drinking and for how long; the GGTP enzyme will usually go above 250 units per liter. Normal amino acids will double in alcoholics. Folic acid will decrease, and uric acid will increase. It takes more than 5 ounces of alcohol a day, on a regular basis, to affect these test values; but the greater the alcohol intake, the higher the test value.

Risk factors: Negligible (see general risk factors for blood testing).

Pain/discomfort: Minimal (see general pain/discomfort factors for blood testing).

Accuracy and significance: The GGT test is considered more accurate than the GGTP but both tests are considered to have an accuracy rate between 40 and 80 percent. Other causes of liver disease can result in false positive tests; some people, on the other hand, can consume a dozen drinks a day and still show negative tests. Questionnaire-type tests are considered more accurate than chemical tests—especially for predicting the possibility of future alcoholism. Patients taking antiepileptic drugs may show a false positive GGT test.

ALKALINE PHOSPHATASE

Alkaline phosphatase is an enzyme normally found in the blood. Different forms of this enzyme are also produced in the intestines, liver, and bone cells. Conditions that stimulate bone cell activity and that deposit excess calcium in the bones create elevated alkaline phosphatase levels in the blood. A single test for alkaline phosphatase is insufficient for diagnosis; it must be evaluated several times. Blood is usually taken from an arm vein for serum examination. All urine passed in an 8-hour period (usually overnight) may also be tested. In certain rare diseases alkaline phosphatase is also observed in white blood cells.

When performed: When cancer is suspected; to differentiate the causes of liver disease; following injury; when parathyroid disease is suspected; to study nutritional problems such as Vitamin D deficiency.

Normal values: Values vary with the kind of test measurement used: 2 to 4.5 Bodansky units; 0.8 to 2.3 Bessey-Lowry units; 3.0 to 13.0 King-Armstrong units. Normal values are higher in children because of bone growth activity.

Abnormal values: Higher than normal values are found with cancerous and noncancerous bone disease, liver disease, blockage of the bile duct system (gall bladder disease), Gaucher's disease (a type of anemia), healing fractures, rickets, leukemia, thyroid gland infection, and hyperparathyroidism; values may also rise during the latter part of pregnancy. Elevated alkaline phosphatase levels are caused by a number of drugs, including male hormones, tranquilizers such as Thorazine, antibiotics such as erythromycin and oxacillin, some antiarthritic drugs such as gold and Indocin, and oral antidiabetic drugs. Birth control pills will also elevate alkaline phosphatase levels.

Lower than normal values are found in patients taking too much vitamin D or too little vitamin C, and in conditions of poor nutrition. Patients taking Atromid-S to reduce blood cholesterol levels have been reported to have falsely lowered alkaline phosphatase levels, which could mask the diagnosis of certain liver diseases; it has also been noted that patients who take Atromid-S have a much greater incidence of gall bladder disease.

Risk factors: Negligible (see general risk factors for blood testing).

Pain/discomfort: Minimal (see general pain/discomfort factors for blood testing).

Accuracy and significance: This is a very generalized test that shows abnormal values in the presence of so many different diseases that it is really used only for screening, supplementation, and confirmation.

ALPHA FETOPROTEIN (Fetal Alpha Globulin)

Alpha fetoprotein is the primary serum protein (see **Albumin/Globulin**) of the fetus during pregnancy; it usually disappears totally from the newborn's blood immediately after birth. Should it reappear in later life, it most likely indicates liver cell pathology. Blood is taken from a vein and the serum is tested. Amniotic fluid (the fluid around the fetus) is also tested.

When performed: When liver disease, especially liver cell cancer, is suspected; when a cancer (most likely from the ovary or testicle) is thought to have spread to the liver; as a means of following the progress of therapy in the treatment of hepatitis; on amniotic fluid, see **Amniocentesis.**

Normal values: Normally no alpha fetoprotein is found in the blood except in pregnancy. During pregnancy up to 2.5 mg per 100 ml may be detected in the amniotic fluid, depending on the month of gestation.

Abnormal values: Any amount found in the blood serum of an adult (young children may still have a trace) is abnormal and commonly indicates a liver cell cancer; however, it can on occasion be found in other cancers and thus is not an absolute diagnostic indicator. It sometimes appears during recovery from hepatitis. When alpha fetoprotein is increased in amniotic fluid, it can indicate a problem with the fetus such as spinal cord defects.

Risk factors: Negligible when blood is tested (see general risk factors for blood testing). With examination of amniotic fluid, see general risk factors for catheter and needle insertion.

Pain/discomfort: Minimal when blood is tested (see general pain/discomfort factors for blood testing). With examination of amniotic fluid for alpha fetoprotein, see general pain/discomfort factors for catheter and needle insertion.

Accuracy and significance: Considered 90 percent accurate in revealing ovarian and testicular tumors, 80 percent accurate for liver cancer, and less than 50 percent accurate for other cancers. When the test is properly performed, any abnormal values found in amniotic fluid are considered very significant. Unfortunately, poor technical procedures lead to false abnormal values.

AMINOACIDURIA

Abnormal amounts of amino acids appear in the urine whenever there are certain inborn (inherited) errors of metabolism. There are nearly 2,000 known inherited diseases of this type (see, for example, **Phenylketonuria**), but only about two dozen have regular test procedures. There are also a few similar conditions that are acquired after birth. Each condition has some unique way of manifesting itself. For example, cystinuria causes kidney stones; alkaptonuria causes a form of arthritis; Hartnup's disease is primarily a skin condition; maple syrup urine disease (so named because the urine takes on a maple syrup odor) can cause convulsions; homocystinuria can bring about eye problems; tyrosinemia causes liver and kidney disease; and histidinemia victims have speech defects.

In most instances, because of the missing enzyme, the kidney cannot handle the faulty metabolism of certain amino acids from proteins that are eaten. There is also a degree of mental retardation in many of these difficulties. Urine and blood may be screened for general amino acid abnormalities, but in most instances tests for specific amino acid excess are performed on the basis of the patient's symptoms.

When performed: Most often on newborn infants, but also on young children (occasionally on adults with appropriate symptoms) who show signs of retardation or other inherited abnormalities. The following states require screening of newborn infants for one or more of the various aminoacidurias: Alaska, Arizona, Colorado, Florida, Georgia, Idaho, Maine, Maryland, Massachusetts, Montana, Nevada, New Mexico, New York, Ohio, Oregon, Texas, Wisconsin and Wyoming; should parents present a written objection, some of these states will waive the requirement.

Normal values: Each of the 29 amino acids and their metabolites has a different normal value. In the blood the levels are usually high at birth and lessen with age. In the urine the opposite is the rule.

Abnormal values: Increased amounts in the plasma and urine not only help diagnose the condition but can also indicate specific dietary treatment, which is usually successful.

Risk factors: Negligible (see general risk factors for blood testing).

Pain/discomfort: Minimal (see general pain/discomfort factors for blood testing).

Accuracy and significance: The tests are extremely accurate in the detection and measurement of amino acids, but they must be carefully correlated with the patient's family history, symptoms, and signs.

(*Note:* For other legally required newborn screening tests see:

Galactosemia, Hemoglobin, Phenylketonuria, Red Blood Cell, Thyroid Function.)

AMNIOCENTESIS

Studying the amniotic fluid (the fluid that surrounds the fetus during pregnancy) is becoming commonplace when it is suspected that a child might be born with an inherited defect. In the United States more than 100,000 children are born each year with some form of developmental disability. The fetus gives off cells while growing, and these cells can be studied directly. The test is usually performed early in pregnancy (after 15 weeks), but it can also be done before delivery to insure that the fetus is sufficiently mature to survive.

After locating the exact position of the fetus, usually with the **Ultrasound** test, the physician places a long thin needle through the abdomen into the uterus and withdraws the fluid.

Many different metabolic conditions can be diagnosed prior to birth (Down's syndrome, **Tay-Sachs Disease,** some malformations). The process is called karyotyping (**Chromosome Analysis**), or comparing the fetal chromosome size, shape, and number to what is known to be normal, thus predicting the genetic status of the unborn infant. Chromosome analysis is also performed from blood samples on young children and adults when there are sex identification problems or a question of an inherited abnormality. The same type of test can be performed on blood cells and other body tissues. (The Tay-Sachs blood-screening test for potential parents can help determine the probability of having children with Tay-Sachs disease.) The test can usually determine the sex of the fetus, but many people do not wish to know this fact before birth.

Amniotic fluid is also tested for **Alpha Fetoprotein** and **Bilirubin.**

When performed: The test is especially applicable to pregnant women over 35 years of age; families who have relatives with metabolic problems; families who have children born with Down's syndrome; and families who have past indications of chromosome abnormalities. It is also used when there have been cases of mental retardation in the family; when there is a question of an Rh problem; to offer genetic counseling early enough in pregnancy; to determine the sex and maturity of the unborn child; and to diagnose the "funny-looking kid" syndrome.

Normal values: Chromosomal analysis shows no defect.

Abnormal values: When chromosomal patterns show either excessive or missing genes; when certain genes are translocated or found on the wrong chromosomes; when chromosomes are broken. More than 180 different metabolic diseases may now be diagnosed through chromosome analysis and additional congenital abnormalities continue to be discovered yearly.

An excess of alpha fetoprotein in amniotic fluid usually indicates a neurological defect; the degree of increase in bilirubin helps predict how serious an Rh baby's condition will be after birth.

Risk factors: Needle injury to the fetus, bleeding and/or infection occur in less than one percent of tests performed. There is a risk of one out of every two hundred children being aborted by the test.

Pain/discomfort: Minimal (see general pain/discomfort factors for catheter and needle insertion).

Accuracy and significance: Generally the test is considered 95 percent accurate in its ability to detect inherited defects in children. Even sex determination is not 100 percent accurate; errors have occurred in one out of twenty tests.

AMYLASE

Amylase (composed of several enzymes used in the digestion of starch) is normally found in very small amounts in blood serum. It is produced in the pancreas, the salivary glands, the fallopian tubes, and mostly in the liver. Blood is drawn from an arm vein and the serum is examined. The urine is also tested.

When performed: When abdominal pain suggests pancreatitis; for mumps, pancreas duct obstruction, acute renal (kidney) insufficiency, and intestinal obstruction.

Normal values: Normal serum levels range from 80 to 150 Somogyi units per 100 ml. Normal urine shows from 1,000 to 5,000 Somogyi units per 24-hour sample.

Abnormal values: Amylase levels are increased primarily with pancreatitis, pancreas duct obstruction, salivary gland or duct problems (mumps), perforated ulcer, intestinal obstruction, and renal insufficiency. Amylase levels may also be elevated by certain drugs, including codeine, a large amount of alcohol, indomethacin (Indocin), meperidine (Demerol), morphine, pentazocine (Talwin), and thiazide diuretics. An elevated amylase level becomes even more specific for pancreatitis if the urine shows an increase in amylase clearance by the kidneys when compared with **Creatinine** clearance. Amylase levels may be lower than normal in hepatitis or liver damage or when there is trauma to or deficient functioning of the pancreas so that it is unable to produce the enzyme.

Risk factors: Negligible (see general risk factors for blood testing).

Pain/discomfort: Minimal (see general pain/discomfort factors for blood testing).

Accuracy and significance: Considered 80 percent accurate. Although amylase is the primary laboratory test to diagnose pancreatic disease, it is known to show false positive results in patients with acute alcoholic intoxication. In order to maintain a high degree of accuracy, should there be any doubt about the diagnosis, the different forms of amylase isoenzymes (the S type from the salivary glands and the P type from the pancreas) must be determined.

ANTINUCLEAR ANTIBODIES (ANA)

Antigens such as bacteria, toxins, tissue cells, or foreign proteins are provocative factors in many illnesses. They induce the body to produce antibodies to fight the antigens. The antibodies attempt to combine with the antigens in order to neutralize them. In certain rare and unique diseases, the body's immune system, whose main function is to resist disease, produces antibodies to parts of the patient's own body. These antibodies are special forms of gamma globulins called immunoglobulins and seem to affect all parts of the body that have nucleoprotein, especially muscles and skin. They are called antinuclear antibodies and are found most commonly in people with systemic lupus erythematosus (SLE); they may also be found in people who have relatives suffering from SLE but who do not themselves have the disease.

Blood is taken from a vein and the serum is examined under the microscope after a fluorescent dye is added. Antinuclear antibodies will appear to fluoresce if they are present. When the ANA test is positive, the serum is then diluted, first in half, then in a 1:4 dilution, a 1:8 dilution, a 1:16 dilution, and so on. The weaker the dilution that fluoresces, the more positive the test.

The lupus erythematosus (LE) cell test is a form of ANA test that is sometimes more specific for SLE. It is considered "positive" when an antinuclear antibody combines with white blood cells and offers a characteristic LE cell picture (grouping) when viewed under the microscope. Several LE cells must be seen to constitute a positive test. Eighty percent of people with SLE have positive LE cell tests.

When performed: The ANA test is used primarily when there is suspicion of systemic lupus erythematosus (SLE). It is also performed when a patient has a variety of unexplained symptoms such as mysterious rash, arthritis, or chest pains that cannot easily be diagnosed.

Normal values: Antinuclear antibodies are not usually found in the blood. Their presence, though, does not always mean disease, as when found in close relatives of people with SLE.

Abnormal values: Abnormal levels are found mostly with SLE, which usually produces the highest titers (the presence of ANA in the weakest dilutions of serum); scleroderma (marked thickening of the skin) and rheumatoid arthritis usually cause ANA to be observed but in much lower titers (very little dilution). Some forms of kidney disease and certain infections of the pleura (lining around the lungs) can cause ANA. Many drugs can cause a false positive test: certain thiazide diuretics, almost all antibiotics (penicillin, Terramycin, isoniazid), some tranquilizers such as Taractin, the oral contraceptive pills, a few drugs used to treat high blood pressure (Apresoline), and procainamide, which is used primarily to treat heartbeat irregularities, but is sometimes used as an unproven youth restorer. The presence of ANA may be masked or hidden (false negative) even with disease if the patient is taking steroid drugs.

Risk factors: Negligible (see general risk factors for blood testing).

Pain/discomfort: Minimal (see general pain/discomfort factors for blood testing).

Accuracy and significance: Although it is not considered a very specific test, it is used to help confirm the diagnosis of systemic lupus erythematosus (SLE). The absence of antinuclear antibodies is probably of greater significance in excluding a diagnosis of SLE. There are many other, much more valuable tests to help diagnose SLE and other unusual skin conditions.

ANTITHROMBIN III

Antithrombin III (ATIII; A-THR3) is one of the body's plasma proteins (a globulin), that slows down or stops the clotting of blood. It is assumed that the drug heparin works as an anticoagulant by activating the body's antithrombin III. In 1965, a deficiency of antithrombin III was discovered in certain young patients who were unusually susceptible to clotting disease, and who suffered and even died from unexplained thrombosis in blood vessels (phlebitis), and blood clots that travelled to the lungs (pulmonary emboli). The condition is believed to be inherited, and the disease can now be treated. The test is performed on blood, most often taken from an arm vein.

When performed: Whenever there are repeated episodes of phlebitis (blood clots in a vein), thrombus (clots in an artery), especially in people under the age of 30, on family members once the condition is diagnosed or suspected; when patients do not react to anticoagulant drugs; prior to surgery.

Normal values: 20–45 mg per 100 ml, or from 70 to 140 percent of the value obtained from a normal control serum.

Abnormal values: Less than 20 mg per 100 ml, or less than 70 percent of a control value.

Risk factors: Negligible (see general risk factors for blood testing).

Pain/discomfort: Minimal (see general pain/discomfort factors for blood testing).

Accuracy and significance: The test is considered quite accurate and very significant, as it can be life-saving, especially when performed for difficulties of clotting following surgery.

B

BICARBONATE (HCO_3)

Bicarbonate (sometimes called carbonates) is the most important buffer compound in the blood. A buffer keeps the **pH** (acid-base balance) of the blood at its proper strength. Bicarbonate is a blood electrolyte that works hand in hand with carbonic acid (from which it is derived as part of the metabolism of food) to help regulate blood pH. There is 20 times as much bicarbonate in the blood as carbonic acid; thus the normal pH is slightly alkaline.

Bicarbonate is easily regulated by the kidney, which excretes it when there is an excess and holds it back when needed; the amount of carbon dioxide in the blood, and the amount breathed out by the lungs, also controls bicarbonate levels. If bicarbonate is lost from the body because of a kidney problem, diarrhea, or other disease, a state of acidosis (too much acid in the blood) exists.

In most instances the bicarbonate concentration is determined by testing for the total amount of carbon dioxide, but at times bicarbonate itself becomes a valuable measurement. The "standard bicarbonate" or base excess or deficit may also be measured, but this is rarely done in practice. Blood is taken from a vein and the serum is tested.

When performed: As a verification of other tests such as the blood gases (carbon dioxide, oxygen, and hydrogen) and the pH; when there is some doubt as to the exact state of the blood pH; to differentiate the type of kidney disease, toxic coma, and certain lung problems.

Normal values: Blood bicarbonate levels normally range from 24 to 26 mEq per liter.

Abnormal values: Bicarbonate is usually increased when there is severe vomiting, when excessive bicarbonatelike products are ingested (antacid preparations for ulcers or burning stomach); when diuretic and steroid drugs are used, and when difficult breathing prevents the release of proper amounts of carbon dioxide. Blood bicarbonate is decreased moderately with rapid breathing (when excessive carbon dioxide is exhaled) and with liver disease; it is decreased markedly with aspirin or other toxic chemical poisoning, with kidney disease, and with diarrhea.

Risk factors: Negligible (see general risk factors for blood testing).

Pain/discomfort: Minimal (see general pain/discomfort factors for blood testing).

Accuracy and significance: Although sometimes performed alone, the test has real significance when it is performed along with the **pH**, thereby increasing the accuracy of a diagnosis of the blood's acidity-alkalinity levels. It is also used to differentiate abnormalities in the acidity-alkalinity relationship of the blood and body fluids, and to detect any abnormality due to a metabolic problem or a respiratory disease. When used in conjunction with **Carbon Dioxide** and **Oxygen,** it is considered extremely accurate in differentiating diseases caused by lung or kidney problems. It is also of great significance in helping diagnose a person in coma, especially when drug overdose is suspected.

BILIRUBIN

Bilirubin is a gold-colored pigment waste product of the body. It is formed mostly from the hemoglobin in red blood cells when they break down at the end of their usual life span (four months). Every day about 7 to 8 g (a teaspoon and a half) of hemoglobin is released from dying red blood cells to make 250 mg of bilirubin. Bilirubin then becomes part of the bile fluid that goes from the liver to the gall bladder to the intestines; almost all of it is normally eliminated by the bowels.

Excessive production or decreased excretion of bilirubin increases the minute normal amounts in the blood, and its unique color, when increased, causes yellow jaundice in the skin and the whites of the eyes. Before it is acted upon by the liver, bilirubin is attached to albumin protein molecules in the blood; in this state it is called indirect bilirubin. After it is acted upon by the liver, the portion no longer bound to proteins is called direct bilirubin. The sum of the two equals the total bilirubin.

Blood is taken from a vein and the serum or plasma is examined. Bilirubin is also measured in the urine (only direct bilirubin is excreted, causing a dark color). Shaking urine in a glass tube will change the normal white color of the foam to a dark yellow or brown if bilirubin is present. Amniotic fluid (the water around the fetus during pregnancy) may also be tested for excess bilirubin (it is normally present in tiny amounts and decreases throughout pregnancy).

When performed: The test is performed primarily to distinguish different forms of liver disease, especially liver cell disease from bile duct obstruction such as from gallstones. It can also help determine the cause of certain anemias. When a patient has gray-white or colorless bowel movements, the bilirubin is measured to ascertain the cause.

Normal values: The total serum bilirubin runs from 0.2 to 1.5 mg per 100 ml. The direct bilirubin usually measures from 0.1 to 0.4 mg per 100 ml; the indirect bilirubin runs about the same but may be slightly higher and still be normal. The urine normally contains no bilirubin. Amniotic fluid usually contains a trace of bilirubin.

Abnormal values: Total bilirubin (both direct and indirect) is increased with liver cirrhosis. When something blocks the flow of bile, such as a gallstone or cancer of the pancreas, the total and direct bilirubin is increased, but the indirect bilirubin usually stays within its normal range. Liver disease from Thorazine and other tranquilizers as well as drugs such as male hormones, some antibiotics, and certain arthritic pain products can cause elevated direct bilirubin: usually the indirect bilirubin stays normal. In contrast, in certain anemias where blood cells break easily such as erythroblastosis fetalis (the anemia most often caused by Rh problems), the total serum bilirubin and the indirect bilirubin are elevated, but the direct bilirubin stays normal. As red blood cells are destroyed, the bilirubin increases in amniotic fluid, and this is a way of following the course of the disease. Fasting or low caloric diet causes a marked rise in serum bilirubin in 24 hours.

Risk factors: Negligible when blood is tested (see general risk factors for blood testing). With examination of amniotic fluid, see general risk factors for catheter and needle insertion.

Pain/discomfort: Minimal when blood is tested (see general pain/discomfort factors for blood testing). With examination of amniotic fluid for bilirubin, see general pain/discomfort factors for catheter and needle insertion.

Accuracy and significance: A bilirubin test is considered a highly accurate and sensitive measure of liver disease. It has little significance in distinguishing between specific liver diseases. To assure an accurate interpretation of the test, the effects of many different prescription drugs on liver function must always be considered.

BIOPSY

Biopsy is the removal of a piece of tissue from the body for detailed, usually microscopic, examination. Examination of isolated cells such as blood cells or those obtained for a bone marrow test or Pap smear (see **Cytology**) are forms of a biopsy. Most often, however, a small piece of tissue is excised with a scalpel. (If the lesion is small, as are most skin growths, the entire mass is removed.) The specimen is sliced to extreme thinness (microtomy), stained, and examined through the microscope.

In needle biopsy, a fine needle is inserted into a body organ, tissue, or suspected lesion and a minute piece is sucked into the needle tip for microscopic examination. This is usually performed under the fluoroscope so as to be precise about the location of the specimen. In most instances a local anesthetic is used. Needle biopsies of the breast, liver, spleen, pancreas, kidney, and lung are regularly performed. Biopsy of the prostate may be obtained during cystoscopy (use of an instrument that allows a direct view of the urethra and bladder). In general, the result of a biopsy of a tumor is reported as benign (noncancerous) or malignant (cancerous). A biopsy may also reveal an infection or foreign body as the cause of the lesion. To correctly diagnose diseases of the fingernails and toenails, which are often the result of a fungus, a nail biopsy is necessary.

(*Note:* a needle biopsy is also known as an aspiration biopsy; when a larger opening is necessary it may be called a punch biopsy. The terms incisional and excisional biopsy refer to whether only a piece of the lesion to be studied is removed, or whether the entire suspected growth is excised. When an endoscope is used to observe the area in question—such as through the cystoscope—the biopsy may be called an endoscopic biopsy; if the surface area is scraped, as when studying the inside walls of the uterus, the term surface biopsy may be used. A percutaneous biopsy is any biopsy obtained by penetrating the skin, most often with a needle.)

When performed: Whenever a suspicious lesion is seen (either directly on the skin or in a body cavity), felt (as in the breast), or noted (by X-ray); whenever there is suspected disease in an organ (such as the liver or lung) that cannot be diagnosed.

Normal values: The very existence of a lesion usually contradicts a normal value, but there are various skin growths such as birthmarks that are not disease related.

Abnormal values: Any biopsy showing pathological cells is considered abnormal. Benign cells can be pathological, or disease related, even if they are not cancerous.

Risk factors: General risk factors include the remote possibility of hemorrhage and the even more remote possibility of infection: much depends on the part of the body being biopsied. With a skin biopsy there is the possibility of a scar. Many doctors feel that, when performing a biopsy on a suspected cancer, unless the biopsy is large enough to be outside the suspicious area, the irritation of the cutting or withdrawal of the biopsy needle may accelerate the spread of the cancer.

Pain/discomfort: Much depends on the part of the body being biopsied and whether anesthesia is used. Biopsies taken from inside the body—the bladder, esophagus, stomach, large bowel, liver, lungs, and bone marrow—are usually uncomfortable procedures, even when anesthesia is employed. Discomfort lasting several days is not unusual following such biopsies. If a patient is particularly apprehensive, a general anesthesia is often administered for the procedure. Biopsies from the skin or surface organs involve little discomfort.

Accuracy and significance: When a biopsy is properly performed, preserved, and handled, its accuracy is near 100 percent. Unfortunately, cancer cells can be missed at times. There are also instances when normal or non-cancerous cells appear as abnormal and cause an erroneous diagnosis. This is not common, but it does seem to occur more often when a frozen specimen is studied. Frozen biopsy specimens are utilized when, during an operation for suspected cancer, the surgeon wants an immediate answer as to just how much surgery he will perform (a report from a routine biopsy takes two to three days).

BLEEDING AND CLOTTING TIME

Although essentially two different tests, bleeding and clotting time are invariably performed together as if they were one. They are crude measures of hemostasis (how quickly bleeding is stopped by normal body responses). More specifically, bleeding time is primarily an indication of the condition of the blood vessels (principally the capillaries) and an indication of platelet function. In addition to clotting factors, the test measures how well and how quickly small arteries and veins will constrict and close off to stop bleeding when injured. Clotting time is a generalized indication of the effectiveness of the many factors within the fluid blood itself (as opposed to the blood vessels) to bring about coagulation (clotting).

The original technique of nicking the earlobe or a fingertip is still used occasionally to measure bleeding time. However, the preferred technique (Ivy bleeding time) is to apply a standard amount of pressure around the upper arm with a blood pressure cuff and then to make two incisions 10 mm (about 7/16") long and 1 mm (1/32") deep on the lower arm. Blotting paper is touched to the cut every 30 seconds until the bleeding stops, at which point the time is noted.

In tests of clotting time, blood is usually drawn from a vein and placed in several narrow glass tubes. Sometimes the tubes are broken apart; sometimes they are tilted. In either case, the time is noted when the blood visibly clots (the cells go from a liquid to a solid state).

When performed: The test is used when there are unusual bleeding tendencies (either inherited or caused by drugs or other diseases); when liver disease is suspected, and whenever a patient is to have a surgical procedure or extensive dental work. The clotting time alone may be measured as a guide to dosage when a patient receives heparin as part of anticoagulant therapy; it may also be used as a test of platelet function (see **Platelet Count**).

Normal values: Bleeding time usually averages 5 minutes; however, bleeding times of up to 10 minutes are still considered within normal limits by some laboratories. Clotting time usually ranges from 6 to 16 minutes.

Abnormal values: Longer than usual bleeding time generally indicates thrombocytopenia (a decrease in the normal amount of blood platelets, which are essential for clotting). It can also mean that the platelets, although normal in number, are not functioning properly. Bleeding and clotting time together are prolonged when there are coagulation defects—either absence of the multiple clot-causing factors normally in blood or interference with one or more of these factors (such as when a patient is given heparin). The clotting time alone is not a specific diagnostic test. It is usually (though not always) increased with hemophilia. Taking large doses of aspirin can cause increased bleeding and clotting times, as can uremia (a form of kidney failure where the by-products of proteins cannot filter through the kidney) and certain kinds of leukemia.

Risk factors: Negligible (see general risk factors for blood testing).

Pain/discomfort: Minimal (see general pain/discomfort factors for blood testing). The incisions are so shallow that they rarely cause pain.

Accuracy and significance: The test is quite accurate in detecting bleeding tendencies; however, it is not sufficiently accurate for consistent use on a patient taking anticoagulant drugs. The test is so non-specific, it is of no major significance in determining a diagnosis.

BLOOD CELL DIFFERENTIAL

Changes in the amounts of *each type* of **White Blood Cell** (leukocyte) and changes in the size and shape of **Red Blood Cells** (erythrocytes) can be of greater importance than changes in the total white and red blood cell counts. Particularly, ascertaining changes in the proportions of the different kinds of white blood cells helps to define different disease processes. The blood cell differential test also distinguishes abnormalities in red blood cells (such as sickling, different forms of anemia, insufficient iron) and will show malaria if present. A drop of blood is taken from the fingertip, earlobe, or heel; or a drop of venous blood taken for other tests may be used. The blood is stained and then examined through a microscope by a hematologist or trained technician. No machine can perform this test.

When performed: When there is an infectious process, an allergy, or a parasitic infestation; with suspicion of any blood disease such as anemia or leukemia.

Normal values: Usually each of the different kinds of white blood cells are found in the following proportions:

Neutrophils:

65% total, with 58% mature neutrophils and 7% young neutrophils (neutrophils are the primary cells that ingest and destroy microorganisms and other toxic disease-producing substances).

Lymphocytes:

27% (lymphocytes represent antibody activity in producing immunity to disease).

Monocytes:

5% (while thought of as old lymphocytes, they represent chronic disease processes in the body).

Eosinophils:

2% (eosinophils are related to allergies and parasitic infestations).

Basophils:

1% (the role of the basophil is still not clearly understood).

Abnormal values: An increased proportion of neutrophils usually indicates poisoning, cancer, hemorrhage, or an infectious process (there are a few exceptions; for reasons still unknown, a virus infection, typhoid fever, and malaria do not cause the expected increase in neutrophils). When most of the neutrophils are young, elevated levels usually reflect leukemia. A decreased amount of neutrophils is seen with spleen disorders, lupus erythematosus, vitamin B_{12} and/or folic acid deficiency, and bone marrow damage from drugs or X-rays. Typhoid and malaria are two infections that cause a decrease in neutrophils. Decreased amounts of all white blood cells may be found in a patient taking steroid drugs.

Lymphocytes are increased primarily after radiation exposure and in hepatitis, herpes simplex and herpes zoster (shingles), infectious mononucleosis, syphilis, and leukemia. They are decreased in lupus erythematosus and other conditions where there is reduced immunity to disease. See **Lymphocyte Typing.**

Monocytes are increased with tuberculosis, cancers, anemias, rickettsial diseases (such as Rocky Mountain spotted fever), and typhoid. A decrease in monocytes is rarely seen.

Eosinophils are increased with asthma, hay fever, and similar conditions, and especially with worm and other parasite invasion. The use of diet depressant drugs such as amphetamines, certain tranquilizers, bulk forming laxatives such as those containing psyllium seeds, and certain antibiotics can also cause a rise in eosinophils. They are decreased with alcohol intoxication.

Basophils may be increased with leukemias and adrenal disease and are sometimes missing with hyperthyroidism and allergies.

Risk factors: Negligible (see general risk factors for blood testing).

Pain/discomfort: Minimal (see general pain/discomfort factors for blood testing).

Accuracy and significance: The test is very accurate when properly performed. However, it is only significant in the sense that it can point toward diagnostic possibilities. For example, a rise in the percentage of eosinophils will not tell the doctor whether the increase is due to allergy, worms, or some other condition.

BLOOD PRESSURE

The term "blood pressure" generally refers to the pressure in the arteries as opposed to the veins. To take one's blood pressure is to measure the pressure (tension) of the blood within the artery walls. (Pressures in the capillaries and veins are quite different.) The end result is derived from a number of factors: the force of each heartbeat, the elasticity or resilience of the walls of the artery, the amount of blood flowing through the arteries at any one time, the viscosity (thickness) of the blood, the number of molecules of various substances (such as protein and sodium) in the blood, the amount of certain hormones and enzymes (such as adrenalin from the adrenal gland and renin from the kidney) circulating in the blood, and the functioning of the autonomic or sympathetic nervous system (over which a person has no direct control) in response to changes in posture, stressful situations, and other stimuli.

The blood pressure is altered during every heartbeat, reaching its highest point when the heart muscle is most contracted (forcing blood into the arteries) and its lowest point when the heart muscle relaxes after each heartbeat. The heart muscle contraction is medically called systole, and the highest point of one's blood pressure is known as systolic. The momentary resting phase of the heart is called diastole, and the low point of one's blood pressure is known as diastolic. The difference between these two pressures is called the pulse pressure.

The measurement of blood pressure is recorded by noting how

high in millimeters (mm) applied pressure will cause a column of mercury (Hg) to rise on a measuring instrument. A cuff or sleeve is wrapped around an extremity (most commonly the upper arm); air is pumped into the cuff to apply a counterpressure to all the tissues surrounding the artery (skin, muscles, etc.). By reading the level of counterpressure on an air pressure dial gauge or directly observing how high the mercury rises, the physician can note when the artery collapses (similar to applying a tourniquet and then releasing the pressure to allow the artery to fill normally); at that point the pressure being applied just exceeds the pressure within the artery. Collapse of the artery is most commonly noted by listening for the cessation of the pulse through a stethoscope placed on the inside of the arm in front of the elbow or by feeling for the pulse until the examiner can no longer feel the beat.

When sufficient pressure is applied around the arm to collapse the artery, the pulse will no longer be heard or felt, giving the systolic blood pressure reading. As outside pressure from the cuff is lessened, the pulse can be heard or felt the instant the artery pressure exceeds that of the surrounding cuff (again the measure of the systolic pressure). The pulse will be heard or felt as long as sufficient pressure is applied from the outside to cause the blood pulsations to rebound off the artery walls. When the outside pressure is low enough so there is no measurable resistance against the artery wall, the pulse will no longer be heard (it will still be felt); this point is noted for the diastolic pressure measurement. Today there are electronic instruments that translate the pulse sounds into light impulses or noises, which are much easier to record.

It is important to measure blood pressure in both arms and both legs; to measure it while the patient is standing, sitting, and lying down; and most of all to measure it when the patient is as relaxed as possible. Most physicians measure blood pressure at the onset of an examination, again about halfway through and as the last procedure (when the patient is most likely to be at ease). Recently, doctors have asked patients to measure their own blood pressure at home (or have a family member test it) during various times of the day and to note activities at the time in order to arrive at the most usual reading. Blood pressure readings must be abnormal on three different days before a diagnosis of hypertension can be made.

Venous blood pressure as opposed to arterial blood pressure is recorded directly by using a manometer, a thin glass tube with measurement markings connected to a needle. The needle is placed inside a vein in the arm, which is kept at heart level (it may also be placed in a neck vein, with the patient lying down); the actual rise of blood in the tube is noted. Vein pressure can be estimated by observing the veins on the back of the hand when the arm is raised. Normally the veins collapse when the hand reaches heart level; neck veins usually collapse when the patient is in a sitting position.

When performed: Arterial blood pressure is routinely measured during a physical examination to detect early stages of hypertension (high blood pressure), a condition that exists in one out of every ten Americans. It is also followed closely in patients who are overweight; patients who have thyroid and other hormone diseases, kidney diseases, or lung diseases; and during pregnancy. During surgical procedures the blood pressure is monitored constantly as a guide to the patient's condition, especially to check for blood loss.

Venous blood pressure is measured primarily in heart disease to determine which side of the heart is in difficulty. It is also measured when blood transfusions are given to make sure the patient does not receive too much blood (which can cause congestion of the lungs) as well as when intravenous fluids are administered to patients in diabetic coma.

Normal values: The most generalized figures given for arterial blood pressure are 120/80, which means the systolic pressure is 120 mm Hg and the diastolic pressure is 80 mm Hg when a person is at rest and relaxed. But blood pressure seems to rise naturally as people get older. Even with age, however, the diastolic pressure should not rise as much as the systolic. A consistent blood pressure of greater than 140/85, regardless of age, should be thought of as a warning sign. Venous blood pressure normally ranges from 40 to 80 mm Hg. The pulse pressure averages 40 mm Hg.

Abnormal values: In general, a systolic blood pressure reading over 150 mm Hg and/or a diastolic blood pressure reading over 90 mm Hg is considered evidence of hypertension. Three out of four people with high blood pressure readings (excluding those obtained erroneously) have essential hypertension (caused by some direct body dysfunction); one out of four cases of hypertension have a secondary cause that can be diagnosed, such as kidney disease, connective tissue disease, nervous system involvement, lung disease, or hormonal problems. Certain drugs, such as those used for asthma, can cause high blood pressure readings.

High blood pressure is more a cause of heart disease than a result of heart problems. When blood pressure is elevated in the arms but normal or low in the legs, or when blood pressure in the right arm is greater than in the left, it usually indicates coarctation (constriction) of the aorta. Hypotension, or low blood pressure, most commonly occurs when a person moves from a sitting to a standing position (postural or orthostatic hypotension). It may also be caused by diuretic and other antihypertensive drugs, by many tranquilizers, by certain Parkinson-type diseases, and, of course, by shock or severe bleeding.

A major cause of erroneous arterial blood pressure readings is faulty measurement technique. Putting the cuff on wrong, not inflating the cuff properly, and failing to hear the proper pulse sounds (either because of inattentiveness or because of other distracting noises) are the three most common reasons for erroneous, usually elevated, blood pressure readings. Performing a single test, on one arm, at the onset of an examination can also lead to inaccurate high blood pressure readings. Failure to take into account any apprehensiveness on the part of a patient will invariably give false results.

Venous blood pressure rises primarily with heart conditions such as right-sided heart failure or heart valve damage to the point that blood cannot easily enter the heart chambers. A rapid fall in venous pressure usually indicates internal bleeding such as from an ulcer.

Risk factors: There is no physical risk in measuring blood pressure with the standard blood pressure apparatus; however, should the machine be improperly calibrated the ensuing treatment, or lack of it, could be incorrect. For the measurement of pressure by a needle inserted in a blood vessel, see general risk factors for blood testing and catheter or needle insertion.

Pain/discomfort: Normally pressure from the measuring cuff is minimal, but over-inflation of the cuff can be uncomfortable. When needles are used to measure blood pressure see general pain/discomfort factors for blood testing and catheter or needle insertion.

Accuracy and significance: Properly performed blood pressure readings are extremely accurate. When the newer electronic blood pressure measuring devices which detect pulse sounds are used—as they are at health fairs, in drug stores, etc.—it should be remembered that loud noises at the time of testing can produce abnormal results. Blood pressure measurements are very significant in following the course of many different diseases, and during pregnancy and surgery.

The latest studies on the accuracy of blood pressure measurements have shown that the test is far more accurate when it is performed at home than when it is performed in a doctor's office; in addition, it usually measures 20 to 30 mm Hg lower than when it is performed by a doctor.

BODY TEMPERATURE

Most people associate the measurement of body temperature with an infection—from a simple cold or pneumonia to abscesses and appendicitis. In actuality, a rise in body temperature (fever) reflects increased metabolic activity; in the case of an infection the elevated temperature indicates increased **White Blood Cell** production and action as they attempt to destroy invading microorganisms—whether they are bacteria, fungi, parasites, or some viruses—along with immune body production usually specific to the cause of the disease. At times, the presence of fever may be the only indication of a hidden illness. Tuberculosis may be present within the body in lesions too small to be detected by any other tests; food poisoning whose symptoms are only a mild annoyance may be accompanied by an elevated temperature; other infections of the gastrointestinal tract such as colitis or diverticulitis may have a fever as their initial warning sign.

At other times, various tumors (cancerous or not) produce a rise in body temperature. Leukemias and cancers of the liver and lung seem to do this most often. Conditions related to **Immunology,** such as systemic lupus erythematosus, as well as other diseases that cause abnormal values in **Antinuclear Antibodies** tests, may also bring about fever. Various forms of arthritis can cause a rise in body temperature before pain is felt in the joints. And disruptions in the hormone system, especially those causing water retention or excretion problems, may alter body temperature.

It is also possible for the body's temperature to drop below normal—this condition is called hypothermia. While a slight drop may routinely occur in elderly people or in those who reside in cold climates, a drop in body temperature can also be present in patients with circulation problems or diabetes and in those who abuse alcohol, barbiturates, and certain tranquilizers. In certain instances, hypothermia can be as dangerous as a high fever.

Body temperature also rises slightly during the menstrual cycle. The basal body temperature test indicates the time of ovulation (when the ovum or egg is released from the ovary ready for fertilization or pregnancy). The body temperature is taken each morning on arising (usually by mouth) and recorded. It usually remains slightly below normal (normal is 98.6° F, or 37° C) until ovulation occurs, when it rises to normal or slightly above and stays elevated until menstruation. Thus, if a woman is having difficulty becoming pregnant, the couple is told to wait for the temperature to rise before having intercourse. The test can, of course, also be used as a contraceptive guide to show when conception would be impossible. The basal temperature test is used in conjunction with the Pap test (see **Cytology**) to study the menstrual cycle phase.

Many prescription drugs can cause a rise in body temperature. (Most doctors initially call this FUO, fever of unknown origin.) The drugs include the amphetamines, numerous anti-cholinergics (used to relax gastrointestinal spasm), a few blood pressure medications, procainamide, and, surprisingly, several aspirin-like products used to reduce pain. An elevated temperature after vaccination and other immunizations is also not unusual. Body temperature is commonly measured by inserting a thermometer in the mouth under the tongue, in the rectum, or under the armpit (axillary). Some new devices measure skin surface temperature and convert it to body temperature.

Temperature may also be measured in the urine. There are times when a patient has a persistent high fever, yet no body pathology is detected. Measuring the temperature of the urine immediately after it is passed will indicate which patients have a false high temperature—that is, which patients are employing devices to deliberately raise the temperature of the thermometer.

When performed: In almost all instances of illness, especially infection, as an indication of the severity of the disease, and to measure the success or failure of treatment. The basal body temperature is measured when patients have fertility problems; when chemical contraception is obviated; and when gynecological problems are suspected. The urinary temperature test is used when patients are suspected of faking fever.

Normal values: Normal body temperature is usually between 98° and 99° F, or around 37° C; there is normally a 1° rise in temperature at the time of ovulation. Normal skin surface temperature is about 86° F.

Abnormal values: Any elevation of body temperature greater than 100° F, failure of the body temperature to rise about 1° in the midmenstrual cycle, and a difference of more than 1° between body and urine temperature are all considered abnormal.

Risk factors: Breakage of the thermometer; the risk is, of course, relative to the thermometer's location. Should breakage occur, the amount of mercury released is not considered very dangerous. If thermometers are not properly sterilized prior to each use, there is the risk of transmitting infection.

Pain/discomfort: Minimal.

Accuracy and significance: Virtually all types of thermometers are sufficiently accurate. When using body temperature readings for ovulation time or birth control, special ovulation thermometers with larger spaces between the pertinent degree divisions, are much easier to read.

BONE MARROW

Red and white blood cells and platelets are produced in the bone marrow. When a disease process affects the bone marrow, there is either an increase or a reduction of these essential blood elements. Also, depending on the nature of the disease, **Iron** may be increased in, or lost from, the bone marrow. A tiny amount of bone marrow can be aspirated (withdrawn) for examination with a syringe and special needle. The most common sites for bone marrow aspiration are the crest of the hip bone and the sternum (breast bone). Bone marrow may also be cultured for infection (see **Culture**).

When performed: When leukemia, certain anemias, blood diseases such as hemolysis (self-destruction of red blood cells) or polycythemia (too many red blood cells), drug toxicity, or tumor growths such as lymphoma, myelofibrosis, and multiple myeloma are suspected; to follow the effectiveness of therapy in these diseases.

Normal values: A normal bone marrow specimen contains 15 different kinds of cells in varying stages of growth and in varying amounts. Normally, a small amount of iron is found in the marrow (detected using a special stain). Examination and determination of the normalcy of the different kinds of cells and the amount of iron must be made by a hematologist.

Abnormal values: Evidence of red cell destruction, presence of sickle or other diseased cells, absence of normal cells, and excess of diseased cells are all considered abnormal. Iron absence is found with iron deficiency anemia (usually due to blood loss); an increase in iron is seen with pernicious and hemolytic anemia and anemia caused by infection.

Risk factors: Negligible (see general risk factors for catheter or needle insertion).

Pain/discomfort: Even with a local anesthetic there is often moderate pain when the bone marrow aspiration needle penetrates the bone surface (see general pain/discomfort factors for catheter or needle insertion).

Accuracy and significance: A bone marrow study is considered far more accurate than a **Blood Cell Differential** study especially to determine the leukemias, and to ascertain the specific cause of anemia. Bone marrow studies are particularly significant in measuring adverse effects of toxic substances, including many of the drugs used to treat cancer.

C

CALCITONIN

Calcitonin is a hormone produced by the thyroid gland. Its principal task seems to be to help the body get rid of excess **Calcium.** It acts in opposition to the parathyroid gland hormone in that it slows down the release of calcium from the bones to the serum. Blood is taken from a vein and the serum is tested. Calcitonin from salmon is even more potent in humans than human calcitonin and is used to treat certain bone disease.

When performed: When X-rays show the bones to be losing minerals; when thyroid cancer or certain adrenal tumors are suspected; to verify high levels of calcium in the blood.

Normal values: From 5 to 300 pg per ml (usually less than 400 pg per ml) is considered normal.

Abnormal values: Calcitonin levels are increased with certain thyroid cancers, stomach cancers, anemia, and kidney disease.

Risk factors: Negligible (see general risk factors for blood testing).

Pain/discomfort: Minimal (see general pain/discomfort factors for blood testing).

Accuracy and significance: The test is only 80 to 90 percent accurate, as it has been known to show normal values in some patients with the type of cancer that produces elevated values. Its significance is in differentiating among various forms of thyroid cancer.

CALCIUM

There are approximately two pounds of calcium in the body at all times, almost all in the bones and teeth. About 0.03 ounce of calcium is taken in each day in a normal diet. This is the bare minimum required to fulfill the body's regular needs, because 80% of ingested calcium is excreted (in urine and sweat and through the bowels). Calcium is needed to maintain many body processes such as muscle contraction and nerve transmission, to keep cells from being destroyed, and to ensure that blood will clot.

The body's calcium need and use are controlled by the hormone from the parathyroid glands (four separate, tiny glands buried within the thyroid gland but distinctly different from it) and almost as much by the amount of phosphorus and vitamin D in the body (see **Alkaline Phosphatase; Phosphorus**). When there is an excess of parathyroid hormone, calcium increases in the blood and phosphorus decreases; with insufficient parathyroid hormone, the opposite occurs. The thyroid gland exerts a serum-lowering effect on calcium through the production of a unique hormone called **Calcitonin.**

Three different forms of calcium are in the blood: the ionized or active form, which comprises approximately half the total amount; 45% in a form attached to the serum protein albumin; and a form attached to phosphates, which comprises about 5% of the total. The usual test for calcium measures all three forms and is called the total calcium (there are special tests to measure only the ionized portion). Blood calcium is measured in the serum from venous blood. It is also measured in the urine (Sulkowitch test), in the feces, and in the spinal fluid.

When performed: The test is used primarily when there are suspected abnormalities of the parathyroid gland; when there are mysterious symptoms such as memory problems, unusual sleepiness, or nerve and muscle problems; and, in contrast, when there is excessive muscle irritability. When a patient has difficulty swallowing, tongue problems, or certain forms of deafness, calcium levels in the blood may aid in discovering the cause. Other gland dysfunctions such as a lack of adrenal hormones or too much thyroid hormone may be diagnosed by testing for calcium. The test is also used when there is suspicion of vitamin D poisoning or unexplained bleeding and to differentiate various bone diseases, including the unique bone problems of women after the menopause; when cancer is suspected.

Tests are now available for measuring **Parathyroid** hormone directly.

Normal values: Normal values in serum range from 8.5 to 10.5 mg per 100 ml (4.25 to 5.25 mEq per liter); in urine, no more than 150 mg in a 24-hour sample; in feces, about 800 mg a day (depending on diet); and in spinal fluid, 4 to 5 mg per 100 ml.

Abnormal values: Serum calcium is increased in hyperparathyroidism, certain bone tumors, and rarefaction or demineralization of bone (osteoporosis); adrenal disease; hyperthyroidism; when too much vitamin D or milk is taken; when too much antacid medication (usually for ulcers) is consumed; when diuretics are taken; and in rare lung diseases. Serum calcium is decreased when the parathyroid gland is inactive or if that gland has been accidentally removed during thyroid surgery; when there is insufficient vitamin D or when vitamin D cannot be absorbed; with kidney disease and certain bone diseases such as rickets; and in nutritional problems when insufficient calcium is eaten or absorbed. When serum calcium levels are lower than normal, total serum proteins (especially albumin) must be evaluated; decreased albumin will give a decreased calcium value (see **Albumin/Globulin**). Cancer is the most common cause of increased serum calcium levels.

Calcium levels in the urine fairly well reflect serum calcium levels, but they are increased when patients are taking certain diuretic drugs (which cause decreased levels in serum). Calcium is increased in feces when there are problems with intestinal absorption. Calcium levels are increased in the spinal fluid with tuberculous meningitis.

Risk factors: Negligible (see general risk factors for blood testing).

Pain/discomfort: Minimal (see general pain/discomfort factors for blood testing).

Accuracy and significance: If correctly performed, the test is about 90 percent accurate in verifying the existence of numerous conditions. (A common error is using improperly cleaned glassware that contains traces of calcium.) As abnormal calcium levels are common to a variety of diseases and nutritional problems, the test's significance is particularly dependent on such factors as the doctor's observations, X-ray findings and corroborative hormone tests.

CALORIC

The caloric test is so named because it uses differences in temperature as the basis for diagnosing ear nerve damage that can cause dizziness.

Dizziness or vertigo can also accompany hearing loss, vision problems, brain disease, or alcoholism. Patients describe feelings of turning, twirling (or things around them twirling), and faintness. Vertigo is most often a result of disease to the vestibular part of the nerve that allows hearing; the vestibular part controls balance. In the caloric test, one teaspoon of ice water is instilled in the ear canal with a rubber syringe (similar to the technique used when washing wax out of the ear). This should cause nystagmus (the eyes move quickly away from the ice water and then slowly back). If nystagmus does not occur, two more teaspoons of ice water are used. Should the eyes still fail to move, four and then eight teaspoons of ice water are used.

At times hot water is used as well as ice water. The hot water should cause an opposite eye movement pattern from the ice water. Performing the test with both hot and cold temperatures will give more accurate results. As a confirmation for vertigo, the Romberg test is used. The patient stands with feet together and eyes closed; with vertigo the patient will tend to fall to one side.

When performed: Primarily when there is dizziness or fainting, especially after ear injury or in ear disease; whenever impaired hearing exists; with patients taking certain antibiotic drugs and with anemias; when psychological problems are suspected; with a comatose patient to determine the extent, if any, of brain damage.

Normal values: Nystagmus should occur after one teaspoon of water is instilled in the ear canal.

Abnormal values: If nystagmus does not appear until after two or more teaspoons of ice water are placed in the ear, the ear nerve may be diseased but the possibility of cure exists. If eight teaspoons of ice water in the ear do not produce nystagmus, it may be assumed that the nerve is permanently damaged.

Vertigo can be caused by any disease or injury that affects the vestibular nerve as well as damage inflicted by many antibiotic drugs (usually when given in large doses for long periods of time). Atherosclerosis of the blood supply to the ear, cholesteotomas (growths), and certain poisons can also cause vertigo.

Risk factors: Negligible. Too much water pressure can injure a previously damaged eardrum, but this rarely occurs.

Pain/discomfort: Minimal, although some patients find cold water in the ear mildly uncomfortable.

Accuracy and significance: Considered quite accurate in differentiating between treatable and permanent non-treatable ear disease.

CANCER

At the present time there is no absolute, or even consistently reliable, test for early cancer detection; nor is there a reasonably accurate test to screen for hidden cancers. If any one test comes close, it is the **Carcinoembryonic Antigen** (CEA), once considered specific for colon and rectal cancers (some doctors think it justifiable for lung cancers), but now considered inadequate by the National Institutes of Health. The **Acid Phosphatase** test for prostatic acid phosphatase (PAP) is considered useful in diagnosing early prostate cancer. Some doctors use the **Alpha Fetoprotein** test to substantiate liver cancers; others use a version of the ferritin (see **Iron**) test that measures isoferritins, to confirm suspicions of liver cancer as well as other cancers. A particular ferritin substance is occasionally found on the T cells and B cells (see **Lymphocyte Typing**) of breast cancer patients; T and B cells are also examined for lymph cell cancers. **Hydroxyproline** tests are employed when bone cancer is suspected, and a few doctors use hydroxyproline measurements for breast cancer evaluation. **Alkaline Phosphatase** values are considered to be of diagnostic aid in bone and liver cancers (or when cancer cells from other parts of the body migrate to the bone or liver, a process known as metastasis); even the enzymes tests used to evaluate **Alcoholism** are considered of value in discovering metastasis to the liver. The alpha-antitrypsin test (see **Albumin/Globulin**) is a generalized, though non-specific, indication of cancer as is the **Haptoglobin** test, another form of globulin. **Lactic Dehydrogenase** (LDH), while non-specific, can offer a clue that cancer may be present somewhere within the body, most likely in the breast, lung, or bowel. **Catecholamines** can signal the possible presence of an adrenal gland tumor or some abnormal nervous system growth.

Some hormone tests can point to cancer. **Calcitonin** values may help diagnose thyroid cancer; human chorionic gonadotropin (see **Pregnancy** and **Testis Function**) and lactogenic hormone (see **Prolactin**) abnormalities are known to result from various tumors; **Gastrin** values are extremely abnormal when certain stomach tumors exist; and antithyroglobulin levels are sometimes used to aid in the diagnosis of thyroid cancer (see **Thyroid Function**). The **Estrogen Receptor** test helps determine which cancers will respond to hormone therapy instead of surgery. **Serotonin**, which some doctors believe is a hormone, is used experimentally as a diagnostic aid for certain cancers. **Glucagon** and **Insulin** tests are performed when there is a suspicion of a pancreas tumor. **Cortisol** measurements can direct attention to the possibility of an adrenal gland tumor, especially when coordinated with a test for **Catecholamines.**

Immunoglobulin tests can offer early warning signs for certain cancers, particularly multiple myeloma.

In addition, there are many new enzyme, protein, antigen, and collagen breakdown products being evaluated as tumor markers (collagen is the matrix of supporting tissue of bone, skin, and other body organs).

At the present time, however, most doctors believe a combination of tests affords a better opportunity for a diagnosis than the use of only one or two tests. There are also other forms of medical testing such as **Radiography, Nuclear Scanning, Ultrasound, Computerized Tomography,** and even variations on the **Agglutination** test that may help detect hidden cancer.

CAPILLARY FRAGILITY (Rumpel-Leede)

In a number of diseases of blood vessels—such as thrombocytopenia (decreased thrombocytes or platelets needed for clotting), disorders of platelet function, scurvy, and purpura—the small blood vessels near the skin surface become very fragile. In the capillary fragility test, a blood pressure cuff is placed on the forearm and inflated until it is approximately midway between the diastolic and systolic pressure—usually from 80 to 100 mm of mercury (see **Blood Pressure**). This pressure is maintained for five to ten minutes. The cuff is removed and the arm is inspected for the number of petechiae (small hemorrhages) that have appeared under the skin in a premarked area.

The petechiometer is a new device now available to measure capillary fragility. A small suction cup is applied to the forearm and pressure, measured and controlled by a gauge, performs the same function as it does in the blood pressure cuff.

When performed: As one of many tests to determine hemostatic function (blood clotting and blood vessel structure).

Normal values: Normally the cuff pressure will not produce petechiae. For some unknown reason, women with red hair are sometimes more sensitive and have a slightly positive reaction without any disease condition.

Abnormal values: The appearance of multiple petechiae indicates weakness of the tiny blood vessels and/or a platelet defect.

Risk factors: Negligible as this is a non-invasive test.

Pain/discomfort: Minimal; some patients find the tightness of the blood pressure cuff uncomfortable.

Accuracy and significance: Although the test indicates susceptibility to spontaneous bleeding under the skin, it is of no major significance as it can not differentiate among defects in the capillaries or platelet disease.

CARBON DIOXIDE (CO_2)

Carbon dioxide (CO_2) and water are end products of oxygen metabolic processes. Carbon dioxide's primary route of elimination is through the lungs (during respiration the blood gives off CO_2 and picks up oxygen); a small amount of CO_2 is changed into bicarbonates and is excreted in the urine. The depth and rapidity of a person's breathing help to control the blood CO_2 levels.

There are several different ways to measure carbon dioxide in the blood. The oldest and probably the most common test (although it is considered the least precise) measures the *carbon dioxide combining power*. A more accurate evaluation is obtained by measuring the *carbon dioxide content;* when performed with the **pH** test, it will also demonstrate the exact amounts of free bicarbonate and carbonic acid in the blood. The preferred method of evaluation is testing for *carbon dioxide tension*, or PCO_2 (sometimes called partial pressure or carbonic acid concentration).

Regardless of how CO_2 is determined, the primary purpose of the test is to measure ventilation, or how well air moves in and out of the lungs. A secondary purpose is to determine what is affecting the acid-base balance or pH (acidity or alkalinity) of the blood, which is an extremely important and very sensitive reflection of potentially disastrous bodily disorders. Blood is taken from either an artery or a vein in a special syringe to avoid any contact with air, and the serum is tested.

When performed: Whenever there are respiratory problems; whenever there is suspicion of acidosis (the pH of the blood too low) or alkalosis (the pH too high), both of which are usually brought about by metabolic or respiratory disorders; when a patient has suffered severe injuries, is in coma, or is severely disoriented; when there are severe muscle cramps, severe vomiting, or diarrhea.

Normal values: Carbon dioxide tension (PCO_2) normally ranges from 35 to 45 mm Hg in arterial blood (slightly lower in women) and 38 to 50 mm Hg in venous blood; CO_2 content, from 19 to 25 mM per liter in arterial blood and 22 to 30 mM per liter in venous blood; and CO_2 combining power, from 24 to 32 mEq per liter in arterial blood and 38 to 50 mEq per liter in venous blood.

Abnormal values: Increased carbon dioxide is found primarily in respiratory acidosis from lung conditions that prevent CO_2 from being exhaled (such as asthma, emphysema, and severe chest injuries) and during anesthesia when the patient rebreathes his own air. It is usually elevated with metabolic alkalosis caused by taking diuretic drugs, steroid hormones, or antacid preparations; with vomiting, intestinal obstruction, starvation; and with hyperactive adrenal glands. Decreased carbon dioxide is found with metabolic acidosis caused by drug poisoning (especially from aspirin and from ammonium chloride that is sold for use as a diuretic without a prescription) and with diarrhea, liver disease, kidney disease, and diabetes that is out of control. It is also lower than normal when respiratory alkalosis exists (most commonly caused by hyperventilation, or deliberate rapid breathing).

Risk factors: Negligible (see general risk factors for blood testing).

Pain/discomfort: Minimal (see general pain/discomfort factors for blood testing).

Accuracy and significance: The measurement of carbon dioxide tension, along with oxygen tension and pH, is considered the most accurate way to evaluate the function of the lung, which is to permit oxygen to reach and saturate the blood. The blood gases are the most significant **Pulmonary Function** tests in diagnosing the body's ability to carry adequate oxygen to the tissues, and to dispose of carbon dioxide as a waste product of metabolism.

CARCINOEMBRYONIC ANTIGEN (CEA)

Originally the carcinoembryonic antigen (CEA) test was used to detect cancer of the colon, but the antigen has since been found to appear with other cancers as well (pancreas, lung, breast, and prostate). Blood is drawn from a vein and the serum is examined. Other body fluids (joint fluid, peritoneal fluid, amniotic fluid) may also be tested.

When performed: The test is performed primarily to follow the course and treatment of patients with known cancers. It is also used to determine the extent of cancer, since CEA can return to normal values following successful surgery. When a cancer patient has a checkup, the level of carcinoembryonic antigen may rise months before new symptoms appear, alerting the doctor to the need for immediate further therapy. The test may also be performed to diagnose certain causes of jaundice.

Normal values: Levels below 2 ng per ml are not considered indicative of pathology. Carcinoembryonic antigen is found in very small amounts in many pregnant women, in infants, and in other normal individuals.

Abnormal values: A CEA greater than 5 to 10 ng per ml is found in a majority of patients with known cancer. Increased values are also found in patients with alcoholic cirrhosis, colitis, ulcers, and emphysema, and in heavy smokers. A subspecies of CEA called CEA-S is specific for gastrointestinal cancers without being elevated for other conditions.

Risk factors: Negligible (see general risk factors for blood testing and catheter and needle insertion).

Pain/discomfort: Minimal (see general pain/discomfort factors for blood testing and catheter and needle insertion).

Accuracy and significance: The CEA test has a high sensitivity rating—it is usually elevated in a cancer patient, particularly one with cancer of the colon—however, it has a low specificity. Less than half the patients with early cancer show a positive test. The test is most useful in following the progress of cancer patients who have had treatment, as it helps evaluate which type of treatment is the most effective. The CEA should not be considered a routine screening test for cancer.

CATECHOLAMINES

Catecholamines are produced by the medulla, or central part of the adrenal gland, as opposed to the outer area or cortex, where cortisone-type hormones originate (see **Cortisol**). Epinephrine (adrenalin) and norepinephrine (noradrenalin) are the two principal catecholamine hormones. They are called pressor amines because of their ability to constrict blood vessel walls, thus elevating the blood pressure. Norepinephrine is also necessary to transmit nerve impulses in the brain.

The two catecholamines can be tested in the blood, but they are most commonly measured in the urine, along with their metabolic end products, vanillymandelic acid (VMA), homovanillic acid (HVA), and metanephrines. Recently it has been found that decreased amounts of norepinephrine in the brain cause patients to experience symptoms of depression; excessive amounts seem to be associated with manic symptoms.

Decreased amounts of norepinephrine in the urine, accompanied by decreased amounts of 3-methoxy-4-hydroxyphenyl glycol (MHPG), another related catecholamine, are considered good evidence for a diagnosis of psychologically caused depression, particularly when exhibited as manic-depression. Increased values point to depression engendered by a physical rather than a psychological condition. There is tentative evidence that decreased MHPG with increased norepinephrine, VMA, and HVA signifies schizophrenia.

When performed: When pheochromocytoma (a tumor of the adrenal gland that causes high blood pressure) is suspected; to assess adrenal function; in certain cases of depression when a specific cause cannot be found; when neuroblastoma is suspected.

Normal values: Urine levels should not exceed 100 mcg per 100 ml in a 24-hour sample. A single urine sample should not exceed 15 mcg per 100 ml. Plasma epinephrine averages 20 ng per 100 ml; norepinephrine, 60 ng per 100 ml. Urine VMA should not exceed 8 mg per 100 ml in a 24-hour sample.

Abnormal values: When total urine catecholamines exceed 200 mcg per 100 ml and/or VMA is greater than 25 mg per 100 ml, disease is present, most likely pheochromocytoma. However, several other nerve tumors can cause increased values (in which case HVA is also increased), as can myasthenia gravis and muscular dystrophy. Certain drugs such as those used to treat depression, aspirin, some antibiotics, and coffee, tea, chocolates, fruits, and vanilla extract can cause false high values. Stress or exercise can increase catecholamines. Increased norepinephrine has been found in autism.

Risk factors: Negligible (see general risk factors for blood testing).

Pain/discomfort: Minimal (see general pain/discomfort factors for blood testing).

Accuracy and significance: Catecholamine measurements are quite an accurate contribution to the diagnosis of pheochromocytoma, but at this time they have little significance in other conditions. The test's accuracy is affected by a variety of foods and drugs, and can also show a misleading value related to the amount of physical activity prior to testing.

CEREBELLUM

The cerebellum is the part of the brain that helps control balance and coordination. Loss of coordinated movements can result from cerebellum disease as well as from certain nerve conditions that cause inability to feel pressure and other sensations. The cerebellum tests help to determine if the problem is in the brain itself, as opposed to the spinal cord and its nerve extensions.

The easiest coordination test is to have the patient stand up with feet together and close his eyes; with cerebellum disease the patient tends to fall. Attempting to walk heel to toe with eyes closed is an extension of the same test. In another simple coordination test the patient may be asked to touch the tip of his nose with his finger (with the arm first extended out); the test is repeated with the eyes closed. Trying to touch the fingers in rapid succession with the thumb is another cerebellum test, as is trying to point to objects with the big toe while lying down.

When performed: In cases of ataxia (loss of muscle coordination or irregular muscle actions); when brain disease is suspected; following head injuries; to differentiate alcoholism, drug, or hysterical reactions from physical disease.

Normal values: Normally patients perform the simple tasks of coordination without difficulty.

Abnormal values: Patients with impaired coordination are unable to perform the simple movements described. Usually, only one side of the body is affected with cerebellum disease; both sides of the body are usually involved with conditions that arise from below the brain level.

Risk factors: Negligible. Attendants should be on hand to prevent injury as a result of a fall.

Pain/discomfort: None.

Accuracy and significance: When all the cerebellum tests are performed in sequence, the test is quite accurate in diagnosing loss of coordination as a specific brain condition.

CEREBROSPINAL FLUID

Testing the spinal fluid—more accurately described as the cerebrospinal fluid, since it surrounds the brain as well as the spinal cord—is a valuable diagnostic aid in many nervous system diseases (infections and brain and spinal cord damage associated with injury or cancer). Many tests may be performed on the spinal fluid; the usual examination consists of measuring the pressure of the fluid within the spinal canal, observing the transparency and color of the fluid, and counting the white blood cells. The most common chemical tests performed on spinal fluid to establish or prove a diagnosis are chloride, sugar, proteins, and quantitative VDRL (Venereal Disease Research Laboratories) reactions to follow the treatment for syphilis. A small needle is placed in the back, between the lumbar (lower back) vertebrae, and the fluid is withdrawn (hence the term "lumbar puncture," "spinal puncture," or "spinal tap"). While the test is most commonly performed with the patient sitting up and bent slightly forward, there are times when the patient lies on his side with an assistant bending the head toward raised knees. The test should not be performed when increased intracranial pressure is suspected.

When performed: Following head or back injury or when such injury is suspected but not proved; when symptoms suggest brain tumor or stroke; when there is a severe infection (virus, meningitis, poliomyelitis, encephalitis) that seems to be affecting the brain or muscles; when there are suspected birth injuries.

Normal values: The spinal fluid has a normal pressure equal to 70 to 200 mm of water (in the sitting position; it is slightly lower when lying down). The fluid should be transparent and without color. There should be no white blood cells in the spinal fluid; however, a cell count of up to 10 is still considered normal by many physicians. Normally the fluid contains 5 to 15 mg per 100 ml of protein, 45 to 80 mg per 100 ml of sugar, and 110 to 125 mEq per liter of chloride.

Abnormal values: The spinal fluid pressure may be lower than normal when there is a spinal cord tumor or shock, or even after fainting. In diabetic coma the pressure is decreased. The pressure is increased following brain and spinal cord injury and in infection.

The color may have a reddish tinge if there is bleeding into the spinal canal following injury or stroke. With infection or with old blood from previous damage, the color may change to yellow or gray.

The cell count rises with infection, tumor, and most conditions that directly affect the brain, spinal cord, and their coverings.

Chemical tests for sugar and chloride are used to differentiate poliomyelitis from meningitis. Protein is elevated in almost all diseases that are reflected in the spinal fluid.

Risk factors: A lumbar puncture (spinal tap) might occasion a hemorrhage in the area of needle penetration, especially if the needle is improperly placed, or the patient moves. Other risks are included in general risk factors for catheter or needle insertion. Approximately one out of every one thousand patients who undergoes cerebrospinal fluid testing suffers nerve paralysis; in most instances the paralysis is reversible.

Pain/discomfort: Minimal. Most patients tolerate needle insertion without anesthesia. Some patients feel that assuming the fetal position, lying on one's side, is the most uncomfortable aspect of the test. There is the possibility of a headache a few hours after the test is completed. Medical opinion on the subject varies; some doctors require bed rest for several hours after the test to help prevent headaches, while others believe the headache seems to occur most often in patients who are told to expect a headache.

Accuracy and significance: When properly performed, the test is very accurate in helping to diagnose brain and spinal cord disease. It is especially significant in determining the specific cause of meningitis and/or encephalitis.

CHLAMYDIA IDENTIFICATION

Chlamydial infections have become so common that knowledgeable doctors are requesting laboratories to perform specific searches to isolate these unique bacteria. Public health officials report that the diseases caused by chlamydial infections are not only extremely dangerous but have reached epidemic proportions in the United States. Unfortunately, unless the doctor is aware of the bacterium and the damage it causes, its diagnosis is missed and the diseases are left untreated. Among the illnesses caused by chlamydia are: trachoma blindness, pneumonia and eye infections in newborn infants, ectopic pregnancy (the fetus develops outside the uterus), lymphogranuloma venereum, generalized pelvic inflammatory disease (a major cause of infertility), spontaneous abortion, psittacosis pneumonia (also called "parrot fever" in the belief that it is spread by pet birds), fatal infections in new mothers immediately after childbirth, and most commonly, non-gonococcal urethritis (NGU) or non-specific urethritis as it was named before the cause was discovered (an infection of the urethra—from which urine is discharged—that is thought to be three times as common as **Gonorrhea**). There are two species of chlamydia; one responds to certain antibiotic drugs while the other does not. Although it is possible to test for antibodies signifying chlamydial conditions through various **Agglutination** and **Complement Fixation** techniques which use blood taken from a vein, the most common method is by **Culture.** Samples are taken from any part of the body with abnormal secretions (urethra, vagina, eye, sputum, even the back of the throat), treated to eliminate any potentially contaminating organisms and then, because these unusual bacteria need body energy to multiply, grown on special cells. A specific diagnosis can take two to three days.

When performed: When a patient's symptoms imply a sexually transmitted disease that is not easily diagnosed, and especially if that patient is in the later months of pregnancy; when flu-like or pneumonia symptoms persist; with eye infections that are not easily diagnosed; following sudden infant death syndrome; when rectal inflammation or itching persists; when undiagnosed vaginitis persists. Many public health officials recommend routine chlamydia cultures for all pregnant women.

Normal values: No growth of the organism on the culture; no evident titer when blood is tested for antibodies.

Abnormal values: Evidence of chlamydial organisms after culturing; antibody titers greater than 1 to 64.

Risk factors: Negligible (see general risk factors for blood testing and for catheter or needle insertion).

Pain/discomfort: Minimal (see general pain/discomfort factors for blood testing and for catheter or needle insertion).

Accuracy and significance: Culture growths, when properly performed, are considered about 90 percent accurate. Antibody observation studies are only about 50 percent accurate.

CHLORIDE

Chloride, a salt of hydrochloric acid, is mostly taken into the body as part of salt (sodium chloride). It is usually tested along with **Bicarbonate, Potassium,** and **Sodium,** since they all act reciprocally to balance the body's acid-base system and control water metabolism. The major concentration of chloride is in the tissues around cells and in stomach secretions (a very dilute hydrochloric acid). The kidney usually excretes about as much chloride as is taken in. Blood is collected from a vein and the serum is examined. Urine and spinal fluid may also be examined for chloride content.

When performed: When dizziness, weakness, or unconsciousness cannot easily be diagnosed; when adrenal disease is suspected.

Normal values: Normal values in the serum range from 100 to 110 mEq per liter (350 to 385 mg per 100 ml); in the urine, from 100 to 250 mEq per 24-hour sample; in the spinal fluid, from 120 to 130 mEq per liter.

Abnormal values: Serum chloride levels are occasionally elevated with kidney disease (but can be normal), dehydration, and aspirin toxicity. They are decreased with vomiting, diarrhea, excessive sweating, diuresis (with or without drugs), heart disease, and diabetic acidosis. Spinal fluid levels are usually decreased with meningitis; urine levels are decreased with hypoactive adrenal disease.

A special test called Robinson-Power-Kepler is used occasionally to help diagnose Addison's disease (inadequate adrenal function). After drinking a great deal of water, patients with the disease excrete higher than normal amounts of chloride in the urine but lower than normal amounts of water.

Risk factors: Negligible (see general risk factors for blood testing).

Pain/discomfort: Minimal (see general pain/discomfort factors for blood testing).

Accuracy and significance: Although the test is fairly accurate in measuring body chlorides, it is of little significance when used alone, because there are so many different conditions that alter chloride levels.

CHOLESTEROL

Cholesterol is an essential body product that is manufactured by many organs such as the liver, the skin, and the intestines. It is not a fat, as is erroneously believed, but is a solid alcohol called a steroid; steroid compounds also include hormones, vitamins, and drugs. It has been estimated that the average person ingests about 600 mg of cholesterol each day. Cholesterol is found in most foods of animal origin; plant foods are usually free of the substance. Cholesterol is indispensable for brain and nervous system growth and development (nerves cannot transmit impulses without it) as well as for the body's manufacture of sex hormones.

Cholesterol measurements are not very specific for diagnosing disease, and for many years the test was virtually abandoned; recently it has had a resurgence as a possible predictor of heart problems. Its actual predictive value has not yet been proved, however, and it is not totally accepted as a reliable heart risk measurement by most scientists and many cardiologists. Cardiac surgeons, who usually treat the most severe heart and artery disease, report that 80% of their patients have normal blood cholesterol levels.

Recently it has been observed that the lower the blood cholesterol levels, the higher the incidence of cancer. It is an epidemiological observation that will take extensive study to document. However, it is known that as blood cholesterol levels are therapeutically reduced, the incidence of gall bladder problems—one adverse effect—increases.

The usual laboratory test measures total cholesterol, or all the cholesterol that is attached to various fats and proteins floating in the blood. However, when it comes to studying heart disease prediction, the specific protein-fat complexes (see **Lipoproteins**) to which the cholesterol is attached are more important. An excess of certain cholesterols—called alpha, or high-density lipoprotein (HDL) cholesterols—is associated with a *decrease* in heart disease. When cholesterol combines with a fatty acid, it is called a cholesterol ester.

Low density or very low density lipoproteins (LDL, VLDL) appear as the "bad" cholesterols and, epidemiologically, they seem to be the ones associated with heart disease.

Blood cholesterol levels will rise almost instantaneously when an individual is frightened, under anxiety, or in pain, and even when an individual is exposed to an uncomfortably loud noise. For example, many income tax accountants have a great increase in their cholesterol levels during the weeks before April 15; the elevated levels return to normal by May 1. Blood is taken from a vein and the serum is examined.

When performed: When there is suspicion of thyroid disease; with liver disease when there is a question of drug damage or hepatitis; with people who have xanthomatosis (yellowish plaques around the eyes, on the eyelids, over the elbows, and on the palms), although more than half of all people with xanthomatosis have normal cholesterol values; to measure the body's reaction to adrenal hormones; to measure an individual's response to stressful situations; as an experimental aid in the prediction of heart disease.

Normal values: Normal serum cholesterol levels range from 150 to 280 mg per 100 ml. These figures are not absolute. Higher values are normally found in older people; and with patients over 50 years of age, most laboratories consider 350 mg the upper limit of normal. Normal values also vary with the technique used (automated testing is considered less accurate and produces higher values).

Abnormal values: Serum cholesterol is increased with familial hypercholesteremia (an inherited trait); with hypothyroidism (cretinism), hepatitis, and kidney disease (nephrosis); and when the flow of bile from the gall bladder is obstructed. Elevated cholesterol levels also result from pregnancy (after the second month); from fear of the test results at the time the test is performed; and from taking male hormones, certain tranquilizers, cortisone products, vitamins A and D, some diuretic drugs, and epinephrine (adrenalin) products such as those used by asthmatics. Eating a great deal of cholesterol within a few hours of the test may have a slight effect on some people, but it is not constant.

Lower than normal cholesterol values are usually found with hyperthyroidism (Graves' disease), cirrhosis of the liver, certain anemias, and severe infections. Taking female hormones, thyroid hormones, aspirin, vitamin C or B_3 (niacin), certain antibiotics, and drugs used to treat diabetes will lower cholesterol values.

Decreased cholesterol esters indicate liver disease (hepatitis or active cirrhosis).

Risk factors: Negligible (see general risk factors for blood testing).

Pain/discomfort: Minimal (see general pain/discomfort factors for blood testing).

Accuracy and significance: Cholesterol measurements are neither very accurate nor considered significant for any one particular disease. So many variables can affect blood cholesterol that, should the blood be tested hourly throughout the day, or even once daily over a month's time, it would not be unusual to find a wide variation in blood cholesterol values. Whenever an HDL cholesterol test is performed, the serum must be packed in dry ice immediately until the analysis is undertaken, otherwise false values will be reported.

CHOLINESTERASE

There are two different forms of cholinesterase: one may be referred to as true cholinesterase, or acetylcholinesterase, and the other as pseudo-cholinesterase. Both enzymes are necessary for proper functioning of the parasympathetic nervous system, which controls the body's involuntary processes that transmit nerve impulses to the heart, gastrointestinal tract, tear ducts, etc. When these processes are reduced or interfered with—either by disease or by inhalation, ingestion, or skin contact with organic phosphate insecticide such as malathion—the patient has increased parasympathetic nervous system activity. Symptoms include increased stomach acidity, increased intestinal motility, erratic pulse and heart rate, difficulty in breathing, increased sweating, salivation, and watering of the eyes.

In almost all instances, pinpoint-sized pupils are an early sign of interference with the parasympathetic nervous system. Severe reactions include headache, muscle twitching, convulsions, and diarrhea. Some physicians believe ingestion of monosodium glutamate can also cause these reactions. True cholinesterase is measured from red blood cells; pseudo-cholinesterase is measured from serum. Both are obtained from blood taken from a patient's vein.

A special test to measure the presence of cholinesterase is the succinylcholine reaction. Succinylcholine is administered, and if cholinesterase is missing the patient will experience severe difficulty in breathing and muscle inactivity. The test is sometimes given by an anesthetist just prior to surgery to make sure that cholinesterase is present. Succinylcholine may also be used to aid in relaxation during surgery.

When performed: When a variety of symptoms that result from excessive parasympathetic nervous system activity are observed (as described above), especially after possible exposure to an insecticide; in certain skin, liver, and kidney diseases.

Normal values: Cholinesterase values in serum average at least 0.5 pH units per hour. In red blood cells true cholinesterase levels should be at least 0.7 pH units per hour. Some laboratories report cholinesterase values in their own units; these may range from 40 to 80 units as a total value.

Abnormal values: Decreased values indicate interference with the enzyme, usually as a result of organic phosphate poisoning. (Some physicians believe that the lower the value, the greater the intensity of the phosphate poisoning.) Cholinesterase may also be decreased during pregnancy and with cancer, liver disease, and certain skin conditions. Rarely, the levels are increased in kidney disease and hyperthyroidism.

Risk factors: Negligible (see general risk factors for blood testing).

Pain/discomfort: Minimal (see general pain/discomfort factors for blood testing).

Accuracy and significance: The test quite accurately evaluates organic phosphate insecticide toxicity. It is especially significant when administered prior to surgery during which certain muscle relaxants are to be used.

CHOLYLGLYCINE (Bile Acid Cholylglycine)

Cholylglycine is a component of bile acids that are made by the liver, stored in the gall bladder, and excreted into the small intestines whenever fats are eaten. The bile emulsifies the fats so they can be absorbed by the bowel. Once these bile acids have performed their function, they travel back to the liver where they are stored or remanufactured as needed. If liver disease exists, however, cholylglycine remains in the blood in larger than normal amounts; what makes this liver test somewhat different from others is that it shows abnormal values very early—even before actual liver disease becomes evident physically. And, it helps to differentiate between the causes of liver disease as the early effect from alcohol is not reflected in this test. Blood is taken from a vein for study.

When performed: When liver disease, or beginning liver involvement is suspected. To help ascertain the cause and extent of liver disease.

Normal values: Less than 70 mg per 100 ml.

Abnormal values: More than 70 mg per 100 ml.

Risk factors: Negligible (see general risk factors for blood testing).

Pain/discomfort: Minimal (see general pain/discomfort factors for blood testing).

Accuracy and significance: Some doctors believe this might be the best test to detect early signs of liver damage. (The sooner such illness is diagnosed the easier it is to treat successfully.) It is also thought that the increase in abnormal values could be a valid indicator of the extent of the liver damage; values of up to 10,000 mg per ml are not unusual and the extremely large range of abnormal values allows a very sensitive way of measuring the degree of the disease.

CHROMOSOME ANALYSIS (Cytogenetics, Chromatin, Karyotyping)

All normal body cells have 46 chromosomes, including a set of sex chromosomes called chromatin cells. In the chromatin test the inside of the cheek is scraped for a minute specimen (called a buccal smear), and the cells are stained and examined under the microscope; these cells will reveal the presence or absence of a particular active sexual identity cell called the Barr body. The normal female cell has one Barr body and no Y-chromatin. The normal male cell shows no Barr body and one Y-chromatin. (The **Amniocentesis** test is a more detailed study of the chromosome makeup of the unborn infant.) Chromosome analysis also includes the evaluation of their number, structure, and the location of specific genes to determine the existence of other genetic problems such as Down's syndrome. In addition to buccal smears, tissue from the skin, lung, ovary, and testicle can be tested, as well as bone marrow. White blood cells (from blood taken from a vein) seem to be the preferred material for study.

When performed: Whenever there is some doubt about the gender of the individual; whenever abnormal sexual development seems evident—either mentally or physically (undescended testicles, abnormal hair distribution, abnormal fat distribution, growth problems, infertility, failure to menstruate, and gynecomastia, or large breasts in a male); whenever a woman has repeated episodes of spontaneous abortion; whenever there is evidence of physical or mental developmental disability in siblings, or in relatives of the prospective parents.

Normal values: There should be no Barr body in the male and one Barr body in the female. Each cell should contain exactly 46 chromosomes.

Abnormal values: Abnormal values include finding only 45 chromosomes with no Barr body and finding 47 or more chromosomes with one or more Barr bodies. Most of these conditions produce physical sexual developmental abnormalities that usually become obvious with growth.

Other abnormalities may be predicted when the genes are incorrectly located on the chromosomes, or a specific chromosome is physically defective (when chromosome number 21 is abnormal it is indicative of Down's syndrome).

Risk factors: Negligible (see general risk factors for blood testing and catheter and needle insertion).

Pain/discomfort: Minimal (see general pain/discomfort factors for blood testing and catheter and needle insertion).

Accuracy and significance: Total chromosome analysis is considered about 95 percent accurate. Accuracy increases when more specific studies are performed. The significance of the tests is relative and depends on the action taken following diagnosis.

COGNITIVE CAPACITY SCREENING

The cognitive capacity screening test aids in making one of the most difficult of all diagnoses: whether ostensible mental illness is organic (caused by brain damage or metabolic problems) or functional (caused by an inability or unwillingness to behave properly). Conventional mental status examinations (simply talking with a patient) may miss mental problems caused by physical disease.

In the cognitive capacity screening test, the patient is asked 30 questions. (For example: "Listen to these numbers—8, 1, 4, 3. Now count from 1 to 10 out loud and then repeat 8, 1, 4, 3." "Take 7 away from 100 and what do you have? Now take 7 away from that answer and keep taking 7 away from each answer.")

This test is becoming more and more important because of the increasing nursing-home population. Some institutions (as well as some public and private mental hospitals) tend to medicate their patients with tranquilizers and antidepressant drugs before determining if the patient's behavior has an organic or psychological basis. Such drugs will make true dementia cases seem much worse than they really are.

When performed: To ascertain a patient's ability to think, reason, and remember; to distinguish between organic dementia and functional delirium; to help diagnose brain pathology.

Normal values: Answering 20 or more questions correctly usually indicates no organic mental disease.

Abnormal values: Fewer than 20 correct answers should cause further investigation into the possibility of brain disease. Answering more than 20 questions correctly and still acting in a bizarre fashion usually indicates a psychotic reaction. Loss of memory for recent events with clear recall of incidents long past is another indication of many forms of dementia, especially Alzheimer's disease (senile dementia).

Risk factors: None.

Pain/discomfort: None.

Accuracy and significance: The test must be performed by someone trained to recognize the influence of drugs and/or malingering.

COLD PRESSOR

Pressor refers to stimulation of the nerves that control the walls of the arteries. When the autonomic nervous system is excited, it causes the arteries' walls to shrink which, in turn, produces a rise in blood pressure. One way to stimulate these nerves is to place the hand in ice water (one degree above freezing) for one minute. Not only will blood pressure increase temporarily, but the pulse rate will also increase and the heart will use more oxygen. This is a normal response. Once the hand is removed from the cold water, blood pressure and pulse quickly return to their previous levels. If the patient has artery disease, usually in an extremity, the blood pressure's return to normal is delayed for a long time. If a patient has some degree of coronary artery disease (i.e., in the arteries that feed the heart muscle), the cold pressor stimulation may elicit evidence of the disease by causing chest pain, or it might produce corroboration from an **Electrocardiogram, Radiography,** or **Nuclear Scanning.** In addition, the test may precipitate heart arrhythmias (disorders in the heart beat such as palpitations). The cold pressor test can, in fact, substitute for the exercise stress electrocardiogram; it is easier than walking on a treadmill or cycling, especially while X-rays or nuclear scanning studies are being done at the same time.

When performed: To note the reaction of a patient's blood pressure to cold as a measure of the body's response to stimuli affecting the autonomic nervous system; to help diagnose particular diseases of the arteries such as Raynaud's phenomenon (spasm of the blood vessels, especially in the extremities, causing numbness); to help ascertain the presence of heart disease; at times the test is performed in association with an **Echocardiogram** to help uncover problems of the heart valves.

Normal values: After the hand is removed from the cold water, the blood pressure should return to its previous level within five minutes; the pulse should return to its usual rate within three minutes. The test should not provoke pain, shortness of breath, dizziness, and any graphic change on the electrocardiograph or X-ray if they are being performed concurrently.

Abnormal values: When the blood pressure and/or pulse take longer than 30 minutes to return to previous levels after removing the hand from the cold water. Any physical or technical evidence of impairment of the heart's circulation, rhythm, or valves.

Risk factors: The test can precipitate serious heart problems, but it happens very rarely. The test should always be performed in the presence of a doctor prepared to cope with any emergency.

Pain/discomfort: Minimal. Some people find it uncomfortable, but not painful, to keep their hand in ice water for a full minute. If heart disease is present, it is possible to bring on severe chest pains, but doctors usually consider this and do not perform the test on those who might have such a reaction.

Accuracy and significance: A number of doctors prefer this test to the stress electrocardiogram which uses physical exercise, finding it more accurate and less dangerous. A few diseases of the blood vessels, some bleeding conditions, and an occasional tumor may cause an abnormal cold pressor response and must be considered by the doctor; workers who use chain saws, jack hammers, and grinders also may show an abnormal response (their constant exposure to vibrations seems to make their skin unusually sensitive).

COLOR BLINDNESS

About one in every 25 men (and one in every 250 women) cannot perceive the difference between red and green. This condition is almost always inherited. Very rarely, people cannot tell the difference between blue and yellow. The color blindness test usually consists of a special color plate made up of various colored dots that form numbers or figures. For example, a triangle or number 7 in red, orange, and yellow dots may be surrounded by many blue, green, and violet dots. The plate is shown to the patient, who is asked to describe the numbers or shapes.

Several different tests of color blindness (Ishihara, Hardy-Rand Rittler, HRR) are used, since people sometimes memorize a particular test in order to pass. Various colored lamps may also be used to detect those who either pretend to be color blind or who try to hide the condition.

When performed: On people whose occupation requires color discrimination (pilots, truck drivers, etc.).

Normal values: No matter how many different colored dots make up a color plate, a normal individual can distinguish the number or figures imprinted within a design of other colors.

Abnormal values: Someone who is color blind will be unable to discriminate a specific number or object among the many colored dots. Color blindness may be a consequence of alcoholism with blue-yellow defects being the most common.

Risk factors: None.

Pain/discomfort: None.

Accuracy and significance: The test is quite accurate; there are sufficiently different forms to counteract any attempt to mislead the doctor.

COMPLEMENT

Serum complements are proteins in the blood that are part of the antigen-antibody system, which both fights and sometimes causes autoimmune disease (see **Agglutination; Antinuclear Antibodies**). There are at least 15 different forms of complement known at the present time; they are usually tested for as total complement, but they can be measured individually. Some forms of complement help neutralize viruses and destroy bacteria; others produce allergic reactions. To give a few examples: complement-1, referred to as C-1, is usually reduced in patients with chronic urticaria (hives, red raised blotches, and itching); a C-2 deficiency points to autoimmune disease (systemic lupus erythematosus or SLE); decreased C-3 values suggest kidney or liver disease; C-4 is used to follow the progress of SLE; decreased C-5 values indicate an inability to fight off infection; the remaining specific complement values are studied in relation to specific disease susceptibility.

The complement decay rate test, also called the complement-1 esterase inhibitor test, is specific for diagnosing hereditary angioneurotic edema (a condition in which the skin, mucous membranes, and body organs, especially the lungs, suddenly swell up and become red). Blood is taken from a vein and the complement is measured from serum.

When performed: To differentiate familial angioneurotic edema from the noninherited allergic form of the disease (a far less serious condition); whenever autoimmune disease such as lupus erythematosus or scleroderma is suspected; in undiagnosed arthritis and kidney disease; when there is an overwhelming infection without a known cause.

Normal values: Total complement ranges from 50 to 100 CH_{50} units per ml. Normal values may vary with the method used. Normal values for individual components of complement (such as C-1, C-2, C-3) vary too widely with each laboratory to list any standard; the reported value is really a relative increase or decrease in the total complement and each component.

Abnormal values: Increased amounts of total complement are found with infections, jaundice, gout, after heart attacks, and sometimes with rheumatoid arthritis. Increased C-3 is found with cancer. Decreased amounts of complement (which are of greater significance) are found in a great many conditions, including chronic kidney disease, severe liver disease, lupus erythematosus, serum sickness (a severe allergic reaction), and myasthenia gravis.

Risk factors: Negligible (see general risk factors for blood testing).

Pain/discomfort: Minimal (see general pain/discomfort factors for blood testing)

Accuracy and significance: Basically, complement testing is in the research and experimental stage, but it is used to evaluate mysterious medical conditions, especially those relating to immunity. Because such a variety of conditions affects the components of complement, the tests are minimally significant except when employed to confirm suspected rare diseases.

COMPLEMENT FIXATION

The complement fixation test, which aids in the diagnosis of many diseases, relies on forms of serum antibody proteins (called **Complement**) being present in the blood to identify the specific disease under consideration. Antibodies are formed when the body is exposed to infections; if the antigens (specific causes) of the disease are mixed with a patient's serum, along with specially prepared sheep red blood cells, the antibodies and the antigens will combine and the blood cells will remain whole. If, on the other hand, the patient's serum does not contain complement antibodies to the disease, the sheep red blood cells will dissolve (a process called hemolysis).

Blood is taken from a vein and the serum is tested. The serum is diluted to the lowest concentration (highest dilution) that will give a positive reaction (no hemolysis) and is reported as that dilution, called titer. The test is related to the **Agglutination** reaction test, except that agglutination depends on the clumping together of the red blood cells as opposed to their staying whole and separate or their destruction. (At times the same disease will give a positive reaction to both the complement fixation test and the agglutination test.)

The precipitin reaction is another form of complement fixation test. It is particularly valuable in diagnosing suspected fungus diseases, especially aspergillosis of the lung (an infection that usually accompanies and aggravates asthma).

When performed: The test is used most often when there is suspicion of a virus-caused disease that cannot be accurately diagnosed. A few bacterial and fungus diseases also show a positive complement fixation test. Some specific diseases that can yield a positive high-dilution complement fixation include:

Blastomycosis
(a fungus-caused lung disease)
Coccidioidomycosis
(a fungus-caused disease that begins in the lung, sometimes called valley fever)
Chlamydia
(see also **Chlamydia Identification**)
Dengue fever
(breakbone fever)
Encephalitis
(also to differentiate the kind)
Gastroenteritis
Gonorrhea
Hemorrhagic fever
Hydatid disease
(echinococcosis)
Influenza
(also to distinguish types A, B, and C)
Legionnaire's Disease
(a pneumonia-like infection)
Lassa fever
(a new African disease)
Meningitis
(primarily virus-caused)
Pneumonia
(primarily virus-caused)

Poliomyelitis
Psittacosis
(a pneumonia-type disease from bird droppings)
Syphilis
Tick fever
Trachoma
Tuberculosis
Venereal Diseases
(now referred to as sexually transmitted diseases or STD's)
Virus Disease

Normal values: Because of possible past unknown or unremembered infections, an unchanging low-titer positive reaction (a reaction in a very strong or slightly diluted solution) to many diseases is not considered unusual.

Abnormal values: A high titer (a reaction in a very weak or highly diluted solution) to a suspected disease, especially a titer that rises even higher (becomes positive in more highly diluted solution of serum) after a week or two, indicates the presence of disease. Although the test is used mostly to diagnose suspected disease, it can also be positive in cases of thyroid infection, gout, and severe allergic conditions. Some of the 15 different forms of complement may be reduced in a variety of diseases, usually of the inherited type, but also with various forms of arthritis, certain anemias, malaria, and systemic lupus erythematosus.

Risk factors: Negligible (see general risk factors for blood testing).

Pain/discomfort: Minimal (see general pain/discomfort factors for blood testing).

Accuracy and significance: A positive test, indicating the presence of specific disease antibodies, is considered 90 percent accurate (there are rare instances when a patient with the disease shows no antibodies, there are also times when a patient with a positive reaction does not have the disease under consideration).

COMPREHENSIVE MULTIPLE TEST SCREENING

One of many terms used to describe a group of tests (anywhere from 12 to 40 different ones) performed at the same time. A doctor may use the term SMA, for Sequential Multiple Analyzer, one of the earliest machines to perform several different tests concurrently. The original machines could complete 12 tests on 60 patients in one hour; today's machines perform 7,200 tests on 240 patients in the same time. Other terms used for comprehensive multiple test screening are chemistry panel, chemical screening, chemical scan, and profile. When chemical screening is ordered it may include any or all of the following tests, depending on the laboratory and its equipment:

Albumin/Globulin ratio plus total protein
Alkaline Phosphatase
Antinuclear Antibodies
Bilirubin, direct and total
Blood Cell Differential
Calcium
Carbon Dioxide
Chloride
Cholesterol plus high-density **Lipoproteins** or HDL
C-Reactive Protein
Creatine Phosphokinase
Creatinine
Gamma glutamyl transpeptidase or GGPT (see **Alcoholism**)
Glucose
HBsAg (see **Hepatitis**)
Hematocrit
Hemoglobin
Iron plus iron-binding capacity and transferrin
Lactic Dehydrogenase
Magnesium
Phosphorus or phosphates
Potassium
Red Blood Cell Count
Red Blood Cell Indices
SGOT and SGPT (see **Glutamic Oxalacetic Transaminase**)
Sodium
T4 and/or T3 uptake (see **Thyroid Function**)
Triglycerides and total lipids (see **Lipids**)
Urea Nitrogen
Uric Acid
White Blood Cell Count

Each of the above tests is described in detail elsewhere in the book. In most instances chemical screening is more in the nature of a survey of a patient's health status than directed toward a specific diagnosis. Because of the automated equipment, when all the tests are performed at the same time, the total cost averages from $6 to $14 depending on the laboratory. Unfortunately, the accuracy for tests performed as a panel is not considered as good as it is when the tests are performed separately. Many studies show that when chemical screening is performed on apparently healthy people, one out of every three persons receives at least one erroneous abnormal test result.

COMPUTERIZED TOMOGRAPHY (CT, CAT)

Tomography (see **Radiography**) is the focusing of X-rays on a specific level or plane of the body (as if one passed a thin piece of photographic paper through, say, the abdomen, and recorded only what was in that layer of tissue that the film touched). All other areas above, below, or to either side of that plane are obliterated. With computerized tomography (CT), the extremely narrow X-ray beam passes through a cross section of the body (or the brain) and is picked up by an electronic instrument called a scintillator rather than being exposed on the usual X-ray film. The scintillator then feeds into a computer exactly what density (thickness or thinness) of tissue the X-rays passed through. The computer prints out the densities as an illustration of that cross section of the body. Bone, which is of the highest density, comes out white in the picture. Liquids and air, which are of the lowest density, come out black. In between are all shades of gray representing various organs and tissues.

Unlike the typical X-ray exposure, the X-ray camera and scintillator rotate extremely rapidly around the body section being photographed so as to include everything in equal focus. CT is sometimes referred to as transaxial tomography or computerized axial tomography (CAT) because it represents a cross section of the long axis (standing-erect position) of the body. To perform CT on the entire head or a particular body section such as the chest or abdomen takes only one second, and the total amount of X-ray exposure is far less than one old-fashioned X-ray picture. CT images may be viewed on a television screen or reproduced as photographs for permanent study.

There are two different forms of CT: brain scanning and whole-body scanning. CT scanning is different from **Nuclear Scanning** in that no radioactive chemicals are injected into the body. The machines used for each type of scanning are slightly different. Both types of scanning require that the patient remain absolutely motionless for accurate results.

There has been some controversy over CT scanning within the medical profession and especially within the insurance industry, which must pay the costs of the tests. CT scanning is relatively expensive compared with other techniques such as regular X-ray. Furthermore, only a few physicians can be considered experts in the field, since the device was first used in 1973. At the same time, costly as these new machines are, they have been shown to eliminate the need for a great deal of "exploratory" surgery (operations simply to help diagnose a disease, not to cure it). CT scans have also demonstrated that certain allegedly therapeutic surgery would be ineffective if performed. There is general agreement that CT scanning can eliminate potentially dangerous and not always rewarding tests, such as pneumoencephalograms and arteriography (see **Radiography**).

Positron emission transaxial tomography (PETT or PET) is similar to CT, but utilizes radiolabeled substances such as glucose to measure some body functions (metabolic rates in different regions of the body that show the effect of treatment in diseases such as stroke).

When performed: The test is performed whenever brain pathology is suspected, especially brain substance deterioration (dementia), as well as after any head injury, especially to detect a subdural hematoma (although this may not show up on a CT scan for several days). It is also used when brain tumors are suspected; sometimes a contrast dye is injected into a neck artery so that the dye will more clearly demarcate the lesion. CT scanning may be used when hydrocephalus (or any increse in cerebrospinal fluid pressure) is suspected.

Body scanning is performed primarily when there are abdominal or chest problems that cannot be diagnosed by the usual tests. A CT cross section can illustrate the size and shape of all the body organs and their relationship to adjacent organs and tissues. Such a test is especially valuable when pancreatic pathology is suspected (tumors, cysts, hemorrhage, edema) and when liver disease is being considered, especially problems with the bile ducts. It is also valuable in detecting kidney masses and how well the kidneys are functioning, particularly when there is suspected disease of the retroperitoneal space between the abdominal organs and the back muscles and spine (abscesses, hematomas, tumors, diseases of the great blood vessels such as the aorta and large abdominal veins, and lymph node and lymph channel blockage).

Abdominal CT scanning has proved especially valuable when a patient has stomach pains and no evident cause can be found. Many doctors now feel that chest and lung diseases that were once very difficult to diagnose (conditions such as sarcoidosis; old, hidden tuberculosis; enlarged arteries and veins) can be detected by body scanning.

Diseases of the extremities (especially bone and muscle) are being diagnosed by CT more and more often as experience lends itself to greater expertise.

Normal values: A CT scan should show no abnormality in the size and position of organs and tissues.

Abnormal values: Only with extensive experience are doctors able to interpret abnormal findings in a CT illustration and then make a specific diagnosis from that finding. For example, when there is evidence of dementia or physical brain disease, a brain scan will show the convolutions between the brain folds to be much wider than normal—something that cannot be detected by any other test. When CT scans are taken at different levels of the brain, the extent of the disease (along with the possibility of successful treatment) can sometimes be determined. In body scanning, an experienced physician can detect minute pathology such as cysts and tumors that would not be revealed by other tests.

Risk factors: The risk of radiation exposure from a CT scan is less than the risk from a series of routine X-ray exposures. However, there is some X-ray exposure and repeated CT scans will allow radiation accumulation. The greatest risk in CT scanning occurs when a contrast dye medium is injected in a blood vessel as part of the scanning procedure. In addition to the general risk factors for blood testing and catheter or needle insertion, there is the rare risk of an allergic reaction to the dye substance.

Pain/discomfort: Some patients find it uncomfortable to lie perfectly still on a hard surface for several minutes at a time; a number of the newer machines, however, require the patient to remain still for only a few seconds. See general pain/discomfort factors for catheter and needle insertion.

Accuracy and significance: While CT scanning is considered the most effective means to diagnose almost all forms of brain disease, there have been reports of false negative tests; a negative result, therefore, should not be considered absolute evidence that brain disease is absent. Total body scans are extremely accurate and are of great significance as as they can eliminate the risks that accompany diagnostic surgery. Many doctors consider CT scanning the most effective way to diagnose the cause of low back pain whether from the vertebrae or the nerves. Of particular significance is the fact that, should the cause of low back pain be demonstrated by CT scanning, it is most often amenable to medical therapy and does not require surgery.

COPPER

Copper is an essential nutrient. The body requires approximately 2 to 5 mg of copper a day. There are many dietary sources of copper (liver, oysters, beans, peas, avocado, whole grains), so deficiency is relatively uncommon. Copper is measured in the blood serum. In the body copper combines with the protein ceruloplasmin, which can also be measured in the serum as an indication of copper content. Copper is sometimes measured in the urine and in hair.

When performed: When there is suspicion of Wilson's disease (heptolenticular or liver degeneration); in anemia and pregnancy; in patients taking oral contraceptives.

Normal values: Normal serum copper levels range from 75 to 150 mcg per 100 ml. Normal ceruloplasmin levels range from 20 to 45 mg per 100 ml or 35 to 65 IU. Normal urine levels of copper range from 15 to 40 mcg in a 24-hour sample.

Abnormal values: Serum copper levels may be increased in cirrhosis of the liver, leukemia, pregnancy, anemia, heart attack, infections, and when oral contraceptive or birth control pills are used. Decreased serum copper levels are found in Wilson's disease and sprue. Increased ceruloplasmin is seen in pregnancy, heart attack, infections, cirrhosis of the liver, and patients taking oral contraceptives. Decreased ceruloplasmin is found with kwashiorkor disease and Wilson's disease and in infants with anemia and hypoproteinemia. Increased urine copper values are also found with Wilson's disease.

Risk factors: Negligible (see general risk factors for blood testing).

Pain/discomfort: Minimal (see general pain/discomfort factors for blood testing).

Accuracy and significance: As almost all the blood's copper is combined with ceruloplasmin, this is the form of copper most commonly measured. Other than its significance in diagnosing Wilson's disease, copper and ceruloplasmin levels vary so much with many different conditions that they are used primarily to confirm diagnoses.

CORNELL INDEX

The Cornell Medical Index Health Questionnaire is a medical history test that the patient fills out at home before his first interview with the physician. In the section related to bodily symptoms, the questionnaire covers eyes, ears, respiratory system, cardiovascular system, digestive tract, musculoskeletal system, skin, nervous system, genitourinary system, fatigability, frequency of illness, and habits. There are also questions about family history, past illnesses, and moods and feelings (depression, anxiety, sensitivity, inadequacy, anger, tension).

When performed: The index is used as a preliminary test to aid in diagnosis of the individual patient as well as in mass screening. It is especially valuable in distinguishing between psychological and physical problems.

Normal values: Interpretations are based largely on the physician's assessment, which includes an interview with the patient and a physical examination along with the Cornell Medical Index. In general, there should be fewer than 25 "yes" answers.

Abnormal values: The "yes" answers form a pattern that indicates the patient's medical as well as psychological problem areas. More than 25 "yes" answers indicate a serious problem; answering both "yes" and "no" to the same question, omitting answers on six or more questions, or adding remarks to three questions or more are all considered indicative of a problem.

Risk factors: None.

Pain/discomfort: None.

Accuracy and significance: The test is considered quite accurate in helping a doctor confirm any suspicion of a psychological origin for a patient's complaint. It is very significant in directing the doctor's attention to the patient's problem.

CORTISOL

Cortisol (hydrocortisone) is manufactured from cholesterol. It is the main glucocorticoid hormone (a hormone with anti-inflammatory and metabolic activity) secreted by the cortex (outside layers) of the adrenal glands. Cortisol not only reduces the body's protective reactions to bacteria, it also acts on blood sugar levels by inhibiting insulin, helps control protein metabolism, redistributes fat in the body from the arms and legs to the torso, and regulates body water distribution by directing the excretion of sodium and potassium. The amount of cortisol secreted by the cortex is controlled (1) by the hypothalamus portion of the brain, which reacts to physical and emotional stress as well as to other observations of the senses such as noise, odors, and light and darkness; (2) by the pituitary gland, which reacts to how much cortisol is in the blood; and (3) as a consequence of any abnormalities within the adrenal glands (such as tumors). Cortisol testing is now used to detect congenital adrenal disease in a new baby. An infant with insufficient cortisol can go into shock and die if he or she contracts any illness, has an accident, or requires surgery. Cortisol measurements may be made from amniotic fluid (see **Amniocentesis**) as a means of evaluating the maturity and effectiveness of a developing infant's lungs.

The adrenal glands normally produce the greatest amount of

cortisol in the early morning and the smallest amount in the evening. When a person's regular hours are changed (as by working nights and sleeping days), the cortisol secretion rates are usually reversed. Thus, when testing for cortisol, it is vital to know the patient's active and sleeping times. It is also important to know the mental state of the patient, since emotions have a strong influence on the adrenal glands. Blood is collected from a vein and the plasma is tested. Urine is also regularly tested.

When adrenal disease is considered, it is usual to perform an adrenal suppression test. A synthetic glucocorticoid drug such as dexamethasone is given to the patient, and cortisol levels are measured for several days afterward. A patient with normal adrenal glands will show a marked reduction in cortisol secretion the next day and for as long as the drug is administered. With Cushing's syndrome, the adrenal suppression test shows that the adrenals do not stop secreting cortisol; and if cortisol is not even slightly reduced after the first two days, an adrenal tumor is usually indicated. The adrenal suppression test (also called the dexamethasone suppression test or the cortisol suppression test) is also used to confirm the suspicion of organic, or physically caused depression. If the secretion of cortisol is not decreased after a patient takes a measured dose of dexamethasone (synthetic cortisone), it is considered to be strong evidence that the patient's depression is severe and distinct from neurosis. The adrenal suppression test is further used to help distinguish between senile dementia and depressive states. An opposite approach, called the ACTH stimulation test, while not as accurate, may also be employed. ACTH (the pituitary hormone that causes the adrenals to secrete cortisol) is injected. If there is no increase in plasma cortisol, an adrenal tumor is indicated.

In the metyrapone test the patient is given the drug metyrapone, which prevents direct cortisol production, in order to determine if ACTH will stimulate the adrenals. The drug is usually given at midnight and cortisol levels are measured the next morning. Normally the drug-induced reduction in cortisol will cause the body's ACTH to stimulate cortisol production; failure to produce cortisol indicates that the problem lies within the pituitary gland rather than in the adrenals. In patients taking birth control pills or other estrogens, this test can be falsely positive. On rare occasions insulin is given to provoke cortisol secretions; a normal response is a large rise in plasma cortisol.

There are several other tests to measure adrenal cortex function. Two that are used frequently are the urinary 17-ketosteroids (17-

KS) and the urinary 17-hydroxycorticosteroids. The latter measures how much cortisol the adrenals are secreting. The former (17-KS), once the most common adrenal test performed, is no longer considered the most reliable measurement of adrenal activity.

When performed: The test is used primarily to diagnose adrenocortical function such as when Cushing's syndrome (excessive adrenal activity) or Addison's disease (inflammation of the adrenal) is suspected. It is also used when there is precocious puberty, hirsutism (excessive body hair), and excessive signs of feminization in men. It is performed on newborn infants if there is a suspicion of adrenal disease. Today it is used quite frequently to aid in the diagnosis of depression.

Normal values: Normal cortisol values in plasma are less than 30 mcg per 100 ml in the morning and less than 10 mcg per 100 ml in the evening. There should be no more than 10 mcg per 100 ml in a 24-hour urine sample.

Abnormal values: Plasma cortisol levels are increased in stress. In Cushing's syndrome normal night and day variations in cortisol levels are lacking. Cortisol levels are reduced with Addison's disease and with excessive androgenic (masculinizing) hormone activity. Urine levels are increased with Cushing's syndrome and with hyperthyroidism and obesity.

Risk factors: Negligible (see general risk factors for blood testing).

Pain/discomfort: Minimal (see general pain/discomfort factors for blood testing).

Accuracy and significance: Cortisol measurements are considered quite accurate and very significant in diagnosing Cushing's syndrome and Addison's disease. The adrenal suppression test is considered 80 percent accurate and rarely shows a false positive result. Although the test requires the patient to take only one dose of dexamethasone the night before blood cortisol is tested, the test is even more accurate when the patient takes dexamethasone four times a day for two days prior to cortisol testing. It is considered very valuable in helping to predict the prognosis or outcome following treatment for depression. As with so many other tests, a negative response to the adrenal suppression test does not rule out the possibility of depression.

COUNTERIMMUNOELECTROPHORESIS (CIE)

Although there are scores of tests to help diagnose the cause of an infection (see **Agglutination, Complement Fixation, Cul-**

ture, Gram Stain), in some instances counterimmunoelectrophoresis is the fastest way to identify certain disease-causing bacteria. While a culture can take days before the germ can be identified, the CIE test can help supply a specific diagnosis within an hour allowing the doctor to prescribe the proper antibiotic drug almost immediately. In addition, the CIE test can be performed even if the patient is already taking antibiotics which normally interfere with culture tests. The test, related to agglutination techniques, detects antigens from a patient's blood, urine, and other body fluids—particularly cerebrospinal fluid—and is of particular value in helping diagnose the cause of meningitis.

When performed: Whenever there is a severe, yet undiagnosed, infection—usually serious enough to cause septicemia (blood poisoning); most often when the patient has pneumonia or meningitis, and especially in children with these infections.

Normal values: No evidence of any bacterial antigens, although this result alone is not absolute proof that the bacteria are not present.

Abnormal values: Evidence of bacterial antigens after laboratory differentiation of possible false positive test.

Risk factors: Negligible when blood is tested (see general risk factors for blood testing). For other body fluid testing, see general risk factors for catheter and needle insertion.

Pain/discomfort: Minimal when blood is tested (see general pain/discomfort factors for blood testing). For other body fluid testing, see general pain/discomfort factors for catheter and needle insertion.

Accuracy and significance: This can be a significant, even life-saving, test, but it is considered 70 percent accurate in diagnosing meningitis and pneumonias, as there are numerous reports of both false negative and false positive results. Most laboratories know how to cope with false results.

C-PEPTIDE

C-peptide (the C stands for "connecting") is a portion of the basic material used by the body to manufacture insulin. The test, employed primarily in patients with diabetes, measures how much (if any) insulin the patient's pancreas can manufacture. Commercial insulin contains no C-peptide; thus a patient taking regular injections of insulin can still be tested to find out if he is producing any insulin of his own. Knowing if a patient is producing natural insulin (even in small amounts) affects the type of treatment for diabetes. Most often urine is tested; blood serum from a vein may also be measured for C-peptide.

When performed: The test is performed at regular intervals whenever diabetes is known or suspected to ascertain body insulin capability. It is also used to detect if a patient is taking erroneous (usually excessive) doses of insulin and to verify suspected hypoglycemia (low blood sugar). Urine testing is preferred with children when blood specimens are difficult to obtain.

Normal values: There are no specific numerical vales for C-peptide. Its presence indicates that the body can manufactue insulin; its absence indicates that there is no insulin production.

Abnormal values: Failure to detect C-peptide afer giving a patient glucose to stimulate insulin production usually indicates diabetes. Lack of C-peptide in the blood can also mean that a patient has taken so much insulin that the pancreas has shut down because it has no need to produce the hormone. Large amounts of C-peptide can indicate overactive insulin-producing cells in the pancreas, which can cause hypoglycemia.

Risk factors: Negligible (see general risk factors for blood testing).

Pain/discomfort: Minimal (see general pain/discomfort factors for blood testing).

Accuracy and significance: The test is considered quite accurate as long as the testing laboratory is aware of the type of insulin a patient is taking (beef, pork, biogenetic). It is of particular significance in helping diagnose hypoglycemia, the excessive use of insulin by a patient who denies it, and the assessment of pancreas secretions after pancreas surgery.

C-REACTIVE PROTEIN (CRP)

C-reactive protein (CRP) is a blood gamma globulin that reacts with certain bacterial substances in many inflammatory conditions. The CRP test is not specific for any one disease. At one time the test was in widespread use in diagnosing and following patients with rheumatic fever; today the erythrocyte **Sedimentation Rate** (ESR), a similar but simpler and less expensive test, is often used in place of the CRP. Blood is taken from a vein and the serum is tested. In a few disease conditions, especially rheumatic fever, CRP may show up in blood serum before the ESR is elevated.

When performed: In conditions causing inflammation and tissue breakdown; to note progress in the treatment of certain illnesses such as rheumatoid arthritis, tuberculosis, and viral infections.

Normal values: C-reactive proteins are not normally found in the blood.

Abnormal values: C-reactive proteins are found in measurable amounts with bacterial and viral infections, rheumatic fever, cancer, arthritis, heart attack, and pneumonia. Aspirin or steroid drugs will mask the appearance of CRP.

Risk factors: Negligible (see general risk factors for blood testing).

Pain/discomfort: Minimal (see general pain/discomfort factors for blood testing).

Accuracy and significance: The test is positive with such a variety of diseases that it can hardly be significant. However, it is still performed to help distinguish infectious from non-infectious conditions.

CREATINE PHOSPHOKINASE (Creatine Kinase, CPK, CK)

Creatine phosphokinase (CPK) is an enzyme that is found predominantly in skeletal muscle, heart muscle, and the brain. When muscle is damaged, CPK leaks out into the bloodstream. When heart muscle is damaged, most commonly after a heart attack, CPK blood serum levels will rise within hours after the attack. Of all the different enzymes that are usually liberated when heart muscle is damaged, CPK is increased most rapidly (within six hours). It is believed that the rise in CPK is proportionate to the amount of damaged heart muscle. There are at least three forms of CPK, called isoenzymes, and they are labelled according to where they are primarily found: heart, muscle, and brain. CPK-1 is the brain isoenzyme. CPK-2, also called CPK-MB, is the heart isoenzyme. CPK-3 is the muscle isoenzyme.

When performed: To verify suspected heart attack; to ascertain muscular disease and to follow the progress of illness; to help discover genetic carriers of progressive muscular dystrophy; to distinguish malignant hyperthermia (abnormally high fever after receiving certain anesthetics) from fever due to postoperative infection.

Normal values: CPK values can vary with different laboratories. Generally, up to 12 Sigma units and up to 50 IU are considered normal in men and up to 80 IU in women. CPK-3 is normally found in serum. No CPK-1 or CPK-2 should be detected.

Abnormal values: Total CPK levels are almost always elevated after a heart attack; CPK-MB is usually present in a patient's blood six hours following a heart attack. The CPK-MB isoenzyme usually disappears within 24 to 48 hours but total CPK's remain elevated for three to four days. When CPK-1 isoenzymes are detected it usually indicates brain or nervous system disease. Total CPK increases are associated with muscular dystrophy, hypothyroidism, alcoholism, crush injury of the muscles, asthma, and other lung conditions that make breathing difficult. Strenuous exercise and intramuscular injections of medicines can also increase total CPK levels but these usually disappear within 24 hours. Prolonged bed rest, not related to illness, will lower CPK levels.

Risk factors: Negligible (see general risk factors for blood testing).

Pain/discomfort: Minimal (see general pain/discomfort factors for blood testing).

Accuracy and significance: Total CPK levels are not too specific because they are elevated in so many conditions. In contrast, CPK-MB is considered the most significant test to diagnose a heart attack. Recently the amount of the increase in CPK-MB has been proportionately related to the extent of heart muscle damage.

CREATININE

Creatinine is the end product of muscle metabolism (not from heart muscle, however). It is formed from creatine, which provides energy for the muscles to function. Both creatine and creatinine come from amino acids which result from the breakdown of dietary protein. Creatinine is often tested along with **Urea Nitrogen,** which is also primarily a measure of kidney function. (Creatinine is considered the better measure of the two.)

Virtually all creatinine is normally excreted by a part of the kidney called the glomerulus, which is the first of six different filter systems the kidney utilizes to retain products the body needs and to dispose of waste material. Although creatinine is frequently measured in blood serum, the most useful measurement is derived from urine.

The creatinine clearance test is performed on a specimen of urine collected over a 24-hour period. (A newer form of the creatinine clearance test requires the collection of urine only over a 5-hour period.) This test measures the glomerular filtration rate (normally about 5 ounces of blood are filtered by the kidneys each minute) and is thus a fairly reliable indicator of how well the kidneys are functioning.

The insulin clearance test is a bit more precise than creatinine clearance but much more difficult to perform. The urea clearance test is less reliable in that it is affected by diet and how much urine is passed. The PAH (sodium p-aminohippuric acid) clearance test is one of many new kidney function tests that work in a similar way to creatinine clearance. Creatine (not creatinine) is sometimes measured in the serum and the urine as a confirmation of creatinine clearance.

When performed: Primarily when there is suspicion of kidney damage; as an aid in the diagnosis of certain muscle diseases, especially those caused by hormone problems; when a liver problem cannot be specifically diagnosed.

Creatinine clearance is especially useful when there is an abnormal urea nitrogen test; the two tests together may help locate the specific area of kidney trouble. It also helps determine if a kidney problem is caused in part by bleeding or by the way protein in the diet affects the kidneys. The creatinine clearance test is of great value in determining the seriousness of kidney disease as well as in measuring the progress of treatment. It is also of special value when compared with the **Amylase** clearance test to diagnose pancreatitis.

Normal values: Blood serum creatinine values range for 0.8 to 1.3 mg per 100 ml. When measured in the urine, creatinine clearance is expressed as the glomerular filtration rate for a 24-hour period. For men, the normal range is between 110 and 170 ml per minute. Women usually have a slightly lower rate (90 ml per minute is still considered normal).

Abnormal values: Elevated serum creatinine along with reduced creatinine clearance indicates a kidney problem. The severity of the disease is indicated by the amount of reduced glomerular flow. When creatinine values are compared with urea nitrogen values, it is sometimes possible to ascertain if the kidney disease is reflecting the blood flow to the kidney or some blockage in the urinary tract between the kidney and the bladder. Serum creatinine is also increased in certain muscle diseases; when there is vomiting or diarrhea; when patients are taking certain drugs such as steroids, barbiturates, and vitamin C; and when large amounts of roast meats (which contain high levels of creatinine) are eaten.

Risk factors: Negligible (see general risk factors from blood testing).

Pain/discomfort: Minimal (see general pain/discomfort factors for blood testing).

Accuracy and significance: All the clearance tests measure kidney function with reasonable accuracy, but the PAH is the most accurate. Creatinine and the clearance tests are significantly helpful in identifying the damaged area of the kidney and, at times, indicating whether the kidney problem is related to circulation or urinary blockage.

CULTURE

The purpose of a culture is to isolate and identify the microbes that cause disease by an infectious process. The science of microbiology (microbial culture) was formerly known as bacteriology. The name was changed after many organisms in addition to bacteria—viruses, fungi, rickettsia, parasites—were found to cause disease. Since virtually every part of the body is subject to infection, the test is performed on many tissues, secretions, excretions, and fluids. Blood, urine, spinal cord fluid, joint fluid, feces, bone marrow, and material from an abscess, ulcer, sinuses, eyes, ears, nose and throat all may be cultured.

Some microbes do damage directly by their presence; others cause illness by giving off a toxic product (botulism toxin). Disease-causing microbes must always be distinguished from nonharmful organisms that normally live in various parts of the body. Thus, while a direct examination on a slide under a microscope may show bacteria, only a culture can positively identify the type of bacteria.

Usually a sample for culture is placed in two or more containers, each with a different medium (an environment that promotes growth)—one to grow organisms in the presence of air and one to grow them without air. Whenever the specimen is taken, absolute sterility must be observed to avoid contamination. If microbes grow in the sample, many other tests are performed to determine whether the microbes are pathological. Usually small bits of paper saturated with different antibiotic solutions are placed on the microbes to find out which drugs are most effective in killing them. This is called the antibiotic sensitivity test. Such testing is especially important today because so many microorganisms have become resistant to antibiotics.

When microbial infection is suspected, it is also common to perform **Agglutination** and **Complement Fixation** tests to confirm the identity of the organism. Viruses can now be cultured by using living cells (such as chick embryos in eggs, guinea pigs, suckling mice, or specially cultured cells). Viruses are then identified through electron microscope examination and one of the numerous Agglutination or Complement Fixation tests (fluorescent antibody, enzyme-linked immunosorbent assay, radioimmunoassay).

When performed: Whenever there are symptoms of infection (usually high fever) and no specific diagnosis can be made. To help learn about the microorganisms that might be prevalent in a community, especially when an epidemic is suspected.

Normal values: There should be no growth of microorganisms from the various tissues, secretions, and body fluids (except for the normal bacteria in the intestines, throat, etc.).

Abnormal values: Any evident growth of pathological microorganisms is abnormal. When any disease-causing microorganisms are found in the blood, septicemia is indicated. Tuberculosis is diagnosed only by applying an acid-fast stain to distinguish the bacteria in the culture.

Risk factors: Normally there is no risk; the patient usually supplies the specimen to be cultured: sputum, urine, pus from a sore, etc. Occasionally **Endoscopy** is required to obtain a specimen. See also general risk factors for blood testing.

Pain/discomfort: None unless the doctor uses a form of **Endoscopy.** See also general pain/discomfort factors for blood testing.

Accuracy and significance: Culture tests to isolate the cause of an infection are considered very accurate, and equally significant when they are used to select the appropriate drug for treatment of a disease. A negative result (no growth of microorganisms) is important as it points to a virus disease. The test can be lifesaving.

CYSTOMETRY

Normally the bladder will hold about 12 ounces of fluid before the urge to urinate is felt. This urge is caused by the pressure of the fluid against the expanding bladder walls. When the exact response to bladder pressure must be determined, or when it is necessary to know if the patient can discriminate between warm and cold temperatures in the bladder, cystometry is performed.

A catheter (very thin tube) is inserted into the bladder through the urethra and attached to a manometer (a graduated glass tube showing the response to pressure measurements). The bladder is then filled, and the patient's response to known pressure (and the amount of fluid) is recorded. A Lewis cystometer produces a graph showing pressure and capacity response. When necessary, the bladder is then alternately filled with warm and cold water and the patient's response to varying temperatures is recorded.

When performed: Whenever a patient has difficulty urinating (voiding), especially when the patient lacks the normal urge to urinate (usually because of bladder nerve disease); with urinary infections; to test the effect of certain drugs on the bladder, especially when such drugs are to be used to extend the capacity of the bladder or to initiate a response in a bladder that overfills.

Normal values: Until the bladder contains almost a pint of fluid, there should be no uncomfortable sensations. Additional fluid normally causes discomfort, along with sweating and flushing, followed by the urge to urinate.

Abnormal values: Failure to feel pressure after 12 ounces of fluid are instilled in the bladder, along with the inability to distinguish betwen warm and cold solutions, usually indicates disease of the nerves to and from the spinal cord to the bladder. With infections, the bladder will feel full with only a small amount of fluid.

Risk factors: Negligible (see general risk factors for catheter and needle insertion).

Pain/discomfort: Minimal (see general pain/discomfort factors for catheter and needle insertion).

Accuracy and significance: This is a very accurate method to determine whether bladder disease is caused by nerve or spinal cord damage, or infection. Many doctors consider it a significant way to measure the effect drugs will have on the urinary system (some drugs, such as codeine and the anticholinergic drugs used to relax the bowel, make it difficult for a patient to urinate).

CYTOLOGY

Cytology tests detect and identify both normal and abnormal cells (especially cancer cells) in areas that cannot be easily and directly examined. Specimens to be examinied may be obtained from body excretions (urine, feces), secretions (sputum, gastric, eye, peritoneal, breast, prostatic, vaginal, and cerebrospinal fluid), and tissue scrapings (uterus, vagina, mouth, nose, throat, bronchi, rectum, stomach, and cysts). The test makes possible very early diagnosis and treatment of cancer. It can also indicate hormone activity in the body, as well as specific infections and the effect of radiation. After the smears are collected and stained, they are examined under a microscope. The unique tissue-staining technique used in the original test was devised by Dr. George Papanicolaou and is still called a Papanicolaou or Pap test by some doctors.

When performed: As a routine or screening test during a physical examination; whenever cancer is suspected; for hormonal assessment; when there is undiagnosed disease in a particular organ or body system.

Normal values: No abnormal cells should be seen in any stained smear.

Abnormal values: Any cancer cell or even a suspicious cell is considered a positive or abnormal result. A positive test is usually repeated. If the second test is still positive a **Biopsy** (the removal of a minute piece of tissue from the suspected organ), X-rays (see **Radiography**), or other appropriate diagnostic tests must be performed to verify diagnosis. Inappropriate hormone influence on cells or evidence of inflammation is considered abnormal.

Risk factors: Negligible. In addition to the general risk factors for catheter and needle insertion, there are those related to **Endoscopy.** When the Pap test is taken, there is the rare risk of infection but, unfortunately, there is the greater risk that it will be improperly performed and fail to indicate pathology.

Pain/discomfort: Minimal. In addition to the general pain/discomfort factors for catheter and needle insertion, there are those related to endoscopy. A Pap smear should cause no pain or discomfort.

Accuracy and significance: When definitive cancer cells are detected, the test is considered close to 80 percent accurate; the problems arise when there are false positive results implying cancer where no pathology exists. The test is equally significant in evaluating particular hormone activities in the body (Pap test), the effects of X-ray treatment on the body, and the diagnosis of exotic diseases. Aspiration cytology is 90 percent accurate in diagnosing breast cancer. Much depends on use of the proper technique to obtain the sample, and on the training and experience of the pathologist who prepares and interprets the specimen under the microscope.

CYTOMEGALOVIRUS (CMV)

This virus is believed to be part of the **Herpes** virus group that causes cold sores, venereal lesions, shingles, and chicken pox, but cytomegalovirus disease can be far more devastating. Although the symptoms of a cytomegalovirus infection can resemble those of infectious mononucleosis, more often than not there are no symptoms. It is thought that if the population was tested for cytomegalovirus, more than 80 percent of its members would show evidence of exposure to this virus. Although CMV can cause diarrhea, it is most serious when it infects a newborn baby. It is believed that close to 5,000 babies are afflicted with this virus each year and suffer blindness, deafness, blood abnormalities, mental retardation, congenital defects, and encephalitis. It has been found in blood, urine, tears, saliva, and semen, all of which can be tested by examining a specimen through a microscope or by culture. More often, blood is taken from a vein and examined for antibodies through tests similar to **Agglutination** (fluorescent antibody), and by **Complement Fixation.**

When performed: As part of the **TORCH** screening panel for pregnant women and newborn infants; when infectious mononucleosis is suspected but remains unproven; following open heart surgery and other surgery requiring a number of transfusions (for unknown reasons, CMV infection commonly occurs after transfusions of large amounts of blood); when nerve or eye disease cannot be diagnosed.

Normal values: It is difficult to stipulate a "normal" value since more than half the population will exhibit a positive antibody test. However, the antibody level should not change if the test is repeated weeks or months later. There should be no cytomegalovirus bodies inside body cells and no live virus should grow on culture.

Abnormal values: A higher titer of cytomegalovirus antibodies in a newborn; a marked rise in the titer (the amount of detectable antibodies) over a period of a few weeks, especially in a pregnant woman; isolation of the virus by culture, or its presence inside body cells.

Risk factors: Negligible (see general risk factors for blood testing).

Pain/discomfort: Minimal (see general pain/discomfort factors for blood testing).

Accuracy and significance: Unless the antibody titers change markedly, or the culture produces the specific virus, the test, while accurate, is of little significance because a positive result is so common.

D

DEPRESSION

Depression is a mental state that can be caused by physical disease, after pregnancy, and with hormone changes, or it can be a personal reaction to an unpleasant situation. The usual symptoms of depression (tiredness, insomnia, lack of appetite, stomach and intestinal complaints, irritability) can mimic a great many other illnesses. Because of the close association between depression and suicide, it is important to diagnose true depression early.

There are several tests in the form of questionnaires that help to make the specific diagnosis of depression. In the Beck Depression Inventory, the patient is asked to select responses from several sets of leading statements. A set of statements may range, for example, from "I am dissatisifed with everything" to "I am not particularly dissatisfied." Proponents of this test claim that it aids not only in diagnosing depression but also in measuring the degree of depression.

A somewhat similar test is the Zung Self-Rating Depression Scale. The patient is asked to evaluate a series of self-descriptive statements such as "Morning is when I feel best" by checking off a column headed "none or a little of the time," "some of the time," "a good part of the time," or "most or all of the time." This test also claims to be able to indicate the degeee of depression.

All such tests are really only screening devices; a positive diagnosis of depression must be based on in-depth doctor-patient interviews. Additionally there are biochemical tests to aid in the diagnosis of depression. Among them are the adrenal suppression test (see **Cortisol**); and the MHPG urine test (see **Catecholamines**). Today, **Thyroid Function** testing for hypothyroidism is all but routine for patients suffering from depression. In a recent survey of patients undergoing psychiatric treatment for depression, more than 10 percent were found to have some degree of hypothyroidism.

When performed: When patients have vague symptoms, especially tiredness, helplessness, or pessimistic feelings; after a stressful situation in a patient's life (loss of a loved one, loss of a job); when a patient is taking certain drugs, especially tranquilizers; when a patient has marital problems; when suicidal tendencies are suspected by the doctor.

Normal values: Most patients rarely select more than two or three statements that indicate depression.

Abnormal values: Four or more statements associated with a depressed state of mind can indicate mild depression; a greater number of such responses can indicate severe depression and potential suicide. Again, such tests should be used only as screening devices and should be followed by detailed interviews with the patient.

Risk factors: Tests in the form of questionnaires have no risks. See general risk factors for blood testing.

Pain/discomfort: There are no pain/discomfort factors associated with the oral tests. See general pain/discomfort factors for blood testing.

Accuracy and significance: Although questionnaires are not regarded as highly accurate, they may assist a doctor in determining the extent of depression. A doctor's training and experience coupled with biochemical tests are more significant in arriving at a diagnosis.

DILATION AND CURETTAGE (D&C)

The D&C is perhaps the most frequently performed test in the diagnosis of gynecologic problems. The examination is usually performed in a hospital or a clinic under general anesthesia. For the dilatation part of the test, dilators of increasingly large circumference are used to create an opening large enough for examination of the cervical canal (the opening in the cervix to the uterus) and the endometrium (lining of the uterus). A curette (spoon-shaped instrument) is used to scrape the endometrial cavity (curettage) for tissue samples, which are then examined under a microscope. Endometrial screening may sometimes be performed by suction collection instead of scraping, and with this method it can be done in the physician's office, without anesthesia, using a jet irrigation and suction technique. (See **Endoscopy** for hysteroscopy following dilatation.)

When performed: When there is abnormal uterine bleeding or discharge; in infertility; in infections; when there is suspicion of anomaly (uterine abnormality); when there is suspicion of fibroids or cancer of the uterus or cervix; to ascertain the phase of the menstrual cycle; to remove polyps; for therapeutic abortion.

Normal values: Normally no malformations, blockage of the cervical canal, cancer cells, or polyps are found. The cells that line the uterus usually show hormone activity that conforms to menstrual cycle changes.

Abnormal values: Abnormal findings include tumor, cancerous cells, or cells in the uterine lining that do not match the expected phase of the menstrual cycle.

Risk factors: There is a minor risk of infection and subsequent bleeding following a D&C. When a D&C is used for an abortion, the risk increases and the procedure can be quite dangerous when attempted on a patient more than four months pregnant. When general anesthesia is administered there is a moderate risk.

Pain/discomfort: General anesthesia can be followed by nausea and vomiting. After a D&C, there is frequently discomfort in the lower abdomen for a few days; there can also be a menstrual-like discharge lasting up to a week.

Accuracy and significance: The test is quite accurate in helping a doctor determine the cause of many different gynecological problems. It is especially significant in determining whether lesions of the uterus and cervix are cancerous or not.

DISPUTED PARENTAGE

In all areas of the United States approximately 17% of all births are illegitimate; in some urban areas more than 50% of all newborn children are illegitimate. In light of recent court decisions giving the same legal rights to illegitimate children that legitimate children have (support, inheritance, and many other benefits), knowledge of parenthood has become important for legal as well as social reasons. There is the need to protect men who are falsely accused of fatherhood and to assure mothers that the children they bring home from the hospital are really theirs.

The term "paternity test" is a misnomer. Disputed parentage tests do not prove whether a man or woman is really the biological parent of a child; rather, they can only help prove that the man or woman *could not possibly be* the biological parent. At this time nearly 100 different tests can be performed, all of which point out that certain of the mother's or father's biological traits were or were not inherited by the child. Some are based on blood types (such as the O, A, B, AB, Rh, and hemoglobin groups); some are based on immunological characteristics that are transmitted from parent to child (such as enzyme defects, various globulin levels, and cell compatibility). See **HLA**.

Sometimes only one test is needed to show that a child could not possibly be the issue of an alleged parent (for example, if an accused father has type AB blood and the child has type O blood). More often than not, however, seven basic tests are performed; it is claimed that these tests offer a probability of exclusion of 93%. After 62 different tests are performed, the probability of exclusion reaches 98%.

When such tests are performed today, an individual must have an instant-development photograph taken of his face and then affix his signature to the back of the photograph along with his thumbprint. This identifying material is attached to the report to show the specific individual on whom the tests were made. (In the past it was not unusual for a man to go to a laboratory, give the name of the accused father, and offer his blood for testing after earlier, private tests confirmed that the substitute man's blood would exclude him from parentage.) With children, photographs and footprints are used for identification. In addition, the tests are performed in two separate laboratories at the same time. Saliva may also be tested as a confirmatory measure, comparing inherited characteristics of the enzymes.

When performed: The test is used most often in legal disputes concerning births out of wedlock. The most common dispute involves a man accused of being the father of a child. In quite a few instances, however, a mother will claim that the child brought home from the hospital is not hers because of alleged child substitution.

Normal values: There are no normal values in disputed parentage tests since, even if all known tests show that a person could be the parent of a child, there is always a small margin of doubt. If, however, the tests show that parentage would be impossible, they are considered completely accurate. (For example, a woman with type A_2 blood could not possibly be the mother of a child whose blood type was A_1B, no matter who the father was.)

Abnormal values: The only possibility of error occurs when the laboratory's testing serum contains traces of other typing factors not noted on the label (this is not a rare occurrence).

Risk factors: Negligible (see general risk factors for blood testing).

Pain/discomfort: Minimal (see general pain/discomfort factors for blood testing).

Accuracy and significance: When the test shows that either the alleged mother or father could not be the biological parent, it is 100 percent accurate. When tests show only the probability of parenthood, the degree of accuracy depends on the number of different tests performed—the maximum accuracy that can be achieved is 98 percent.

DRUG ABUSE

Until recently, it was difficult to test for narcotics such as marijuana, cocaine, codeine, heroin, morphine, methadone, and dilaudid. It was almost as difficult to detect other drugs sometimes used illegally, such as the amphetamines, barbiturates, and some tranquilizers, especially when they were used to produce exhilaration, deliberate delirium, or oblivion. Today there are quick and simple tests that can reveal the presence of such dangerous drugs in the urine. Requiring no skilled personnel, the tests can be performed in schools, factories, and at home, as well as in the doctor's office or laboratory. Their primary use is to screen and they have proven extremely effective. When there are legal implications, however, many laboratories resort to biochemical blood or urine analysis, both of which are more complicated procedures. There is a difference between **Drug Monitoring** and testing for drug abuse. Drug monitoring is used to determine the optimum dose of a therapeutic drug in order to avoid adverse effects; it is also employed when there is doubt that a patient is taking the prescribed drug.

When performed: When a doctor suspects a patient is illicitly using drugs that might themselves be the cause of an illness, or are producing signs and symptoms that might obscure an underlying disease; to detect criminal activity; to prevent potentially dangerous actions such as driving a car or operating hazardous machinery while under the influence of mind-altering drugs; to explain irrational behavior or sudden personality changes.

Normal values: No evidence of any illegal or unprescribed drug.

Abnormal values: Any evidence of drug abuse. Urine tests are basically qualitative; further technical measurement of the amount of a drug in the body is possible.

Risk factors: None with urine testing (other than possibly providing self-incrimination).

Pain/discomfort: None.

Accuracy and significance: Extremely accurate, with a range of 95 to 99 percent depending on the drug being tested for and the amount of urine available for testing.

DRUG MONITORING

Most prescribed drugs are quite potent; the range of safety between the amount of a drug that is therapeutically effective and the amount that is toxic is very narrow. In addition, there are times when a prescribed drug seems to have no effect, either because of some idiosyncrasy in the patient's metabolism or because the patient is not taking the drug as prescribed. It is known that two out of three patients do not properly follow directions for a prescription drug, and one out of three patients never even have the prescription filled.

Anticonvulsant drugs such as Dilantin (for epilepsy) fluctuate greatly in the body, and it takes only a minute overdose to cause severe damage. Gentamicin (an antibiotic) can cause deafness unless it is monitored carefully. Anticoagulant drugs must also be monitored regularly (see **Prothrombin Time**), as must drugs used in the treatment of arthritis such as salicylates (aspirin), which can cause shock, coma and markedly lower blood glucose levels. Patients taking digitalis preparations (digoxin, digitoxin) are monitored regularly because an overdose can cause fatal irregular heartbeats. Lithium, used to treat manic-depressive illness, can be extremely toxic if blood levels get too high; at the start of treatment, this drug is monitored at least three times a week to avoid convulsions, a dangerous decrease in white blood cells and coma.

Toxicology involves not only testing for overdose of a drug but also monitoring for the optimal therapeutic effect. Antibiotic drugs, psychotherapeutic agents such as tranquilizers and antidepressants, and vitamins are also monitored regularly. In most instances blood is taken from a vein and the serum is tested. Urine, body tissues, and even hair or nail shavings are sometimes tested. Drug monitoring is not identical to **Drug Abuse** testing; in most instances a patient is not unconscious and is able to cooperate.

When performed: To assure that therapeutic blood levels are reached; to prevent toxic reactions from drugs *before* symptoms develop; to detect overdose or abuse of a drug; to determine why a patient does not respond to a drug.

Normal values: Normal values are those that produce a therapeutic effect without causing toxicity. When theophylline drugs (for asthma) are used, they must reach a certain level in the blood before they are effective; less than the required amount in the blood is the same as no drug at all.

Abnormal values: A detectable amount of drug greater than that needed to produce a therapeutic effect is considered abnormal. For example, when Dilantin is prescribed, the drug is given in dosages to produce a blood concentration of from 10 to 20 mcg per ml. Should the blood levels go above 20 mcg per ml, toxicity will occur. Although the therapeutically effective dose of a drug may vary with the size of an individual, the amount of a drug in the blood that can cause toxicity usually remains consistent.

Risk factors: Negligible (see general risk factors for blood testing).

Pain/discomfort: Minimal (see general pain/discomfort factors for blood testing).

Accuracy and significance: While drug monitoring can fairly accurately determine the amount of a drug in the patient's body at the time of blood testing, the significance of the test depends on when the patient took the last dose. The "trough" level of drug monitoring ascertains whether the patient has a therapeutic amount of the drug in his system at all times; the blood sample for testing is taken within 30 minutes before the next dose is due. In contrast, the "peak" level of drug monitoring determines whether the amount of the drug in the patient's system has reached a toxic or dangerous level; the "peak" level is usually tested for immediately after the patient takes the medicine—the exact time depending on the doctor's knowledge of the metabolism of the drug being measured. It should be noted that the blood levels of a drug do not necessarily reflect the amount of that drug taken by a patient. Many variables (absorption, interaction with other drugs, metabolism, kidney function) affect exactly how much of a drug enters, and stays in, the bloodstream. Drug monitoring is also significant in determining a patient's compliance with a doctor's orders.

E

ECHOCARDIOGRAM

The echocardiogram is considered by many physicians to be almost equal in value to the standard **Electrocardiogram** (ECG). Echocardiography is based on the principles of underwater detection (sonar) that the Navy developed during World War II.

When a sound wave is directed into the heart at various locations, the echo, or rebounding sound wave, graphically reflects each part of the heart off which it bounces (see **Ultrasound**). Analysis of the echo images allows a three-dimensional "visualization" of the heart, the heart valves, the muscular structures, and even the blood as it passes through. The technique is similar to fluoroscopy, but with far more detail and with no radiation exposure (the sound waves used to obtain the echoes have never been shown to be harmful).

A transducer (an instrument that can transmit energy into sound and also simultaneously receive sound and translate it back into energy that can be visualized) is rubbed over the heart area of the chest. (Usually a coating of mineral oil is applied to the chest to prevent air from seeping between the instrument and the body.) The transducer can be directed to any specific heart area, and the recorded echo patterns detail the opening and closing and condition of the heart valves. Echocardiograms can also indicate the size of each heart chamber, whether there are any masses in the heart, and especially whether there is excess fluid in the sac around the heart (pericardial effusion)—usually the result of infection or irritation from disease adjacent to the heart.

When performed: To diagnose heart valve disease, enlarged heart, heart tumors, and especially congenital heart defects in infants; when pericardial effusion is suspected; in instances of chest pain, fever, and fainting that cannot be diagnosed; to follow the progress of patients with heart valve replacements.

Normal values: Extensive experience is required to interpret echocardiograms, and great skill and knowledge of heart anatomy are needed to direct the sound waves properly. Thus normal values depend primarily on the technique of the test and the ability of the cardiologist to read the results. Multiple layers of thick and thin lines reflect the echoes from the various layers of heart structure that receive the sounds. There are specific measurements in centimeters (cm) for each area—such as the thickness of the heart wall or the heart chamber (when filled and when empty)—as well as normal expectations of how much blood the heart should hold and eject each time it beats. The difference between normal and abnormal may, however, be only a slight variation in the thickness of one sound wave lasting less than 0.1 second.

Abnormal values: A cardiologist can detect a defect in the opening and closing of a heart valve as well as structural defects in all areas of the heart. The picture of an abnormality can help indicate when certain kinds of treatment will be successful.

Risk factors: None.

Pain/discomfort: None.

Accuracy and significance: A number of doctors believe the echocardiogram reveals more and is slightly more accurate than the standard ECG. However, most doctors choose to confirm a suspected abnormality appearing on an echocardiogram with a Holter monitoring test or **Nuclear Scanning**. The echocardiograph is particularly significant in detecting fluids in the sac around the heart (pericarditis); fluid should never be found around the heart.

ELECTROCARDIOGRAM (ECG)

The electrocardiogram or ECG (formerly known as the EKG because of the original German spelling of the word: *Electrokardiagramma*), is a graphic measure of the heart's muscular activity and a reflection of the self-generated electrical impulses that pass through the heart muscle, causing contraction and relaxation. Various electrodes called leads are placed on the body, usually one on each wrist and ankle and one on the chest that can be moved over the entire heart area. (The leads are metal contacts capable of detecting electrical activity within the body; they do not give off any electricity or have any activity of their own.)

By employing any two electrodes and greatly magnifying the activity they detect, the physician can obtain a diagrammatic representation of the heart's activity. If, for example, the lead from the right arm and the left leg are used, the ECG will largely reflect the activity of the right side of the heart; the same results will be obtained if the movable chest lead is placed to the right of the sternum (breastbone). Use of the various leads in different combinations offers many different "views" of the heart; 12 different "views" are considered standard or routine.

The recorded electrocardiograph shows the rate and regularity of the heart's rhythm; it can also show the force or effectiveness of each heartbeat; the extent and location of any heart muscle damage (both old and new), and the effect of certain drugs. Unfortunately, the ECG can also give false readings; that is, the graph may show what seem to be abnormalities when the heart is normal, or it may fail to reveal heart damage when present. It is not a perfect test and is usually accompanied by several other tests for confirmation of a diagnosis.

For example, when the ECG appears to be normal but the patient has complaints referable to the heart, a stress ECG (sometimes called a treadmill test, an exercise ECG, or a dynamic exercise ECG) may be performed. With the ECG leads in place, the patient walks on a treadmill at a set speed and incline (or operates a stationary bicycle); the ECG is recorded while exercising. Normally no change is observed other than an expected increase in the rate of the heart. But in some patients the extra physical activity cuts down the amount of oxygen reaching the heart muscle, and this shows up on the ECG. The test is stopped immediately if oxygen shortage occurs.

The oldest type of exercise test is the Master two-step (devised by Dr. Arthur Master), in which a patient walks up and down two steps for a specified number of times while the ECG is recorded. This is still an effective test, but it has been replaced by the more impressive treadmills. The stress ECG is considered by some physicians to be a fair predictor of future heart problems. But many physicians feel that the test has no value. Studies have shown that two out of three patients without symptoms who take an exercise ECG may have a false positive result; that is, heart disease may be indicated erroneously. Many doctors believe the **Cold Pressor** test to be as effective as the physical exercise stress test in measuring a patient's response to a burden on the heart.

Another form of heart stress testing is the quiz electrocardiogram. While the ECG is being recorded, the patient is asked questions that both threaten his ego and provoke anxiety. Changes in the ECG during the questioning period can indicate emotionally caused heart disease.

A more recent innovation of the ECG is the Holter monitoring test, in which the patient wears a tiny, portable ECG recording machine (sometimes combined with a tiny voice tape recorder) for 24 hours and notes (or records) any unusual stresses during the day as well as all normal activities (eating, going to the bathroom, etc.). This test can isolate previously hidden heart disease and, of even greater importance, can help indicate causative factors such as personality problems. Holter is also called Ambulatory Electrocardiography Monitoring (AEM) or Dynamic Electrocardiography.

Another new method of testing heart function is the SHK-STI (Spodick-Haffty-Kotilainen measurement and calculation of the **Systolic Time Intervals**). The patient wears an earpiece containing a photoelectric cell that measures the velocity of the blood entering and leaving the ear at the same time that chest electrodes are recording the ECG. These measurements of how well the heart is functioning can be made over a 24-hour period and can be correlated with normal physical activity and exercise.

When performed: The test is performed whenever heart disease is suspected and often as a routine checkup. (It is advisable to have at least one ECG before the age of 40 in order to note any changes that may occur at a later date.) It is also performed whenever a patient complains of shortness of breath, intermittent chest pain, or "palpitations," and when patients are taking drugs such as digitalis or diuretics (which tend to cause potassium changes that can severely affect the heart's activity).

Normal values: Each lead of the ECG has a fairly normal but slightly different pattern. The rate of the heart should be between 70 and 100 beats per minute (athletes may have normal rates of 50), and the pattern should be regular (no extra or missed beats).

Abnormal values: Extensive training and experience in interpreting ECGs allow the physician to detect even a slight variation from normal or expected patterns. The changes may indicate a muscle defect (either damage or insufficient oxygen), or they may reveal nerve conduction changes, which can come from damage to the heart arteries that bring oxygen to the heart muscle or damage to the muscle itself (from the aging process or from old infections). Enlargement of the heart, congenital defects, and valve disease may also be indicated by the ECG.

Risk factors: See general risk factors for electrical instruments. Although the American Medical Association states that a physician need not be present during a stress electrocardiogram test, the risk of adverse effects associated with the test (collapse, exacerbation of existing heart disease, stroke, and heart attack itself) are such that a patient should insist on the presence of a physician to handle any emergency.

Pain/discomfort: There should be no pain or discomfort while a standard ECG is performed; some patients find it uncomfortable to lie still for prolonged periods of time. It is possible to have chest pain while undergoing a stress electrocardiogram.

Accuracy and significance: When the ECG is used as a screening device to detect heart disease in patients without symptoms, it is only considered moderately accurate. The standard ECG may also miss existing heart disease if the pathology exists in unusual areas of heart muscle, or if the problem is related to the heart valves. For patients with obvious heart disease, the ECG is considered 90 percent accurate in locating the problem area. Thus far, the stress ECG is not considered sufficiently accurate to serve as a precise diagnostic technique. The Holter monitoring test is probably the most accurate ECG test as it functions for a long enough period of time to reveal heart rhythm abnormalities that could be overlooked in the 10 to 15 minutes of a standard ECG.

(*Note:* See also **Echocardiogram**; **Pulse Analysis**; **Radiography**; **Systolic Time Intervals**.)

ELECTROENCEPHALOGRAM (EEG)

The electroencephalogram is a graphic recording of the minute electric current given off by brain cell activity. The current is amplified, translated into wavy lines (waves), and recorded on paper. The waves represent intermittent brain cell activity; the height of the waves as well as the distance between each peak depends on body activity (for example, blinking or opening and closing the eyes can create seemingly abnormal waves). The waves can also show hyperactive brain cell activity as seen with epilepsy and interference with brain cell activity as seen with tumors.

From 10 to 24 electrodes are applied to the scalp in specific positions to aid in locating any abnormal lesion that might be reflected on the electroencephalograph. The patient lies quietly with eyes closed and no body movement. At times the patient is told to breathe fast and deeply, as this seems to amplify EEG waves.

The waves of brain activity recorded on the electroencephalograph are classified by Greek letters (alpha, beta, etc.). The biofeedback machine is essentially an electroencephalograph constructed to detect only alpha waves.

When performed: Whenever any nervous system or brain disease is suspected; whenever there are brief episodes of unconsciousness or fainting; following head injury; whenever a patient has suffered a convulsion; when there are persistent episodes of narcolepsy (falling asleep in the midst of one's usual activities); when alcoholism is suspected.

Normal values: Alpha waves (with a frequency of 8 to 15 cycles per second) and beta waves (with a frequency of 16 to 30 cycles per second) are normally found in all individuals. The strength of the wave (the distance above and below the base line) is also important in making a diagnosis.

Abnormal values: Theta waves (with a frequency of 4 to 8 cycles per second) may be found in some normal individuals, but they should not make up more than 10% of the overall recording. An excess of theta waves can indicate a brain tumor, brain damage following a head injury, epilepsy, or stroke.

Delta waves (with a frequency of less than 4 cycles per second) are indicative of a very serious condition (severe injury, brain abscess, brain tumor, or massive brain hemorrhage). Severe infection (encephalitis) can also cause delta waves.

Other wave patterns are specific for epilepsy; often the type of epilepsy can be determined by the electroencephalograph. Specific brain wave values can indicate brain tissue atrophy secondary to alcoholism.

Risk factors: None.

Pain/discomfort: Some patients find the tiny needles that are pressed into the scalp quite uncomfortable; newer non-penetrating electrodes are now available. Many patients find lying still for a prolonged period of time uncomfortable, and some find the necessity to be in an isolated and darkened room somewhat stressful.

Accuracy and significance: The EEG is considered extremely accurate for the detection of epilepsy and a number of other brain activity disorders. It is considered of particular significance when the recording shows no abnormalities despite a patient's complaints. Some patients seem to have epilepsy but really do not; they have what is known as pseudoepilepsy. Patients suffering from hysteria, or who pretend to have epilepsy as a means of dependence or for whatever other reason, can manifest some of the symptoms of epilepsy (they may complain of losing consciousness or fainting), yet their brain wave pattern recorded by the EEG while they are pretending to show symptoms remains normal. This is how doctors differentiate pseudoepilepsy from actual epilepsy.

ELECTROMYOGRAPHY (EMG)

Electromyography is a diagnostic neurologic test to study the potential (electrically measured activity) of muscle at rest, the reaction of muscle to contraction, and the response of muscle to insertion of a needle. The test is an aid in ascertaining whether a patient's illness is directly affecting the spinal cord, muscles, or peripheral nerves.

The patient lies at rest while the peripheral nerves in various areas are stimulated through electrodes, and the electrical activity in muscles and nerves is recorded. In needle electromyography, a small needle is inserted into the muscle and the patient is observed for electrical activity in the muscle at rest, on insertion of the needle, and during muscle contraction. The test is sometimes employed as a measure of the muscle tension produced by nervous stress; usually the muscles of the forehead are tested, since they can indicate relaxation or generalized body tension.

Electromyoneurography is the combined use of electromyography and neurography, which applies the procedures of electromyography to nerves instead of muscles. The two tests offer a more precise means of finding the exact location of nerve damage or disorder.

When performed: To aid in the diagnosis of diseases affecting the muscles, peripheral nerves, and spinal cord; to detect "hysterical" weakness and paralysis.

Normal values: Normally when the muscle is at rest, no electrical activity is observed. When muscles contract, the electromyograph shows a smooth graphic wave-like representation of each contraction; the graph lines are amplified with the increase in strength of each contraction.

Abnormal values: Muscle disease produces a spiked wave pattern; the shape of the spike depends on the particular disease. Muscle weakness produces a diminished wave. With myasthenia gravis, the waves disappear after a few minutes. Nerve involvement as opposed to muscle involvement usually shows a decreased frequency of contractions.

Risk factors: Negligible. See general risk factors for catheter and needle insertion and electrical instruments.

Pain/discomfort: Needle insertion, usually performed without local anesthesia, can be quite uncomfortable and, at times, even painful.

Accuracy and significance: The test is considered quite accurate; it is difficult for a malingerer to pretend to have muscle pathology when muscles respond to electrical stimulation.

ENDOSCOPY

More than 100 years ago a doctor put an open tube into the esophagus of a patient and, using the light from an oil lamp, was able to inspect the esophagus walls. This was the first instance of endoscopy—direct observation of a body organ or cavity. Since that time, the simple, open tubes have been replaced by far more intricate "scopes"; the latest, called fiberoptic endoscopes, can bend light rays so that the doctor can see around corners and obstacles and pinpoint the exact location of any pathology.

The endoscope is now used to examine the esophagus, the stomach, and even the intestines. The instrument is usually equipped not only to allow for observation but also to pump air into the cavity so as to extend the walls and make observation easier; to wash away anything that may obstruct the view (such as blood when looking for a bleeding ulcer); to suction out suspected material for **Cytology** tests; and to take a **Biopsy** specimen for testing. For examination of the upper gastrointestinal tract, the patient usually swallows the tip of the instrument (after the throat has been sprayed with local anesthesia); the swallowed tip carries the narrow tubing along with it.

A similar type of instrument used to detect lung disease is called a bronchoscope; the bronchoscope is usually equipped with a whirling brush at the tip to pick up bronchial cells under a thick mucous layer for microscopic study. Use of the proctosigmoidoscope in the rectum and large bowel is yet another form of endoscopy. Newer colonoscopes can reach as far as five feet into the lower intestinal tract.

At times a direct incision is made in the skin and an endoscope is inserted to view the area beneath. When this is done in the portion of the chest just above the breastbone, it is called mediastinoscopy. This form of endoscopy enables the physician to view the bronchi from the outside, the large blood vessels as they enter and emerge from the heart, and the lymph nodes in the area (which are especially diagnostic when looking for certain tumors).

When the incision for an endoscope is made over the abdomen, it is called peritoneoscopy or laparoscopy. Direct examination of the abdominal cavity offers a unique way of testing the liver for size, growth, and clotting defects, and for obtaining a tissue specimen. With abdominal endoscopy it is also possible to see the gall bladder, pancreas, and spleen, along with the ovaries and outer surface of the uterus. A culdoscopy, which uses an endoscope inserted through the posterior vaginal wall, allows a doctor to view all the female reproductive organs (ovaries, tubes, and outside wall of the uterus). A colposcopy, on the other hand, uses a special endoscope fitted with magnifying lenses for a more extensive examination of the cervix and vagina.

Hysteroscopy is an endoscopic test that allows direct examination of the inside of the uterus. Cystoscopy refers to direct examination of the inside of the bladder; vaginoscopy offers a more detailed scrutiny of the vagina than can be obtained by the usual techniques. Recently the endoscope has been adapted to look into joints; knee endoscopy allows a specific test to evaluate meniscus cartilage or ligament tears of that joint. (Doctors can now perform corrective surgery on the knee through the endoscope.) In almost all instances, endoscopy is performed in conjunction with X-rays (see **Radiography**).

Fetoscopy allows an endoscope, called a fetoscope, to be inserted directly through the abdomen and uterus to observe the developing fetus directly. This process is usually performed during the 18th to 20th weeks of pregnancy. While fetoscopy carries with it the greatest risk to the developing infant, it can reveal defects undetectable by other means and can also be used to treat some of those defects prior to birth.

When performed: When X-rays show suspected lesions in an area that can ultimately be viewed directly by an endoscope (such as bleeding stomach ulcer or liver abscess); when congenital malformations are suspected in various organs, especially the esophagus; when growths, abscesses, or inadequate functioning of an organ is suspected; whenever a biopsy is needed to confirm a diagnosis; when there is abdominal or chest pain that cannot be explained; following trauma when internal injuries are suspected.

Normal values: When an organ (or the surface or lining of an organ) is viewed directly, it should appear normal to the examining physician. Normal values are based primarily on extensive experience (only a trained eye can spot a pinpoint lesion or ulcer).

Abnormal values: Evidence of tumor, abscess, blocked or nonfunctioning ducts, infection, or hemorrhage is considered abnormal.

Risk factors: Generally, when endoscopes are inserted into normal body openings, the risks are minimal. However, there is a possibility of infection because of the difficulty in sterilizing an endoscope. Not only can infections be passed from one patient to another, but bacteria are apt to multiply on endoscopes even when they are not in use. If previously detected pathology is present, there is the slight risk that the endoscope might perforate, rupture, or tear and cause bleeding of the organ being examined. When endoscopes are inserted through a surgical incision, the above risks still apply in addition to the routine risks of surgery (wound healing, wound herniation, and anesthesia). The more appliances (brushes, biopsy cups, crushing clamps) that are attached to, or manipulated through an endoscope, the greater the risks.

Pain/discomfort: Most patients find endoscopy uncomfortable, even with local anesthesia. When surgery is part of endoscopy, there is often post-operative pain in addition to the aftereffects of anesthesia.

Accuracy and significance: Endoscopy is considered one of the most accurate of all medical tests because of the opportunity to view the disease site directly. Most doctors consider endoscopy far more significant than radiography.

ESTROGEN (Estradiol, Estrone, Estriol)

Estrogens are really several different female hormones composed of estradiol (the most potent), estrone, and estriol. All the estrogens are manufactured principally by the ovaries, but small amounts can come from the adrenal glands and even, in men, from the testicles. Usually the total amount of estrogens is measured in the urine; individual components may also be tested. Estradiol can be measured in blood plasma taken from a vein. Estrogen production is controlled by the pituitary gland and responds not only to pregnancy and phases of the menstrual cycle but also to stress (anxiety) situations.

When performed: When little or no ovary function is suspected; when pituitary gland dysfunction is suspected; during pregnancy; when certain inherited sexual dysfunctions are under consideration; when a woman has excessive menstruation that cannot easily be explained; in cases of infertility.

Normal values: Nonpregnant women usually secrete from 10 to 60 mcg of total estrogen per 24-hour urine sample during the first two weeks of the menstrual cycle; this amount rises to about 100 mcg per 24 hours of urine during the last two weeks of the cycle. In pregnant women 24-hour urinary estrogen may rise to 40,000 mcg. Children secrete less than 1 mcg per day. After menopause 1 to 20 mcg per day is normal. Men normally secrete up to 20 mcg in a 24-hour urine sample.

The normal range of plasma estradiol varies with phases of the menstrual cycle. During the first 10 days it averages 50 pg per ml; during the last 20 days it averages 125 pg per ml. Men normally average 20 pg per ml at all times.

Abnormal values: Elevated urinary estrogen levels can result from ovarian tumors, excessive pituitary activity (which can also come from hypothalamic pathology), adrenal hyperactivity, liver disease, and certain inherited chromosomal abnormalities. A decreased amount of estrogens can be found when a patient takes female hormones (which stop body manufacture of estrogens), with problems during pregnancy, with decreased pituitary activity, and with ovarian failure. Severe dieting lowers estrogen levels.

Usually, when abnormal values of estrogens are discovered, specific tests for the various components of estrogen are performed to ascertain the cause. (When a patient takes diethylstilbestrol, for example, the estriol portion of estrogen decreases.) Recently estrogen measurements have also been taken in men; an elevated level (especially of plasma estradiol) with reduced testosterone (see **Testis Function**) seems to be a risk factor in heart disease.

Risk factors: Negligible (see general risk factors for blood testing).

Pain/discomfort: Minimal (see general pain/discomfort factors for blood testing).

Accuracy and significance: Estrogen testing, particularly when the various components are measured, is considered quite accurate in evaluating ovary function. It is also a significant test in aiding in the diagnosis of sexual dysfunction and infertility.

ESTROGEN RECEPTOR (ER)

Some cancers of the breast, uterus, ovary, skin, lymph nodes, and stomach "respond" to and can be treated by certain hormones. It is of great advantage to know which cancers will react to hormone therapy. Two out of three cancer tissues that will absorb estrogens (and an even higher ratio of tissues that also absorb progesterones—progesterone receptor) can be treated by various forms of hormonal manipulation and antiestrogen drugs in place of surgery. The Estrogen Receptor test measures the response of a tumor to estrogen stimulation.

In the estrogen receptor test, a tiny specimen of body tissue (see **Biopsy**), usually breast, is studied to see how responsive it is to estrogens—how it reacts (grows or diminishes) to the hormone's activity in the body. This test is a particular measure of whether a tumor is hormone-sensitive and thus whether it would be of value to have the patient's adrenals or pituitary gland removed (or destroyed by radiation) as part of therapy.

When performed: To ascertain if a cancer can be treated with hormones; when a patient has a metastatic (spreading throughout the body) cancer whose source cannot be located but the cancer itself can be biopsied to indicate if it is treatable by drugs; to show which cancer patients will not benefit from certain surgical procedures such as removal of the pituitary gland or adrenal glands; to indicate which cancer patients might benefit from chemotherapy.

Normal values: There are no normal values for this test; when more than 3 femtomoles of the protein estrogen receptor are found in a cancer, it is considered positive or hormone-receptive.

Abnormal values: A negative response, or failure of the tissue to indicate the presence of estrogen receptors, usually means that hormone treatment will not work and that chemotherapy should be tried.

Risk factors: As with any biopsy there is the slight possiblity of hemorrhage and/or infection.

Pain/discomfort: Minimal as a local anesthetic is commonly used.

Accuracy and significance: The test is approximately 60 percent accurate in predicting which breast cancers will respond to hormone therapy (only about one out of three breast cancers respond to hormones). Should the progesterone test be positive, the accuracy rate increases to 80 percent. There is, however, the rare patient who has a negative estrogen receptor test, yet still responds to hormone therapy.

F

FECES EXAMINATION

The average adult excretes approximately 100 to 300 g (3 to 10 ounces) of fecal matter per day, of which about 70% may be water. The feces (stool) can offer valuable diagnostic clues to diseases of the bowel, the blood, and the metabolic system, and especially to infectious processes that cannot be diagnosed.

Many tests can be performed on the feces. The usual examination consists of noting the color and the presence or absence of blood and mucus, and then making a microscopic search for parasites (worms, amoeba) and their eggs (ova) and a culture for bacteria. On occasion, the amount of fat is measured after a patient is given a high-fat diet for three days. Patients should not brush their teeth or eat meat for three days prior to the test, since any traces of blood from the gums or from rare meat in the feces can cause a false positive reaction.

The Scotch tape test is used to find worms that come out of the bowel at night (particularly pinworms). A piece of Scotch tape is wrapped around a pencil, sticky side out, and touched to the anal area after the body has been warmed, usually under a blanket. The tape is then placed on a glass slide and examined under the microscope.

The **String** test, **Agglutination** and **Complement Fixation** are also tests to help diagnose parasitic disease. (See **Parasite**.)

When performed: As a routine or screening test to detect unsuspected (very early stage) gastrointestinal disease; in an undiagnosed infection (diarrhea); when there is an undiagnosed metabolic difficulty (weight loss); as a verification of gall bladder disease.

Normal values: The normal color of feces (although a great deal depends on diet) ranges from light to dark brown. Microscopic examination should show a predominance of partly digested foods and only a rare blood cell or shred of mucus. Less than 25% of the feces' dry weight should be fat. No parasites or their eggs should be present.

Abnormal values: When there is gall bladder or liver disease, the feces acquire a gray to gray-white color. If there is bleeding high up in the bowel (from the esophagus to the small intestine), the feces have a black, tarry appearance; if the bleeding is near the rectum, red blood may be seen. Yellow-colored feces are seen with certain digestive diseases, especially of the pancreas (sprue). Following a bout of food poisoning, the feces may acquire a greenish hue. Beets can color the stool red. Silver-colored feces, sometimes described as "stainless steel," suggest cancer in or near the pancreas.

Any amount of blood (even occult: not visible but measurable) in the feces is abnormal. Its presence indicates bleeding somewhere in the gastrointestinal system and can mean cancer, infection, anemia, or injury to the bowel.

It is abnormal for more than 25% of the solid part of the stool sample to be fat. Increased amounts of fat in the feces are seen with pancreatic disease, biliary tract obstruction, and problems of intestinal absorption.

An increased amount of mucus is seen in many gastrointestinal conditions, especially infection, dysentery, colitis, fistula, and pancreatic disease.

Microscopic examination of the stool sample can show a specific parasite or its egg that may be causing unknown fever, weight loss, and unusual fatigue. Worm infestation can cause asthmatic symptoms.

Risk factors: None.

Pain/discomfort: None. Some people find it disturbing to collect a stool specimen.

Accuracy and significance: When properly performed all tests on feces are quite accurate. Parasites can be missed by a careless technician. Any abnormal finding in feces is considered significant.

FIBRINOGEN

Fibrinogen (Factor I), a plasma protein manufactured in the liver, is one of the 12 known primary factors essential to the clotting of blood. After a patient suffers an injury that causes bleeding, thromboplastin is given off by damaged tissues and combines with prothrombin and calcium in the body to form thrombin. The thrombin then combines with fibrinogen to make the fibrous substance that allows clot formation. Inability to form fibrinogen may be inherited or acquired from disease. Blood is taken from a vein and the plasma is tested.

When performed: When a coagulation defect (inability of the blood to clot) is suspected; with excessive unexplained black-and-blue areas or mucous membrane bleeding.

Normal values: Normal fibrinogen levels range from 200 to 500 mg per 100 ml or 0.2 to 0.5 g per 100 ml.

Abnormal values: Deficiency of fibrinogen (hypofibrinogenemia) may be congenital as well as acquired from liver disease, vitamin B deficiency, and certain bone cancers. Fibrinogen levels may be elevated in nephrosis and multiple myeloma. In pregnancy and in certain severe infections, the levels are slightly higher than normal.

Risk factors: Negligible (see general risk factors for blood testing).

Pain/discomfort: Minimal (see general pain/discomfort factors for blood testing).

Accuracy and significance: Because abnormal fibrinogen values appear in a variety of conditions, the test is only significant when determining the cause of coagulation problems.

FLUORESCEIN EYE STAIN

Fluorescein, an orange-colored dye, is used in testing for abnormalities of the cornea (the surface over the pupil and lens of the eye). The dye is dropped onto the eye and allowed to spread over the surface. Sometimes individual sterile strips of paper containing the dye are used instead of liquid fluorescein to avoid the possibility of bacterial growth in the bottled solution. The dye will lodge in any irregularities on the cornea, the rest will wash away with tears. When ultraviolet or "black" light is then directed on the eye, the fluorescein will glow green and so indicate any abnormalities such as scratches, ulcers, foreign bodies (even as small as an eyelash hair), and various infectious diseases that can cause physical damage to the corneal surface.

Most eye injuries and other problems can be observed directly by the physician when the ultraviolet light is directed on the eye; in addition, a biomicroscope or "slit lamp" may be used to obtain a greatly magnified view of the eye surface. The biomicroscope is also used for more detailed examination of the structures of the eye.

At times the gonioscope (a special instrument to examine the surface of the eye) is used, with or without fluorescein eye stain.

When performed: Whenever any injury to or infection of the eye is suspected, especially when a superficial examination shows no evidence of trauma; during and after the fitting of contact lenses to make sure that tears pass normally under each lens; before applying cortisone to the eye.

Normal values: If there is no break in the surface of the cornea either from disease or injury, the fluorescein stain will wash out with tears and will reflect no damage when subjected to ultraviolet light.

Abnormal values: Any break in the smooth corneal surface will show a greenish fluorescence when viewed under ultraviolet light. From the size, shape, and location of the dye, the physician can usually make a specific diagnosis.

Risk factors: None.

Pain/discomfort: Should the fluorescein stain touch the skin surface around the eye, it might leave a slight discoloration which is temporary.

Accuracy and significance: The test is extremely accurate in detecting the smallest of eye surface injuries and is particularly valuable in the fitting of contact lenses.

FOLATES (FOLIC ACID)

Folates, of which folic acid is but one version, are essential to prevent anemia. Large amounts are found in beef, green vegetables, liver, nuts, oranges, and yeast. They become reduced primarily from an inadequate diet, but also from alcoholism and certain drugs such as birth control pills. The body stores of folic acid last for only a month or two, and folate deficiency can often be diagnosed before anemia is apparent. Blood is drawn from a vein and the serum is examined.

When performed: When folic acid deficiency, especially in pregnancy, or megaloblastic anemia (abnormally large but undeveloped red blood cells) is suspected; when the tongue is smooth and enlarged.

Normal values: Normal folic acid levels range from 5 to 25 ng per ml of serum.

Abnormal values: Decreased folic acid levels in the serum are found in malnutrition, pregnancy, anemia, alcoholism, and intestinal diseases characterized by malabsorption of folic acid (such as celiac disease and sprue).

Risk factors: Negligible (see general risk factors/for blood testing).

Pain/discomfort: Minimal (see general pain/discomfort factors for blood testing).

Accuracy and significance: Blood serum folate measurements are reasonably accurate; however, when there is doubt in relation to clinical findings, folate measurements of red blood cells usually resolve the question. The test is significant in distinguishing the difference between folic acid and vitamin B_{12} deficiency. If anemia is treated without determining this difference, damage to the nerves can occur.

FUNDOSCOPY

The fundus, or black part of the eyeball, is examined by using an ophthalmoscope. The primary area examined is the retina (which receives images and transmits them to the brain); this is also the only area of the body where blood vessels (small arteries and veins) can be seen directly. The optic disc—the point where the optic nerve enters the brain from the eye—is also examined; the appearance of the edge or margin of this small, circular area is important in the diagnosis of many different diseases. Usually a tiny beam of light is projected through the pupil onto the back of the eyeball; the area is viewed through a variety of ophthalmoscopic lenses to focus upon the particular object being studied (blood vessel, retina, nerve).

When performed: Usually part of any routine physical examination by a physician as well as any eye exam by an ophthalmologist; when eye disease such as glaucoma is suspected; whenever diabetes, atherosclerosis (artery disease), or hypertension is suspected; when brain lesion or brain disease is considered; following head injury; to corroborate certain infections and malignancies.

Normal values: The optic disc, the retina, and the blood vessels should appear normal to the doctor. Specific terms are used to indicate the presence or absence of disease (such as stages of high blood pressure, diabetes, or the protrusion of the optic disc).

Abnormal values: Abnormal values depend on the degree of disease observed through the ophthalmoscope and are usually rated from I to V, depending on severity.

Risk factors: None.

Pain/discomfort: None.

Accuracy and significance: This is one of the most valuable tests a patient undergoes. It is extremely significant for it can reveal the first signs of heart and blood vessel disease (especially high blood pressure), brain disease, diabetes, and, of course, specific eye conditions.

FUNGUS

Diseases caused by fungi (molds and yeasts) are called mycotic. They can cause localized problems such as the tiny, itching white patches that sometimes appear in the mouth, throat, or vagina; or they can be the basis for extremely serious, sometimes fatal systemic body infections such as coccidioidomycosis and cryptococcosis, histoplasmosis, aspergillosis (an allergic-type chest infection often confused with asthma), and blastomycosis (a fungus disease of the skin, bones, and urinary system). Ringworm is a fungus disease; common forms include athlete's foot and, when in the groin, "jock itch."

The easiest way to test for a fungus is to take a scraping or smear from the affected area and examine the specimen under the microscope; each fungus has a characteristic appearance. All take on a blue color when studied with the **Gram Stain** test. Some of the ringworm fungi will fluoresce (give off a greenish or brownish glow) when examined with Wood's light (ultraviolet rays), especially those on the scalp or under the nails.

When systemic illness or a blood infection is suspected, the blood from a vein is cultured to isolate the causative organism; it can sometimes take weeks before definitive growth of the disease-causing organism is seen. In rare instances, specimens thought to contain fungi are injected into animals to observe the effects (fungi develop much faster in animals than in humans). A specimen from the animal can then be tested to determine the kind of fungus growth.

One other way of diagnosing fungus disease is through **Complement Fixation**; when this method is employed several blood samples are taken two weeks apart.

When performed: Most commonly on areas of itching skin, especially the scalp; with persistent vaginal discharge; with persistent lung infections; with undiagnosed generalized infections, especially meningitis.

Normal values: Normally fungi are not found in or on the human body. On occasion, a nondisease-causing fungus may be isolated from the mouth or vagina. Such infestations usually do not last very long.

Abnormal values: The isolation of any pathological fungi from the skin, hair, or blood or under the nails is considered abnormal. Fungus diseases may be confirmed by **Skin Reaction, Agglutination,** and **Complement Fixation** tests.

Risk factors: Negligible (see general risk factors for blood testing).

Pain/discomfort: Minimal (see general pain/discomfort factors for blood testing).

Accuracy and significance: Culture tests for fungus are considered the most accurate, but there is a prolonged wait for results. Blood testing, while limited in its accuracy (many people with an infection do not show a positive blood test; some people who have undergone prior skin testing for fungus can show a positive blood test without having the disease), is valuable when time is of the essence. Many doctors do not consider skin testing a valuable aid to diagnosis.

G

GALACTOSEMIA

Galactosemia is an inherited defect in one part of carbohydrate metabolism. Galactose is a form of sugar found in milk, sugar beets and seaweed. There are two forms of the disease, both due to the lack of an enzyme needed to change galactose either to glucose or some other substance. One form causes vomiting and diarrhea in the newborn baby, followed by liver disease, mental retardation, and cataracts if not diagnosed and treated early enough. The second form causes cataracts only. Once diagnosed, the treatment is to eliminate galactose from the diet.

Blood is taken from the infant, usually from the umbilical cord at birth.

When performed: When newborn infants show nutritional problems or gastrointestinal symptoms. Galactosemia testing of newborn babies is required in more than half of the United States; the exceptions are: Alabama, Arkansas, Delaware, Hawaii, Illinois, Indiana, Iowa, Kansas, Louisiana, Michigan, Mississippi, Missouri, Nebraska, New Jersey, North Dakota, Pennsylvania, South Carolina, South Dakota, Tennessee, Vermont, Virginia, Washington, and West Virginia; some states suspend the regulation if the parents object to such testing.

Normal values: Detection of the appropriate enzymes.

Abnormal values: Failure to detect the appropriate enzymes.

Risk factors: Negligible when blood is tested (see general risk factors for blood testing).

Pain/discomfort: Minimal when blood is tested (see general pain/discomfort factors for blood testing).

Accuracy and significance: The routine screening tests are quite accurate; however, some techniques are so sensitive they may show a rare form of galactosemia that causes no symptoms.

GASTRIC ANALYSIS

Gastric analysis is performed primarily to determine whether the stomach secretes hydrochloric acid (as it normally should); the test also shows whether the stomach produces the necessary digestive enzymes and whether it contains any cancer cells. Water, electrolytes, hydrochloric acid, mucin, pepsin, **Gastrin,** and a substance called intrinsic factor that is necessary to absorb vitamin B_{12} are all components of gastric secretions. When a patient is at rest, only small amounts of acid are secreted. The sight and smell of food, as well as actual food intake, can cause the stomach to secrete acid.

A tube is passed through the nose or mouth and into the stomach. The gastric fluid is withdrawn by suction continually for one hour. (The patient should not eat or take any medication for 12 hours prior to the test.) If at the end of one hour there is still doubt about whether acid is being secreted, an injection of histamine may be given to stimulate maximal acid production. One hour later, the gastric fluid is again tested. A tubeless method of analysis (which is not as exact but more comfortable for the patient) may be performed by having the patient swallow a dye (Diagnex blue) and noting the color of the urine.

The stomach fluid of newborn infants is sometimes examined within 6 hours after birth to help diagnose the respiratory distress syndrome (breathing difficulty). The presence of lung fluid in gastric contents is considered positive for the disease.

When performed: Whenever there is an undiagnosed anemia or repeated stomach infections (gastritis); when certain vitamin deficiencies are suspected; when searching for stomach cancer; when tuberculosis is suspected but the tuberculosis bacteria cannot be found.

After ulcer surgery, insulin is sometimes injected into a patient to see if stomach acid is still being secreted. Normally insulin causes acid to appear, and absence of acid is a measure of the success of the surgery, which should have prevented acid formation. This is called the Hollander test.

Normal values: The average gastric hydrochloric acid output is 1.25 to 4 mEq per hour, but it can go as high as 12 mEq per hour and still be normal. Normal gastric secretory volume (all components) is between 50 and 100 ml per hour.

Abnormal values: Acid secretion is elevated in duodenal ulcer and in Zollinger-Ellison syndrome (gastrin-secreting tumor). In gastric cancer and anemia, less than the normal amount of acid (or no acid) is secreted. A new finding indicates that an increased amount of **Lactic Dehydrogenase** in the gastric fluid seems to be a sign of stomach cancer.

Risk factors: Virtually none; even the passage of the tube into the stomach rarely causes any complications.

Pain/discomfort: Some patients find the insertion of the tube into the stomach quite uncomfortable.

Accuracy and significance: Although gastric analysis reveals the presence or absence of stomach acid, the test is not definitive and does not differentiate among the numerous stomach disorders. However, it can be extremely significant if cancer cells are found. (*Note:* Gastric analysis should not be confused with a stomach contents examination. A stomach contents exam is occasionally performed [after washing out the stomach] to ascertain a poison or drug. It is commonly performed on a deceased person to help determine the time of death based on food contents and the degree of digestion.)

GASTRIN

In addition to acid and enzymes, the stomach produces a hormone called gastrin. This hormone, first provoked by eating food, causes the stomach lining to secrete hydrochloric acid. Gastrin also causes the pancreas to produce insulin and enzymes and the liver to produce bile, all of which aid in digestion. Finally, gastrin increases stomach and intestinal muscle activity, helping to move food down the intestinal tract. There are several other stomach hormones, but gastrin is the only one regularly tested for at this time. Blood is taken from a vein and the serum is measured.

When performed: When there are severe, seemingly incurable ulcers of the stomach and intestine; in cases of suspected pernicious anemia.

Normal values: Normal values range from 0 to 300 pg per ml; the amount seems to increase naturally as a person gets older and may reach 700 pg per ml.

Abnormal values: With the occasional exception of the elderly, any test value over 500 pg per ml is considered a sign of disease. When a stomach ulcer is responding to treatment, gastrin levels will be normal; but in patients with Zollinger-Ellison syndrome (tumors that secrete gastrin and cause multiple ulcers) gastrin levels may rise to 300,000 pg per ml. To affirm the diagnosis, a trace of very dilute hydrochloric acid is given. With Zollinger-Ellison syndrome, the gastrin level stays the same; with anemia, it decreases markedly after the acid reaches the stomach.

Risk factors: Negligible (see general risk factors for blood testing).

Pain/discomfort: Minimal (see general pain/discomfort factors for blood testing).

Accuracy and significance: There is some question as to normal gastrin values as patients with certain anemias and peptic ulcers not located in the stomach can show a slight rise in gastrin levels. In fact, the test is significant only when confirming the Zollinger-Ellison syndrome.

GASTROESOPHAGEAL REFLUX

It has been reported that more than one out of ten people suffer from gastroesophageal reflux, or acid reflux as the condition is also known. When stomach acid regurgitates or flows back into the lower portion of the esophagus, it causes a burning sensation in the chest just behind the sternum or breastbone. This is commonly called heartburn or pyrosis, and the pain can be so severe that sometimes it is mistaken for a heart attack. The two conditions must be differentiated in order to provide proper treatment. It is thought that the lower esophageal sphincter (LES)—a sphincter is a band of muscles that opens and closes entrances to body cavities—loses the ability to stay closed under pressure from the stomach's contents; this allows the acid to enter the esophagus and irritate the lining, which is insufficiently coated (as is the stomach) to protect itself from the acid's effect. If the burning symptoms, sometimes described as cramping, sharp pain, or simply as pressure, are due to gastroesophageal reflux they seem to be aggravated by lying down and relieved by standing up, seem to be more frequent at night, and usually occur within an hour after a heavy meal. Furthermore, the regurgitation of stomach acid can produce a cough or difficulty in breathing should the acid seep into the windpipe. Another term for the condition is hiatal hernia, where an ostensible defect in the diaphragm allows the upper portion of the stomach to enter the chest area.

There are a variety of tests to diagnose gastroesophageal reflux. The most common is the standard acid reflux test (SART). For this, a measured dose of hydrochloric acid (approximating normal stomach acid) is put into the stomach and a **pH** measuring electrode placed in the lower esophagus. The patient is asked to cough, take very deep breaths, and bear down as if having a bowel movement; the patient repeats this process in different positions (standing, sitting, reclining). If acid is detected in the lower esophagus, gastroesophageal reflux is considered a good possibility. Another, somewhat similar, test is 24-hour esophageal pH monitoring, where the electrode is left in place day and night to observe the esophageal reaction to eating and other usual activities. This test is almost always performed in a hospital so the patient can be observed each time there is pain. Scintiscanning (see **Nuclear Scanning**) is a means to observe the esophageal sphincter in action. The patient swallows radioactive liquid which is then scanned in the sphincter as pressure is put on the abdomen. **Endoscopy** and **Biopsy** of the esophageal surface are other tests to measure the direct effect of acid on the esophageal lining. **Radiography,** in which barium is swallowed and observed in the stomach while the patient is placed in an upside-down position, is one of the older diagnostic techniques.

Another, older test, not as efficient, but still in use, is the acid infusion or Bernstein test. For this, a weak dilution of hydrochloric acid—similar to normal stomach acid—is instilled into the esophagus. The onset of pain similar to the heartburn originally complained of reveals the esophagus' abnormal sensitivity. However, the test does not prove the existence of gastroesophageal reflux. When acid is placed further down the gastrointestinal tract, usually by a tube just past the stomach, it is the Palmer test, designed to help diagnose ulcers. In the past, when doctors operated on patients to cut the vagus nerve that controls stomach acid secretions, insulin was injected into the patients to determine if the surgery was successful. Insulin made the acid flow again if all the vagus nerve fibers were not severed. This is known as the Hollander test. Today, many of these tests have been replaced by the **String** test.

When performed: To diagnose heartburn; to differentiate among the possible causes of chest pains (usually by performing the test along with the **Electrocardiogram, Radiography,** and **Endoscopy**); to help determine the cause of anemia (the reflux irritation sometimes causes internal bleeding); where repeated bouts of a pneumonia-like condition cannot be diagnosed; in infants who do not develop normally.

Normal values: A pH measurement greater than 4 in the esophagus at all times; no evidence of a weak lower esophageal sphincter; no visible evidence of stomach contents (radioactive or radioopaque material) seen in the esophagus; no evidence of ulceration or erosion when viewed by endoscopy.

Abnormal values: A pH measurement less than 4 (showing extreme acidity) in the esophagus at any one time, especially if apparent after eating greasy or spicy foods, after the consumption of alcohol, after having pressure applied to the abdomen, while lying down or during sleep; X-ray evidence of hiatal hernia; direct, endoscopic evidence of irritation to the esophageal lining.

Risk factors: Aside from the usual risks associated with radiography, biopsy, endoscopy, and nuclear scanning (all of which are noted in the descriptive section of each test), there is the slight risk that the acid solution will precipitate the perforation of an existing ulcer, or cause a hemorrhage should the esophageal lining be sufficiently eroded. Then too, there is the remote possibility that the swallowed electrode may break or become detached, possibly necessitating surgery for recovery.

Pain/discomfort: Some people find it difficult to swallow the electrode, but this is usually overcome by anesthetizing the back of the throat. There may be some discomfort when pressure is applied to the abdomen or when the body is positioned upside-down. Should the test cause pain, it is similar in intensity to the heartburn for which the tests are performed.

Accuracy and significance: While the 24-hour esophageal pH monitoring test is considered the most accurate, nearing a rate of 95 percent, the standard acid reflux test is between 80 and 90 percent accurate. Nuclear scanning is as accurate as acid testing but requires a physician and a highly trained technician to be effective. Of course, if a lesion is found, direct observation is 100 percent accurate. Radiography is only considered to be from 60 to 80 percent accurate. Despite the tests' degree of accuracy, there are doctors who doubt that gastroesophageal reflux is the single, direct cause of heartburn.

GENETIC DISORDER SCREENING

At the present time, almost 2,000 different inherited diseases or traits (exhibited by carriers of genetic diseases who do not usually show signs of the disease) are known. Many of these disorders reveal themselves as metabolic defects that interfere with normal body enzyme chemistry; they may also be the consequence of the lack of one or more enzymes necessary for the proper development or function of organs or tissues. Genetic screening tests try to uncover individuals who have a greater than average risk of passing on an inherited condition. Prior to the wide application of genetic disorder screening by doctors and the passage of state laws requiring prenatal testing of pregnant women, more than 100,000 children with congenital defects or genetic disorders were born each year in the United States alone.

Genetic screening may be performed on either parent-to-be (or even on a relative of a parent-to-be) prior to pregnancy; on the mother-to-be or on the fetus during pregnancy; and on the newborn infant before an inherited disorder can take effect. Sometimes a detailed family history can offer clues leading to the discovery of a potentially dangerous genetic disease or trait, the confirmation of which, through testing, can help prevent a subsequent birth defect or disorder and even allow future normal childbearing.

In addition to genetic defects that are metabolic, abnormalities of the fetus can also come from hormonal disorders, infectious diseases, toxic drug influences and even certain kinds of malnutrition suffered by a mother during pregnancy. Chromosomal disorders may arise from exposure to X-rays, excessive use of drugs, and infections; in some instances genes are missing or present in excess, located at the wrong site within the chromosome, or defective in some way.

There are a great many different tests to uncover genetic or prenatal disorders; some are required by law, others are available upon request. The most common ones are described under their own names:

Alpha Fetoprotein
Aminoaciduria
Amniocentesis
Amniography (see **Radiography**)
Bilirubin
Chlamydia Identification
Chromosome Analysis
Cortisol
Cystic Fibrosis (see **Sodium; Sweat**)
Cytomegalovirus
Fetoscopy (see **Endoscopy**)
Galactosemia
German Measles (see **Rubella**)
Hemophilia (see **Partial Thromboplastin Time**)
Herpes
Measles
Muscular Dystrophy (see **Creatine Phosphokinase**)
Phenylketonuria
Sickle Cell Anemia (see **Hemoglobin**)
Syphilis
Tay-Sachs Disease
Thalassemia (see **Hemoglobin**)
Thyroid Function
Toxoplasmosis
Ultrasound

A computerized system containing information on more than 1,000 known birth defects has been established at the Massachusetts Insitute of Technology/Tufts New England Medical Center in Boston. Its services are available to any physician who desires diagnostic techniques, treatments, and prognostic information.

GLUCOSE (Sugar)

The glucose test measures the amount of glucose floating free in the blood or excreted by the kidneys into the bladder. The test is really a measure of how well the body handles carbohydrate metabolism (the breakdown of starches such as vegetables as well as all the various sugar products in the foods we eat). Glucose is the primary fuel or energy source for all the body tissues. It may be burned directly or converted into fat and stored for later use as fatty acid energy. Glucose is stored primarily in the liver and, in small amounts, in other tissues. A uniform blood glucose level is generally maintained in the body through insulin secretion (which decreases it), despite variations due to dietary increase in sugar and energy expenditure. Blood is taken from the vein to assess the level of glucose in serum; glucose may also be tested in whole blood or plasma, in urine, or in spinal fluid.

In preparing for the glucose tolerance test (GTT), the patient eats his usual amount of carbohydrate for several days. Then he fasts for eight to 12 hours prior to the test. First, a fasting blood glucose and urine glucose are measured. Then the patient is given 100 g of glucose in water or soda to drink. Thirty minutes afterward both the blood and urine are again examined for sugar levels. Glucose testing after eating is called postprandial. Every hour thereafter for the next five hours, urine and blood samples are taken to determine how long it takes the body to metabolize the 100 g of glucose. Sometimes the spinal fluid and joint fluids are tested for glucose. (Before more sophisticated methods of medical laboratory testing were developed, doctors used to taste their patient's urine for sugar.)

Today an increasing number of physicians no longer require their patients to fast for eight to 12 hours prior to the glucose or glucose tolerance test. The results seem no less accurate as long as food is not ingested for two hours prior to the test.

When performed: The fasting blood glucose is performed when there is dizziness, weakness, excessive thirst, excessive urination, or any other symptoms and signs suggesting diabetes. The test also helps diagnose hormone disorders, pancreatic disease, certain brain and spinal cord diseases, and many hereditary conditions. A single postprandial test may be performed as a confirmatory measure.

The glucose tolerance test is performed when the fasting and/or postprandial glucose determinations are borderline and diabetes or other disease is still being considered.

The urine examination for sugar is a routine screening test for diabetes as well as for suspected kidney, liver, or hormone disease.

Normal values: Fasting blood glucose levels normally range from 80 to 120 mg per 100 ml of serum, 60 to 100 mg per 100 ml of whole blood. Postprandial levels should not exceed 180 mg per 100 ml.

During the entire five to six hours of the glucose tolerance test, the peak should remain below 180 mg per 100 ml, and after two hours the levels should return to the same as for fasting.

In the urine sugar test, normally no sugar or only an insignificant trace should be detected, even after a high-carbohydrate meal. However, in some individuals who have a low kidney threshold, sugar may be detected in the urine without the presence of disease.

Abnormal values: The fasting blood glucose level is increased (hyperglycemia) with diabetes, Cushing's syndrome (pituitary disease), many endocrine problems, liver disease, and diuretic therapy. The level is decreased with pancreatic disorders, excessive insulin, and glycogen storage disease.

In order to justify a diagnosis of hypoglycemia as a disease condition, blood glucose levels must be less than 40 mg per 100 ml of serum in at least three different instances at the identical time the patient is having symptoms (sweating, palpitations, weakness, bizarre behavior). Alcohol intake may cause temporary hypoglycemia, as will fasting, liver disease, and certain cancers.

In the glucose tolerance test, levels are elevated for more than two hours with diabetes mellitus and decreased with pancreatitis, excess insulin production, and hypoglycemia.

Elevated levels of glucose in the urine may be caused by diabetes mellitus, liver disease, hyperthyroidism and other hormone disorders, pregnancy, brain injury, and excessive ingestion of sugar. In meningitis spinal fluid glucose is decreased; with joint infections joint fluid sugar is decreased.

Risk factors: Negligible (see general risk factors for blood testing).

Pain/discomfort: Minimal (see general pain/discomfort factors for blood testing).

Accuracy and significance: Although glucose measurements can be affected by numerous foods and drugs (oral contraceptives may alter glucose values for several days), the test is considered sufficiently accurate to be the definitive diagnostic test for diabetes. It is particularly significant in determining true hypoglycemia, but only if symptoms occur at very low blood sugar levels. It is a very valuable test in helping to diagnose the type of spinal fluid infection.

The accuracy of the glucose tolerance test, however, can depend more on the values a doctor decides are normal and abnormal than on the biochemical measurements. Many doctors now believe a value greater than 180 mg per 100 ml is not necessarily abnormal and is actually a false positive result. They contend that normal values can reach 270 mg per 100 ml and that only when values exceed that amount should a diagnosis of diabetes be made. Using these new upper limits of normal, false positive tests that may occur when a patient is under emotional stress are almost always eliminated.

At the present time it is considered sound medical practice to confirm a suspected diagnosis of diabetes with the **C-Peptide** test.

Further confirmation is obtained through the **Glycohemoglobin** test.

GLUCOSE 6-PHOSPHATE DEHYDROGENASE (G6PD)

Glucose 6-phosphate dehydrogenase is an enzyme normally found in red blood cells. In people with a deficiency of this enzyme (an inherited condition), red blood cells are no longer protected from oxidation, causing hemolysis (destruction of red blood cells and subsequent separation of hemoglobin), which can lead to anemia. The deficiency is more frequent in Blacks, Orientals, and Caucasians from the Mediterranean area, and more serious in men than in women. Blood is taken from a vein and tested. It may simply be screened for the presence of G6PD, or the quantity of G6PD may be measured precisely. Either test can still miss the deficiency in some women.

When performed: In undiagnosed hemolytic anemia; before administration of antimalarial drugs, sulfonamides, and nitrofurans.

Normal values: Glucose 6-phosphate dehydrogenase should normally be found in significant amounts in red blood cells: 120 to 280 units per billion cells.

Abnormal values: Glucose 6-phosphate dehydrogenase deficiency, while not usually serious or chronic, can at times be fatal. It does not show itself until the patient ingests drugs or foods that precipitate the hemolytic anemia, which can then cause hemoglobinuria, jaundice, fever, and renal failure. Some of those drugs are Primaquine (for malaria), aspirin, sulfa products, nitrofurans, vitamin C, certain antibiotics, some worm medicines, inhalation of naphthalene (moth repellent), and eating fava beans—but only in people born with a G6PD deficiency.

Risk factors: Negligible (see general risk factors for blood testing).

Pain/discomfort: Minimal (see general pain/discomfort factors for blood testing).

Accuracy and significance: The test is very accurate and will detect approximately 90 percent of those who have an inherited deficiency of this particular enzyme. It is especially significant in screening individuals who should take prophylactic drugs against malaria, and those who persistently suffer from anemia after taking a variety of medicines.

GLUTAMIC OXALACETIC TRANSAMINASE (SGOT)

Serum glutamic oxalacetic transaminase (SGOT) and serum glutamic pyruvic transaminase (SGPT) are enzymes present primarily in the heart and liver. (There are tiny amounts in the kidney, lungs, brain, and a few other body tissues.) These enzymes are unique in that they are released into the blood when there is heart muscle damage, liver cell destruction, or rickettsial (extra-large-size bacteria) infections. Blood is taken from a vein and the serum is tested.

When performed: When there is suspected heart damage; to follow the progress of a patient after a heart attack; in certain types of liver disease; when there is an unexplained infection.

Normal values: Normally there are less then 30 SGOT units per ml and less than 25 SGPT units per ml in the blood serum.

Abnormal values: Serum levels of SGOT and SGPT are elevated following a heart attack and reach their peak in 24 to 48 hours after the onset of illness. With heart disease, SGOT levels are higher than SGPT levels. Serum levels return to normal four to six days after the attack. In some acute heart disease (other than heart attack), the peak levels are reached in 72 hours. In liver disease (infectious hepatitis and cirrhosis) SGPT levels are higher than SGOT levels. Because a few other conditions such as pancreatitis, infectious mononucleosis, and certain muscle diseases can also cause an increase of these enzymes in the blood, they must always be evaluated along with the patient's symptoms.

Risk factors: Negligible (see general risk factors for blood testing).

Pain/discomfort: Minimal (see general pain/discomfort factors for blood testing).

Accuracy and significance: The enzyme measurements are still routinely performed, but they reflect so many different conditions they are no longer considered as significant in evaluating heart disease as they once were; **Creatine Phosphokinase** and **Lactic Dehydrogenase** are more accurate and specific.

(Note: The newer name for SGOT is aspartate amino transferase [AST]; SGPT is now called alanine amino transferase [ALT].)

GLYCOHEMOGLOBIN

The glycohemoglobin test measures the percentage of hemoglobin molecules that have glucose (sugar) attached to them. The greater the amount of glucose in the blood, the greater the percentage of glycosylated hemoglobin (also known as Hb Ala-c). The test is of particular value in monitoring a patient with diabetes to ascertain that the patient's blood sugar level is properly controlled; thus it is also a measure of the success or failure of treatment.

Initially the glycohemoglobin test is usually performed along with the **Glucose** tolerance test; but it may be substituted for that test after a treatment regimen has been established, since it requires far less time and far fewer blood samples from the patient and since the patient need not fast beforehand. Glycohemoglobin measurements indicate blood sugar activity during the six to eight weeks prior to the test, whereas the glucose tolerance test measures only blood sugar levels at the moment. At the present time, the glycohemoglobin test is usually performed every two months in order to provide the physician with data to help control the diabetic patient. Blood from a vein is examined.

When performed: The test is used primarily to measure the control (proper treatment) of a patient with diabetes; it not only helps reveal difficulties in sugar utilization, but can also reveal patients who ignore their prescribed treatment. Sometimes the test is used to measure the body's carbohydrate metabolism.

Normal values: Patients without diabetes, and patients with the disease who are responding to treatment average from 2% to 7.5% glycohemoglobin.

Abnormal values: Patients who have uncontrolled diabetes or who are receiving inadequate treatment will have glycohemoglobin values greater than 7.5%. Values in excess of 9.2% indicate definite improper control of a diabetic condition. Rarely a patient with a known hemoglobin disease, but without diabetes, will have elevated values.

Risk factors: Negligible (see general risk factors for blood testing).

Pain/discomfort: Minimal (see general pain/discomfort factors for blood testing).

Accuracy and significance: Some doctors believe the test to be of sufficient accuracy to replace **Glucose** as a way to follow the progress of patients with diabetes. The test has not, however, been in use for a sufficient length of time to allow it to replace diagnostic glucose measurements. False positive results have been known to occur, although these are primarily due to laboratory carelessness.

GONORRHEA (GC, CLAP)

Gonorrhea is primarily an infection of the urethra (the passageway that carries urine from the bladder to outside the body), and is one of the most common communicable diseases in the United States. (By law, all instances of gonorrhea must be reported.) Other parts of the body that can become infected with gonorrhea are: the rectum, the throat, the eyes (the disease can cause ulcers on the eye surface) and any and all of the genital or reproductive organs (a common cause of infertility or sterility). Arthritis is the most common late complication of gonorrhea; heart disease, meningitis, and skin lesions are also known to follow this disease. In men, the most frequent symptom is a burning during urination followed by a cream-colored or yellow discharge from the end of the penis; the onset of pain is usually 24 to 72 hours after being infected. Although women can have similar symptoms, more often than not they are unaware they are infected. Gonorrhea must be differentiated from non-gonococcal urethritis, a similar condition caused by Chlamydia. (See also **Chlamydia Identification.**) While the incidence of chlamydial infection is probably greater than that of gonorrhea, it is not required that chlamydial infections be reported to health authorities. The diagnosis of gonorrhea is usually made by the **Gram Stain** test of the discharge from the male urethra; the bacteria that cause the disease are easily seen inside **White Blood Cells** and appear as distinct pairs resembling tiny bookends. **Culture** helps to confirm the diagnosis; although there are a few **Complement Fixation**-type tests, they are not thought to be too accurate. Today, many forms of the gonorrhea germ are resistant to a number of different antibiotics, making culture-sensitivity tests particularly important to successful treatment. Patients with gonorrhea must be tested monthly for **Syphilis** for a minimum of six months after the infection is diagnosed.

When performed: When a man has any penile discharge, undiagnosed throat or rectal infection, or pain in or near the testicles; on women with an undiagnosed vaginal discharge or undiagnosed abdominal pains. On patients known to have had sexual contact with suspected carriers of the disease.

Normal values: No gonorrhea bacteria should be found.

Abnormal values: Any evidence of the gonorrheal bacteria on a gram stain or culture.

Risk factors: None.

Pain/discomfort: None.

Accuracy and significance: The gram stain is considered sufficiently accurate to begin treatment, but the diagnosis should be verified with a culture test.

GRAM STAIN

The Gram stain test (named after Dr. Hans Christian Gram, a Danish physician) is used primarily to distinguish various bacteria under the microscope that would otherwise be impossible to identify. Sputum, joint fluid, spinal fluid, urine, sinus discharge, urethral discharge, vaginal fluid, and exudates (ooze) from infections can all be examined in this manner. When the specimen takes a gentian violet (bluish purple) or safranin (red) stain, the morphology (size, shape, and form) of bacteria is more easily visualized and aids in both diagnosis and treatment. (Certain bacteria such as tuberculosis germs will not show up on the Gram stain and need special dyes.)

When performed: The test is used primarily to evaluate and distinguish infectious organisms in various body fluids and to aid in the precise choice of therapy. Certain antibiotics are effective only against Gram-positive organisms; other antibiotics are effective only against Gram-negative organisms.

Normal values: Normally no pathological bacteria are observed after staining.

Abnormal values: Gram-negative organisms stain an orange-red color and are usually representative of coliform-type (intestinal and urinary tract) diseases. Gram-positive organisms stain a bluish purple and are usually representative of streptococcal and staphylococcal (upper respiratory tract and abscess) diseases.

Risk factors: Negligible. If joint or **Cerebrospinal Fluid** is withdrawn for examination, see general risk factors for catheter and needle insertion. In most instances the patient furnishes the specimen to be examined.

Pain/discomfort: None if the patient furnishes the specimen. See general pain/discomfort factors for catheter and needle insertion if joint or cerebrospinal fluid is to be examined.

Accuracy and significance: Although the test is valuable as a rapid differentiation among bacterial infections, it is basically only a screening procedure that helps the doctor select an antibiotic before receiving the results of a **Culture** test. In many instances instability of the chemical solutions used to stain the specimen causes up to 40 percent false positive results. When the Gram stain is used to diagnose bacterial pneumonia, about half the tests show false negative results.

GROWTH HORMONE

A pituitary gland hormone called somatotropin or human growth hormone (HGH) controls the height an individual attains. It is, of course, essential for normal growth. Testing for growth hormone offers the earliest indication of generalized pituitary problems. Blood is taken from a vein and the serum is tested. Several tests must be taken at different times before true values can be determined. At times it is necessary to give the patient a large amount of insulin (to produce hypoglycemia, or low blood sugar) to obtain accurate results. Today drugs are available to stop excessive growth hormone secretion (preventing gigantism, or abnormally tall individuals) as well as drugs to allow normal growth hormone secretion (preventing dwarfism).

When performed: The test is used whenever gigantism (acromegaly) or dwarfism is suspected. The earlier the test is performed and the abnormality revealed, the easier and more effective the treatment. The test is given, too, when hyperactive children take stimulant drugs such as dextroamphetamine or methylphenidate (Ritalin); these drugs seem to retard growth.

Normal values: Newborn infants usually have higher levels of somatotropin than adults (over 30 ng per ml); children generally average from 1 to 15 ng per ml; women average up to 30 ng per ml; and men usually range below 10 ng per ml. It is normal for growth hormone levels to increase after insulin is given and to decrease to near zero after a large amount of glucose (sugar) is consumed.

Abnormal values: Lower than normal values are found with dwarfism; elevated values appear with gigantism. Values may also be elevated with diabetes, in stressful situations, following surgery, and with infections. Taking female hormones will cause a rise in growth hormone levels.

Risk factors: Negligible (see general risk factors for blood testing).

Pain/discomfort: Minimal (see general pain/discomfort factors for blood testing).

Accuracy and significance: The test is reasonably accurate in conditions that raise growth hormone levels. There are times, however, when conditions that reflect little or no secretion of growth hormone may make it impossible to evaluate the level of growth hormone in the blood. When this occurs, other hormones and/or chemicals can be injected into a patient to see if they will stimulate sufficient growth hormone for measurement. The accuracy of the growth hormone test can be affected by the time of day the blood is taken and the test may thus require multiple samples for greater significance.

H

HAPTOGLOBIN

Haptoglobin, a plasma globulin (see **Albumin/Globulin**), is a direct measure of hemolysis in the body. Hemolysis means a markedly increased breakdown of red blood cells and the liberation of **Hemoglobin** into the plasma; it can come about from disease, from certain inherited conditions, from certain drugs, and after snakebite. When hemolysis occurs, the red blood cells do not last as long as they should, and this usually (but not always) results in anemia. Blood is taken from a vein and the serum is tested.

When performed: When anemia is present, especially when it is thought to be from an inherited condition such as thalassemia (Mediterranean or Cooley's anemia) or from Rh problems; when it is suspected that certain environmental factors (chemicals, drugs, or physical injury) are causing anemia; in severe infections; with liver disease.

Normal values: Normal haptoglobin levels range from 50 to 150 mg per 100 ml of serum.

Abnormal values: As red blood cells are destroyed, the hemoglobin that is released combines with haptoglobin; thus reduced levels of haptoglobin indicate hemolysis, no matter what the specific cause. Decreased values of haptoglobin are also found in liver disease and with infectious mononucleosis. Certain severe infections, tissue damage such as with heart attack, and cancers cause increased haptoglobin levels.

Risk factors: Negligible (see general risk factors for blood testing).

Pain/discomfort: Minimal (see general pain/discomfort factors for blood testing).

Accuracy and significance: Although the test accurately indicates the breakage of the body's red blood cells, its significance is not great enough to allow a specific diagnosis. The value of the test lies in confirming the susceptibility of red blood cells to breakage.

HEARING FUNCTION

Sound is heard in two ways: by its intensity or volume (loudness) and by its tone, which depends on how fast or how slowly it vibrates. In tests of hearing ability, both factors are measured. In addition, patients are tested for the ability to hear sound by two different means of conduction: air conduction (sounds heard through the ear canal) and bone conduction (sounds detected by the bones around and behind the ear).

The simplest measures of hearing ability are the whisper and voice tests, in which the doctor, sitting about 20 feet away from the patient, whispers and then says numbers out loud while the patient listens with one ear covered. In the ticking-watch test, the physician notes how far away from the ear the watch is still heard.

The most precise hearing test is measured by the audiometer, a machine that puts out sounds of various tones and intensities (volumes). Pure tones vary from 64 cycles per second, or cps (very low, bass-type tones) to almost 12,000 cps (extremely shrill or high-pitched tones). The human ear can usually detect sounds from 16 to 16,000 cps (although some people can hear up to 20,000 cps). Many animals can hear tones of 50,000 cps, beyond the range of human hearing.

The intensity (volume) of sound is expressed in decibels (db). A whisper measures about 20 db. Background noise in the average home runs about 50 db; in an office, about 60 db. Loud classical music rates 80 db, rock music is more than 120 db, and a jet engine ranges from 140 to 180 db. Usually sounds greater than 130 db will cause pain.

For the air conduction part of the test, the patient wears earphones from the audiometer and listens to sounds of designated tones and intensities or to spoken words (sounds may also be broadcast through a speaker in a soundproof room). An attachment from the earphones is then applied to the bone behind the ear and hearing is tested via bone conduction. How well the patient hears sounds through air conduction is an indication of ear drum and middle ear function as well as ear-nerve disease. Bone conduction ability tests the function of the inner ear. **Tuning Fork** tests may also be used to survey hearing problems and to confirm bone or nerve deafness.

Most doctors recommend that an audiometer test be performed **before** any ototoxic drug (ear-nerve damaging) is administered in order to detect any deafness that might result from the medication.

The Lombard test helps to detect faked hearing loss. While wearing audiometer earphones, a patient reads from a book; after a minute or two, a noise from the audiometer is sent to each ear. If hearing is normal, the reader's voice will become louder. Patients with true hearing loss will not raise their voices while reading.

When performed: Whenever there is difficulty in hearing, usually due to ear infection, an inherited condition, or excessive exposure to loud noises (as in certain occupations); following head injury.

Audiometer tests are now being performed in schools to screen out children with hearing loss at an early age.

Whenever ototoxic drugs are administered (antibiotics such as kanamycin, neomycin, ganamycin, and streptomycin; diuretic drugs such as Lasix; and even when large doses of salicylates are administered).

Normal values: For screening purposes only, two pure tones of 256 cps and 4,096 cps (encompassing the range of normal speech sounds) at 5 to 10 db are transmitted through the earphones (air conduction). Should the patient have difficulty in hearing either of these sounds, a more detailed audiogram is performed. Normally, an individual can hear lower tones (64 cps) at 1 to 2 db, higher tones (11,584 cps) at about 10 db, and all pure tones in between at 10 db or less. Air conduction hearing is usually better than bone conduction hearing.

Abnormal values: The inability to hear pure tones below 10 db indicates inner-ear or nerve damage. There are many different kinds of deafness; some people lose only the ability to perceive high tones or low tones; some lose only air or bone conduction hearing. Following injury or excessive noise exposure, high-tone hearing is usually lost. When deafness is inherited, hearing for the entire range of tones is missing. Following infection, the speech range is most commonly lost. Certain antibiotic drugs cause nerve deafness; if the drugs are not used over too long a period of time, hearing may return, but in some instances the medication can cause permanent deafness.

Risk factors: None.

Pain/discomfort: None.

Accuracy and significance: Hearing function tests, when properly performed with properly calibrated equipment, quite accurately diagnose the degree and specific location of a hearing problem. The Lombard test is particularly significant in revealing malingerers.

HEMATOCRIT

The hematocrit shows the percentage of blood cells (mostly red blood cells) comprising the total blood volume. A blood sample from a vein is centrifuged (the solid matter is forced to the bottom of a specially marked tube, leaving the clear plasma in the upper section). In a sense, the test measures the viscosity (thickness) of the blood as well as the amount of fluid in the blood. Many doctors feel the hematocrit test is a better measure of anemia than the **Hemoglobin** test, especially if the patient's diet includes normal amounts of iron.

When performed: In diagnostic screening for anemias and dehydration; to follow the course of therapy for anemias and hemorrhage.

Normal values: Normal hematocrit readings range from 40% to 55% (slightly lower in women).

Abnormal values: Low hematocrit readings (decreased percentage of total cells) are found in red blood cell anemias, immediately after hemorrhage, and whenever there is excessive fluid intake. High hematocrit readings are found in severe dehydration and polycythemia, angina, and after surgery, trauma, or burns.

Risk factors: Negligible (see general risk factors for blood testing).

Pain/discomfort: Minimal (see general pain/discomfort factors for blood testing).

Accuracy and significance: Basically the test screens for indications of anemia. The patient's fluid intake for several hours prior to the test must be considered as either dehydration or an excess of liquid can produce false values. An abnormal result should be followed by more appropriate tests; on its own, a hematocrit value has no real significance.

HEMOGLOBIN

There are many different forms of hemoglobin in the blood; these forms are usually measured together as the total hemoglobin. Hemoglobin is an iron protein substance manufactured inside newly forming red blood cells and stored there for the life of the cells. Because of its unique affinity for oxygen, its task is to pick up oxygen as the red blood cells pass through the lungs and deliver that oxygen to tissue cells throughout the body.

The amount of oxygen the blood can carry depends not only on the amount of hemoglobin present but also on its effectiveness. Exposure to toxic substances can alter the hemoglobin molecule; carbon monoxide gas will easily replace oxygen attached to hemoglobin and form carboxyhemoglobin, preventing any vital oxygen from reaching tissue cells. Carboxyhemoglobin turns the blood (and sometimes the skin) a brilliant red. The Katyama test distinguishes between carboxyhemoglobin and hemoglobin.

Methemoglobin forms when the red blood cells are exposed to certain drugs (especially non-prescription ones such as phenacetin and other aspirin substitutes) or to large amounts of nitrates that are used to treat heart disease and as food preservatives. Methemoglobin picks up oxygen but will not release it to the tissues, making the skin appear bluish. Aspirin-substitute drugs and certain laxatives containing sulfur can cause sulfhemoglobin; this differs from methemoglobin only in that it cannot be treated and stays in the blood until the red blood cells break down. Fetal hemoglobin is the oxygen-carrying iron in the fetus; it almost disappears in adulthood but remains in large quantities when there are various blood diseases. Hemoglobin S is associated with sickle cell anemia; when detected it usually indicates an inherited inability of red blood cells to carry sufficient oxygen to body tissues. There are several specific screening tests to help diagnose sickle cell anemia (Sickledex, Sickle-I.D. System, Sicklequik); these tests may also uncover a sickle cell trait in carriers of the disease (while it is believed that more than 50,000 people in the United States have sickle cell anemia, it is also estimated that more than 2.5 million Americans carry the sickle cell trait without showing any signs of the disease). Sickle cells may also be observed through the microscope during the **Red Blood Cell** test; they resemble a farmer's sickle. Abnormally shaped sickle cells can also plug up tiny arteries in the hands, feet and abdomen, causing inadequate circulation and producing excruciating pain. Hemoglobin A or A-2 may be increased or decreased in the presence of one of the two forms of thalassemia (sometimes called Mediterranean anemia, because it was first discovered in people living adjacent to the Mediterranean Sea, or Cooley's anemia, after Dr. Thomas Benton Cooley, a form of erythroblastic anemia, indicating the type of red blood cells involved), an inherited disease in which hemoglobin is not properly or adequately formed; the condition can cause stillbirth and severe blood problems in later life.

Iron in the diet is the primary source of hemoglobin; replacement iron is necessary when there is blood loss such as with injury or menstruation.

Whenever there is a decreased amount of hemoglobin in the body (the blood carries less oxygen), the heart usually compensates by increasing its effort to circulate blood (the pulse rate becomes more rapid). Only one drop of whole blood, which can be taken from the fingertip, earlobe, or heel, is needed for the test. Hemoglobin can, of course, be evaluated from blood taken for any other procedure. It is also looked for in urine as an indication of bleeding or poisoning.

When performed: Primarily when there is suspicion of anemia, no matter what kind or what the cause; to aid in the diagnosis of many inherited conditions; to distinguish certain poisonings from disease; as an indication of how much blood has been lost after injury or surgery. A few states require newborn babies to be tested for sickle cell anemia; these include Arizona, Colorado, Georgia, Louisiana, New Mexico, North Carolina, and Wyoming (see **Red Blood Cell**).

Normal values: Total hemoglobin levels for men range from 14 to 18 g per 100 ml; for women, 12 to 15 g per 100 ml. Up to 1% carboxyhemoglobin or fetal hemoglobin may be present, but no more than 0.1% of methemoglobin or sulfhemoglobin should be detected. The urine should contain no hemoglobin.

Abnormal values: Serum hemoglobin is sometimes increased when red blood cells are suddenly damaged or destroyed, as with sickle cell disease or the Rh anemia of infancy. Polycythemia (a disease characterized by excessive red blood cells) may show increased hemoglobin.

Hemoglobin values are decreased in almost all forms of anemia, especially those associated with iron deficiency. Symptoms of anemia usually do not appear until the hemoglobin level goes below 8 g per 100 ml. Hemoglobin is decreased in leukemia, after hemorrhage, and in pregnancy (especially after delivery, when there is loss of blood).

Heavy cigarette smoking may cause carboxyhemoglobin values up to 20%, markedly reducing the amount of normal hemoglobin. Thus the test is often used as a check on people who smoke but who deny the fact.

Risk factors: Negligible (see general risk factors for blood testing.

Pain/discomfort: Minimal (see general pain/discomfort factors for blood testing).

Accuracy and significance: Total (undifferentiated) hemoglobin is simply a screening test for anemia and, on its own, has no specific significance. However, tests for particular forms of hemoglobin are very accurate and can be life-saving.

HEPATITIS

Hepatitis is an acute and extremely serious infection of the liver primarily caused by several liver-specific viruses. It can also come from parasites, bacteria, drugs, alcohol, and some metabolic disorders. Different viruses, such as those that cause infectious mononucleosis, and those known as **Cytomegaloviruses** that produce congenital defects and encephalitis, can also cause hepatitis.

Depending on which strain of hepatitis-specific virus inflames the liver, the condition is called type A, or infectious hepatitis, or endemic hepatitis, when type A virus is at fault; when type B virus is the culprit, the disease is usually referred to as type B or serum hepatitis. There is a third form of hepatitis, called non-A, non-B, that seems to occur largely after blood transfusions. (It is not labelled type C because it is thought that more than one new virus is responsible.) Type A hepatitis is commonly spread by contaminated feces that pollute water supplies and foods, particularly shellfish that are eaten raw. It can also be communicated from person to person but it is rare to find a type-A hepatitis carrier similar to the typhoid carrier. Type A, which strikes children and young adults most frequently, is not as serious a disease as type B. One injection of type-A-specific immune serum, gamma globulin, prior to possible exposure to the virus can prevent the illness. Type-B hepatitis, on the other hand, is a very severe disease that can occur at any age. Although symptoms may not appear for months following exposure and infection, they can be so slight they are easily overlooked. Most often the disease is acquired from contact with infected blood (or from improperly sterilized needles, or other medical instruments that have had contact with infected blood). Type-B hepatitis is easily transmitted through sexual contact. There now is a vaccine to help protect against hepatitis-B. It is easy to have hepatitis and not know it. At first, the signs and symptoms resemble influenza. If there is no evidence of jaundice and the urine does not turn dark, the condition can come and go without being diagnosed. This is potentially dangerous as even a mild case of hepatitis can lead to severe liver damage months or even years later. There are several specific antigen and antibody tests for hepatitis (to understand the antigen-antibody testing principles, see **Agglutination**). When the tests are performed as a panel, they reveal: whether the patient has been exposed to hepatitis; the specific type of hepatitis virus; whether the infection exists at that moment; whether the disease is in an early or late stage; whether the patient is a carrier; whether recovery is taking place. The tests examine blood from a vein for:

HAV (hepatitis A virus)
HAVAb (hepatitis A antibody)
HAVAb-M (the specific immunoglobulin M hepatitis antibody)
HBcAb or Anti-HBc (hepatitis B-core antibody)
HBeAg (hepatitis B-core antigen)
HBsAb or Anti-HBs (hepatitis B-surface antibody)

HBsAg, formerly called Australian Antigen, or AU (hepatitis B-surface antigen)

The terms core and surface refer to the body and the outer layer of the hepatitis virus. Tests for the specific virus in the feces are also performed.

When performed: When undiagnosed flu-like illness persists; when unexplained jaundice and/or dark urine is observed; to distinguish between the various types of hepatitis; to protect against subsequent chronic liver disease such as cirrhosis or cancer; to detect carriers of the disease (food handlers, blood donors, medical staff personnel, and patients with certain inherited metabolic defects).

Normal values: No antigen or antibodies of the hepatitis virus should be present; when antibodies alone are detected, it is usually indicative of an inactive hepatitis infection, but additional tests must be performed to ascertain if the patient is a symptomless carrier. No virus particles should be found in the feces examination.

Abnormal values: The detection, along with the quantity, of hepatitis antigens and/or antibodies reveals that the disease is, or was, present; the specific type of causative virus; the stage of the disease (even if in the incubation period before symptoms appear); and whether a carrier state exists. Virus particles are most often found in the incubation period.

Risk factors: Negligible (see general risk factors for blood testing).

Pain/discomfort: Minimal (see general pain/discomfort factors for blood testing).

Accuracy and significance: The tests are considered 95 percent accurate. However, as with many tests to diagnose infection, failure to detect any hepatitis antigen or antibody is not conclusive evidence that the disease is not present.

HERPES

There are several different but related herpes viruses. The first, and probably the best known, is herpes simplex I (or herpes virus hominus type I). It is the cause of the common cold sore (fever blister) that frequently appears on the lips, in and around the mouth, and sometimes in the throat. Most often, those who acquire a herpes simplex I infection do so before the age of five and then have recurrences throughout their lives. In most instances the sores heal within a week or two. Herpes simplex II (herpes virus hominus type II) causes sores similar to cold sores but they are almost always in, on, and around the genital organs and urinary passageways. Today, herpes genitalis, as herpes simplex II is also known, is considered one of the most potentially dangerous sexually transmitted diseases (formerly called venereal diseases). Not only can it cause spontaneous abortion, especially in the first months of pregnancy, but it can also cause terrible damage to the newborn infant (congenital malformations, nerve and brain infections, skin conditions of such severity that they are usually fatal, and myriad eye problems). It is also believed that herpes simplex II may cause cancer of the cervix. The third herpes virus is varicella-zoster virus (VZV) and is the cause of chicken pox as well as herpes zoster, better known as shingles because of the narrow layers of blister-like skin eruptions that appear around the trunk or extremities of the body when the virus travels down the nerves to the skin surface. While chicken pox is commonly a disease of childhood, herpes zoster is largely a disease of late middle age. Next there is herpes virus simiai, primarily the cause of a disease in monkeys in captivity, but a condition that can bring on encephalitis and herpes zoster-like symptoms in humans if they are bitten by infected monkeys. Other viruses thought to be part of the herpes family include **Cytomegalovirus,** and the Epstein-Barr virus that causes **Mononucleosis.**

While scrapings from skin lesions can be examined under the miscroscope to reveal specific cell characteristics, and it is also possible to culture and identify the virus, the most common tests to aid in diagnosis are those blood tests (usually from a vein) related to **Complement Fixation** and **Agglutination** that detect specific antibodies for each type of virus.

When performed: When a patient has blister-like lesions around the genitals; when there is undiagnosed fever, lymph gland swelling, or an unusual pattern of skin eruptions; as part of the **TORCH** screening panel for pregnant women and newborn infants; in instances of unusual nerve or eye disease.

Normal values: No, or very low, amounts of herpes antibodies. No change in antibody amounts (titers) when the test is performed in two stages two to three weeks apart, the second test being conducted well after the onset of suspicious signs and symptoms. No isolation of the virus.

Abnormal values: Large amounts of the specific antibodies, especially an increased amount after several weeks; any physical evidence of the virus, such as its culture.

Risk factors: Negligible (see general risk factors for blood testing).

Pain/discomfort: Minimal (see general pain/discomfort factors for blood testing).

Accuracy and significance: Considered extremely accurate if antibodies are found, and particularly if the antibody level increases within a few weeks. Skin lesion examinations are considered about 80 percent accurate when the virus is isolated from a cell culture, and almost as accurate when cell changes induced by the virus are seen.

HLA (HL-Antigen, Histocompatibility Antigens)

Some white blood cells (leukocytes) and platelets contain antigens (disease-causing material) that initiates the formation of antibodies (disease-fighting material). These antigens are called human leukocyte locus A, or HLA antigens. (Originally only one antigen location was discovered on a gene and it was called A; since then additional HLA antigens have been found on locations other than "A.") Antileukocytic antibodies can be tested for by **Agglutination** or **Complement Fixation**, or by combining the suspected blood serum with lymphocytes (a particular type of **White Blood Cell**) and noting if the lymphocytes are destroyed, indicating the presence of an HLA antibody.

The test is also used to determine histocompatibility, or whether the cells of tissues and organs from one person will "take" when transplanted into another person. There are many different HLA antigens (approaching 100 at present), and the closer the donor-recipient agreement of HLA's, the better the chance that a transplant will not be rejected. Blood is taken from a vein for testing.

When performed: Primarily prior to any organ transplant operation (kidney, heart, or skin grafting); prior to some blood transfusions; with undiagnosed high-fever illnesses, arthritis, and anemia; as part of the many **Disputed Parentage** tests (each person inherits four basic HLA antigens).

Normal values: There are no specific normal values; either the various HLA antigens are present or they are not.

Abnormal values: The greater the number of HLA typing dissimilarities, the less the chance that an organ transplant will take or that a skin graft will heal properly.

Different HLA antigens have been associated with certain diseases. HLA-B27 is found in almost all cases of ankylosing spondylitis (an arthritic condition primarily of the sacroiliac joint and the spine); Reiter's syndrome (a disease, primarily found in men, that is characterized by an infection of the urethra with a discharge from the penis and an infection of the eye and the joints); in certain forms of arthritis in children prior to adolescence; and in a particular form of joint pain that occurs along with an infection of the bowels. A positive HLA-B27 is rarely found with true rheumatic disease. HLA-B13 and HLA-B17 (and occasionally HLA-B27) are usually found in patients with the arthritis of psoriasis. HLA-B7 is increased in patients with pernicious anemia. HLA-A2 is increased in patients with myasthenia gravis. HLA-B8 seems to be associated with dermatitis herpetiformus and systemic lupus erythematosus; it is also positive in many hormone disorders (thyroid, adrenal, and in diabetes). Recently it has been found in patients with myasthenia gravis and hepatitis.

Risk factors: Negligible (see general risk factors for blood testing).

Pain/discomfort: Minimal (see general pain/discomfort factors for blood testing).

Accuracy and significance: While HLA detection and typing can be of considerable value in tissue transplant matchings and in helping solve disputed parentage cases, it has no real significance in the specific diagnosis of any one disease. Some 20 percent of the population seems to have a positive HLA-B8 test without any evidence of disease. However, there are doctors who believe a positive HLA-B27 is 90 percent accurate in diagnosing ankylosing spondylitis and Reiter's syndrome.

HYDROXYPROLINE

Hydroxyproline is an amino acid (one of the basic building blocks of proteins). It is unique in that it exists mostly in collagen, a substance found in bone and in slightly smaller amounts in the skin. While hydroxyproline levels are primarily an indication of a bone condition or bone disease, the test is also to search for certain inherited conditions. Although hydroxyproline can be found in the blood, the test is most often performed on urine.

When performed: When defects of bone metabolism are suspected (usually increased production or increased reabsorption of bone substance); after bone fractures; to follow the treatment of Paget's disease (an inflammation of the bones that causes deformation and bowing of arm and leg bones); to help diagnose rickets (vitamin D deficiency) and to follow the results of treatment; to aid in the diagnosis of certain inherited conditions such as Marfan's syndrome (a disease whose major feature is abnormally long bones).

Normal values: Total hydroxyproline levels range from 10 to 75 mg in a 24-hour specimen of urine.

Abnormal values: Increased amounts of hydroxyproline in the urine are found in most conditions where excessive bone structure is being made or repaired (fractures in children during normal growth, Marfan's syndrome, Paget's disease, and certain hormone problems). A decrease in hydroxyproline levels during treatment for certain bone diseases indicates successful therapy.

Risk factors: Negligible (see general risk factors for blood testing).

Pain/discomfort: Minimal (see general pain/discomfort factors for blood testing).

Accuracy and significance: Only in the first few months of life is a blood test more accurate than a urine test. After that period urine tests quite accurately detect abnormal levels of hydroxyproline. The test is quite significant in helping diagnose inherited defective metabolic diseases.

I

IMMUNOGLOBULIN (Ig)

Immunoglobulins (Ig) are the blood protein antibody particles (gamma globulins) of the body. They react with, protect against, and help destroy antigens, which can cause illness. An antigen may be a microorganism (bacteria, virus, fungus), a chemical, or a toxin given off by an invading microorganism. Usually antibodies are specific; that is, they react only to a particular disease-causing substance (either a new substance or one that has previously attacked the body). Antibodies come from lymphocyte (white blood) cells.

Five major immunoglobulins can be tested for in the blood (a sixth disappears after birth); they are known by letters of the alphabet. IgG (immunoglobulin G), the most abundant type, responds to any foreign-body invasion and can also cause Rh anemia problems. IgA protects against virus and bacterial infections and can cause transfusion reactions; IgM is another response to infection; it also reacts to arthritis and is the primary complement antibody (see **Complement Fixation**); IgE is involved in allergic reactions such as asthma, hay fever, and skin rashes (see **RAST; Skin Reaction**); IgD can be isolated, but its action is still not understood.

The presence of immunoglobulin is the basis on which **Agglutination** tests determine specific diseases. Immunoglobulins are measured individually primarily for purposes of research; they can, however, confirm diagnostic suspicions. Blood is taken from a vein and the serum is tested. Immunoglobulins are also tested in **Cerebrospinal Fluid.**

(*Note:* Cryoglobulins are immunoglobulins that precipitate only in cold temperatures and are present primarily with blood vessel diseases.)

When performed: When excessive gamma globulins (hypergamma-globulinemia) are found, as with leukemias, certain cancers, kidney problems, parasitic infections, and chronic infections; after surgery for cancer as a guide to progress; when multiple sclerosis is suspected (see **Albumin/Globulin**).

Normal values: Normal serum levels for the five major immunoglobulins are as follows:

IgG: 500 to 2,000 mg per 100 ml
IgA: 50 to 400 mg per 100 ml
IgM: 50 to 200 mg per 100 ml
IgE: 0.01 to 0.10 mg per 100 ml
IgD: 0.5 to 5 mg per 100 ml

Abnormal values: Immunoglobulins are increased as a result of infection, allergy, and various autoimmune conditions in which the body in essence turns on itself and causes illness (as in systemic lupus erythematosus). After cancer surgery, an increase in immunoglobulins is usually a good prognostic sign. Immunoglobulins may be decreased with certain leukemias, cancers, and other conditions where immunity is lacking.

Risk factors: Negligible (see general risk factors for blood testing).

Pain/discomfort: Minimal (see general pain/discomfort factors for blood testing).

Accuracy and significance: Immunoglobulins exist in such minute quantities they are difficult to measure. Furthermore, they respond to such a variety of infections and other diseases that, at present, their significance is of more academic than practical value. Yet, in certain conditions they help confirm diagnoses of suspected illnesses. Immunoglobulins, when measured in the spinal fluid, are considered 90 percent accurate for the early diagnosis of multiple sclerosis; however, the same immunoglobulins can also appear with several other diseases.

IMMUNOLOGY

With the advent of new technology in laboratories, many doctors now order "immunological" testing. This is a general term for a variety of tests designed to help diagnose three categories of disease. First, there are the tests to uncover the cause of an infection such as **Agglutination** and **Complement Fixation;** the immunological process is to detect the antibodies the body makes to attack the disease-causing antigens. (Such microorganisms as bacteria and viruses contain antigens.) When a specific antibody to a disease antigen is discovered in the blood, it pinpoints the germ to be treated. Next are the immunology tests that encompass allergies—to food, pollen, dust, animals, chemicals, and drugs (see **RAST**). Last are the tests for those diseases doctors label autoimmune, in which the body tissues or cells produce their own "antigens" followed by antibodies which attempt to heal but may, in fact, cause greater damage than good. The **Antinuclear Antibodies** (ANA) test is a classic example of this immunological phenomenon, and systemic lupus erythematosus is considered the archetypal disease consequence.

As diagnostic skills become more sophisticated, scores of symptoms once attributed to viruses and unknown causes are now understood to be the consequences of immunological deviations. Bone aches, nerve pains, joint pains (some forms of arthritis are considered common immunological conditions), a multitude of skin conditions, especially mysterious rashes, rare forms of thyroid gland inflammation, certain kidney failures, unusual susceptibility to infections, a few anemias, odd muscle weaknesses, and even inexplicable stomach pains are but a few of the bodily characteristics that can now be attributed to immunological conditions. Today it is incumbent upon the doctor to search for the immunological cause of disease when no other diagnosis is possible.

There are any number of immunology tests to ascertain if any circulating immune complexes are at work within a patient's body; the Raji-cell assay, the polyethylene glycol (PEG) assay, the C1q solid-phase assay are among the terms used to describe exotic testing for auto-antibodies (those manufactured by the body which then attack the body and cause illness). Other immunology tests described elsewhere in the book include:

Agglutination
Antinuclear Antibodies (ANA)
Complement
Complement Fixation
C-Reactive Protein
HLA
Immunoglobulin
Lymphocyte Typing
RAST
Rheumatoid Factor
Skin Reaction
Thyroid Function

Immunological tests are proliferating so rapidly it is difficult to keep abreast of them; many are tried and proven useless. However, if immunology testing is ordered, it is reasonable to assume a doctor is considering one of the autoimmune diseases as a diagnosis, or is looking for a condition in which the body actually turns on itself and attacks certain of its organs, just as if some outside cause of disease were doing the same thing.

IMPOTENCE (Male)

Although most male impotence (inability to achieve an erection of the penis) is thought to be of a psychological nature, in a substantial number of instances the problem has an organic (physical) basis or is caused by taking certain drugs. Alcohol, many medicines that treat high blood pressure, many tranquilizers, and most hormones can cause impotence and/or loss of libido. Specific drugs reported to cause loss of sexual desire and impotence in men and frigidity in women include guanethidine (Ismelin), methyldopa, clonidine (Catapres), rauwolfia, and reserpine compounds, phentolamine, tolazoline, phenoxybenamine, propranolol (Inderol), Aldactone, and thiazide diuretics (for treating blood pressure and circulatory problems); the benzodiazepines and other minor tranquilizers such as Dalmane, Librium, Valium, Serax, and Tranxene; the phenothiazines and other major tranquilizers such as Mellaril; monoamine oxidase inhibitors, tricyclic drugs, and lithium (for treating depression); anticholinergic drugs (for treating and relaxing irritable stomach, bladder, and bowel as well as for glaucoma and parkinsonism); certain antibiotic drugs such as nitrofurantoin and ethionamide and parasite-killing drugs such as thiabendazole; drugs used to attack cancer cells; almost all narcotics; marijuana; and methadone.

Most tests for impotence are based on the principle that it is normal for a man to have penile erections during deep sleep, and that the ability to do so is a fairly reliable indication that failure to achieve erection when awake is probably psychogenic. Before therapy can be administered for impotence, it must be determined if the cause is physical or psychological. While this is obviously important for education regarding human sexuality, it is particularly important subsequent to injuries to the genital area. After "straddle"-type accidents, many men feel the obvious physical damage has left them impotent; once they are made aware that they still have erections, albeit during sleep, they usually recover completely. Other situations necessitating some form of impotency test include a potential lawsuit in which the wife of a patient claims the doctor's treatment—be it surgery or medication—caused the couple to suffer "loss of consortorium," or the inability of the spouse to perform sexually.

One specific test requires the patient to spend at least three consecutive nights in a laboratory that has facilities for measuring REM (rapid eye movement), levels of sleep (the deepest stage) as well as nocturnal penile tumescence (swelling). Electrodes are placed on the head and are attached to silicone rings around the penis; measurements are made thoughout the night during sleep. (See also **Plethysmography** and **Thermography.**)

Recently a penile tumescence monitor has been introduced that allows a patient to take the portable typewriter-sized machine home, place the sensor rings around the penis at bedtime, and detect the number, size, and duration of any erections that occur during the night. The erections are recorded on a graph which is sealed inside the machine. Later, a doctor can present the observations to the patient, together with appropriate explanations and reassurances. Some doctors use the machines in their offices to evaluate the effects of drugs on erectile failure. Many doctors, when faced with impotent patients, use a simple screening test prior to involved laboratory measurements. They advise the patient at bedtime to encircle the flaccid penis with a strip of postage stamps perforated along the side of the stamps and fasten the first and last as an overlap. The test is usually carried out for three successive nights. If the stamps come apart at the perforations during sleep, it can be assumed an erection occurred and there is no organic or physical basis for the impotence. Alcohol or sleeping medications must not be used prior to performing the postage stamp test; these drugs tend to prevent REM levels of sleep, during which nocturnal erections are most apt to occur.

When performed: When impotence cannot be diagnosed; prior to surgical penile prosthesis implant insertion; following head, spinal cord, or back injuries; during the rehabilitation of some sex offenders.

Normal values: Most men have several penile erections during the night when in deep stages of sleep, especially while dreaming. Such a response indicates no physical pathology or disease as a cause of impotence.

Abnormal values: Failure to show any penile response after three days of testing indicates some physical basis for impotence. Normally the number of nocturnal sleeping erections decreases in men over 50, but total absence indicates a drug, nerve, blood vessel, or spinal cord problem.

Risk factors: Most measuring instruments operate on such low voltage that no real risks are involved.

Pain/discomfort: Some men find it embarrassing to participate in all-night laboratory situations. Other men undergo extreme anxiety prior to, and during the test.

Accuracy and significance: The test is considered extremely accurate in detecting nocturnal erection. Its significance lies in helping to differentiate between physical and psychological impotence.

INSULIN

Direct measurement of insulin in the blood is primarily an indication of the ability of the pancreas to secrete this hormone (the stomach can also secrete a very small amount) in response to carbohydrate foods, certain amino and fatty acids, and certain other hormones and drugs.

The patient is asked to fast for 12 hours before the test. Blood is taken from a vein and the serum is tested. At times, the patient is then given a measured amount of glucose (sugar) and the blood insulin is measured every half hour for three to four hours. The test cannot be performed on a patient taking insulin injections. The **C-Peptide** test can distinguish naturally produced insulin from injected, commercially produced insulin.

It is now possible to test for insulin antibodies (these are **Immunoglobulins**) to determine if a patient is inherently resistant to insulin and requires an unusually large amount of injected insulin.

When performed: When diabetes is suspected; when physical growth problems are evident; as an indication of whether certain oral antidiabetic drugs will work; when pancreatic disease, especially tumor, is suspected.

Normal values: After a 12-hour fast, the amount of serum insulin normally measures from 5 to 30 μU per ml. After glucose is given, blood insulin levels usually rise to more than 200 μU per ml within an hour and return to normal after four hours.

Abnormal values: Insulin levels are increased with an insulinoma (a tumor of insulin-producing cells), obesity, liver disease, and acromegaly (abnormally enlarged bones). Certain hormone drugs will also raise insulin levels. Insulin is lower than normal with diabetes, following surgery, after a heart attack, and when certain other hormones are absent from the body. Patients under emotional stress will also have reduced amounts of insulin secretion.

Risk factors: Negligible (see general risk factors for blood testing).

Pain/discomfort: Minimal (see general pain/discomfort factors for blood testing).

Accuracy and significance: The test is very accurate in helping diagnose an insulinoma (pancreatic cancer). Its particular significance is in helping a doctor differentiate among the various types of diabetes (juvenile, adult-onset). Insulin antibody tests are of particular value in patients whose diabetes is unstable.

IRON

While the iron test is performed primarily to measure the amount of iron in the body, it is more a measure of the total iron-binding capacity, or the iron's availability to pick up oxygen from the lungs and deliver it to body tissues. Body iron is affected by pregnancy, blood loss, hemoglobin destruction, anemia, deficient iron in the diet, and poor intestinal absorption of iron even when dietary amounts are adequate. An average, balanced diet supplies about 10 mg of iron each day, but no more than 10% of that iron is normally absorbed by the intestines to be utilized. At the same time, the body loses about 1 mg of iron a day (through urine, feces, and sweat). Fortunately, the body usually has a large store of excess iron. Blood is collected from a vein and either the serum or plasma is tested. When repeated iron tests are performed, it is essential that the blood samples be taken at the same time of the day. Iron values are usually highest in the morning, after sleep, and may be half the morning's value by evening. These findings are reversed for people who work nights and sleep days.

Other measures of blood and body iron are the serum iron-binding capacity (transferrin), or the specific amount of iron that can be carried in plasma; and the ferritin level, or the amount of iron stored in the body (primarily in the bone marrow). A patient can have a normal amount of iron, but that iron may not carry and deliver a sufficient amount of oxygen to the tissues.

When performed: In searching for the specific cause of an anemia; when there is unexplained weakness and persistent tiredness; when the patient has a swollen, smooth, painful tongue; when monitoring patients on hemodialysis; when certain vitamin and other food deficiencies are suspected.

Normal value: Iron levels generally range from 75 to 175 mcg per 100 ml of serum. Normal values may vary depending on the laboratory's technique. The values may be slightly lower in women and children. Total iron-binding capacity ranges from 200 to 400 mcg per 100 ml. Serum ferritin ranges from 200 to 400 ng per 100 ml.

Abnormal values: Low blood values are found with anemia, infection, cancers, and pruritis (itching skin); after surgery, and in patients taking steroid drugs. Oral contraceptives, estrogens, or excessive dietary iron intake especially from iron-fortified foods may give elevated values. Extremely high levels of iron and iron-binding capacity are found with hemochromatosis, an inherited intestinal iron absorption disease that can cause sufficient iron accumulation in the body so as to be fatal before the age of 30. Total iron-binding capacity is usually increased only with an iron deficiency anemia; it is normal or decreased with other anemias. Total iron-binding capacity and transferrin may be artificially increased by birth control pills or other female hormones. Decreased ferritin is found with iron deficiency but not with anemia of infection; increased ferritin is found with excessive iron intake.

Risk factors: Negligible (see general risk factors for blood testing).

Pain/discomfort: Minimal (see general pain/discomfort factors for blood testing).

Accuracy and significance: Iron measurements alone are adequate for screening for anemia. In most instances, however, doctors make use of all the iron tests to reach a specific diagnosis.

K

KETONES (Ketone Bodies)

Ketones (two different acids and acetone) are produced in the body when glycogen (a form of carbohydrate) is not available to be utilized for energy. The body then draws upon its fat deposits, which are improperly oxidized and which then produce excessive amounts of ketones in both the blood and the urine. When insulin is absent or not immediately available to metabolize carbohydrates (as in diabetes), fats will be burned for body energy, creating more ketones than the body can utilize. Blood plasma from a vein is examined; urine is usually examined at the same time.

When performed: Especially when a patient is in a coma; to diagnose diabetic acidosis; when there is a question of toxemia in pregnancy; with hyperthyroidism and other metabolic abnormalities.

Since ketones are a "desirable" side effect of the no- (or very low) carbohydrate, high protein and fat weight-loss diet, they are constantly tested for in the urine by the dieter as an indication that excessive body fats are being metabolized.

Normal values: Ketones are not usually detected in the blood; however, up to 3 mg per 100 ml is considered within normal limits. There are very few ketones in the urine (125 mg per 24-hour sample, an amount that would not be detected by the usual urine acetone tests).

Abnormal values: More than 3 mg per 100 ml of serum is considered excessive. In diabetic acidosis, levels over 100 mg per 100 ml may be reached. Excessive ketones are found in the blood and urine in metabolic disorders, in starvation, and after a few days on a no-carbohydrate diet. They are also found in the urine with an inherited condition called maple syrup urine disease (the urine smells like fresh maple syrup) and with another inherited condition called renal glycosuria (the kidneys excrete sugar even though the blood sugar is normal). There may be a false elevation of ketones after administration of the bromsulphalein test.

Risk factors: Negligible (see general risk factors for blood testing).

Pain/discomfort: Minimal (see general pain/discomfort factors for blood testing).

Accuracy and significance: Because ketones are found in so many abnormal conditions, they are significant only as a screening mechanism. They can be of value in following the progress of a diabetic who is unregulated.

L

LACTIC ACID

Lactic acid is an end product of sugar metabolism. When the body increases lactic acid production or fails to excrete lactic acid, the condition is called lactic acidosis (usually a complication of kidney, heart, or liver disease).

Lactic acidosis is characterized by a marked "anion gap." Normally the amount of sodium plus the amount of potassium in the blood (anion group) equals the total amount of chloride and bicarbonate in the blood (cation group). When the difference between the two groups is greater than 30 (that is, when the cation group is decreased), an anion gap exists and is an ominous sign of lactic acidosis. Blood is taken from a vein and the whole blood is tested.

When performed: When there is rapid deep breathing, somnolence, stupor, or coma; when metabolic acidosis is suspected; when an anion gap exists.

Normal values: Lactic acid levels from 5 to 20 mg per 100 ml.

Abnormal values: Elevated blood lactic acid is indicative of lactic acidosis. It can also result from exercise, anemia, leukemias, diabetes mellitus, the taking of certain drugs such as epinephrine for asthma or phenformin for diabetes, and salicylate (aspirin) intoxication.

Risk factors: Negligible (see general risk factors for blood testing).

Pain/discomfort: Minimal (see general pain/discomfort factors for blood testing).

Accuracy and significance: Although the test is fairly accurate in revealing excessive lactic acid in the blood, that is about all it does. It is used primarily in hospital and emergency situations on patients who are extremely ill. It is more a means of recording a patient's progress than an aid in diagnosing any specific disease.

LACTIC DEHYDROGENASE (LDH)

Serum lactic dehydrogenase (LDH) is an enzyme found in many body organs and in red blood cells, which when damaged or diseased release the enzyme into the blood serum. LDH acts as a catalyst in carbohydrate metabolism. There are five different forms (isoenzymes) of LDH, concentrated in varying amounts in such organs as the heart and liver and in the muscles.

Most commonly the total LDH is measured; occasionally the different forms of LDH are tested to help ascertain the location and sometimes the extent of body damage. Blood is taken from a vein and the serum is examined. LDH is also measured in spinal fluid, in pleural (lung) fluid, and in the urine, where it is sometimes used as a screening test for kidney and bladder cancer.

When performed: When there is suspicion of a heart attack or cancer; to diagnose anemia; to aid in determining if a mother is carrying a child with an Rh problem; to distinguish hepatitis from other liver diseases; to aid in the diagnosis of pulmonary embolism.

Normal values: Normal LDH levels range from 200 to 600 units per ml of serum or up to 250 IU. Because different laboratories use so many different methods of testing, normal values may vary greatly.

Abnormal values: Lower than normal values of LDH may be found after excessive X-ray exposure. Increased values are found after a heart attack. LDH levels do not become elevated as rapidly as certain other enzymes tested for when heart disease is suspected (see **Creatine Phosphokinase** and **Glutamic Oxalacetic Transaminase**). When elevated, LDH levels persist much longer. Extremely high values of LDH are found with hepatitis, infectious mononucleosis, and anemias caused by deficiencies of vitamin B_{12} or folic acid. Elevated LDH levels are also seen with leukemia and other cancers, but the test is not specific enough to be the sole basis for diagnosis.

Elevated levels of certain isoenzymes of LDH indicate heart disease; others point to liver problems and are more disease-specific. When total LDH levels are elevated, an LDH heat fractionization test is sometimes performed. After LDH is subjected to high heat, only the heart-produced isoenzymes remain, helping to pinpoint the diagnosis.

LDH levels are increased in the spinal fluid following a stroke and with meningitis. In chest conditions that cause the surface of the lungs to give off fluid (pleurisy), the fluid has high LDH levels. With a urinary tract infection or a growth anywhere from the kidney to the bladder, urine LDH levels are elevated.

Risk factors: Negligible (see general risk factors for blood testing).

Pain/discomfort: Minimal (see general pain/discomfort factors for blood testing).

Accuracy and significance: Although blood levels of LDH increase with a variety of diseases, this test is most commonly used, together with other enzyme tests, to confirm the diagnosis of a heart attack. Its significance is really in helping to determine the cause of chest pain. Isoenzyme determinations are somewhat more specific but still cannot offer a definitive diagnosis.

LACTOSE TOLERANCE (Intestinal Disaccharidase Deficiency)

Lactose is a type of sugar found in milk and milk products, including commercial yogurt, some soft (not hard) cheeses, and many different prepared foods such as bakery products that contain milk solids, baby foods, commercially prepared desserts, soft drinks, soups, and even frozen French-fried potatoes. Many drug preparations use lactose as a binder. Some people do not have sufficient lactase (an enzyme) to break down milk sugar; as a result, they have many different symptoms (mostly gastrointestinal cramps, bloating, and diarrhea) after drinking milk or eating milk products. Because lactose is broken down in the making of hard cheese, this food is usually tolerated by patients with milk intolerance. Intolerance to milk sugar is not an allergy, and the symptoms are not the same as an allergic reaction to milk protein. Usually the symptoms are as a result of ingesting an increased quantity of milk (people without lactase can usually drink a little milk or cream in coffee or on cereal). The condition is found most commonly in Orientals, Arabs, blacks, Italians, and Ashkenazi Jews.

In the lactose tolerance test, a patient is given a measured amount of a lactose solution to drink after a fasting blood sugar test (see **Glucose**) has been performed. An hour or two later another blood sugar test is performed.

A newer and somewhat different way to diagnose lactose intolerance as well as related problems of carbohydrate malabsorption is through a breath-hydrogen analysis. This is of particular value when testing children as it seems more of a game than a test. Instead of being stuck with a needle for blood measurements, the child blows into a balloon and the breath is then tested for its quantity of hydrogen gas. Breath is tested before and after the patient has had a drink of sugar water (sucrose). If the sugar is not absorbed normally, excessive hydrogen forms, indicating the enzyme deficiency as intestinal disaccharidase deficiency (disaccharides are forms of sugar).

When performed: When a patient complains of persistent abdominal or gas pains, especially if the patient's intake of milk has increased.

Normal values: Blood sugar rather than lactose itself is measured. Normally after a patient drinks the lactose solution, the blood sugar will rise at least 40 mg per 100 ml within an hour or two.

Abnormal values: Failure of the blood sugar to rise more than 20 mg per 100 ml after drinking the lactose solution is indicative of lactose intolerance. Elderly patients with certain bone diseases may also show an abnormal result, as will some patients who have recently had gastrointestinal surgery or who have an "irritable" bowel.

Risk factors: Negligible (see general risk factors for blood testing).

Pain/discomfort: Minimal (see general pain/discomfort factors for blood testing).

Accuracy and significance: Although the measurement of blood sugar is the most common way to diagnose the inability to digest various forms of sugar, it is now considered an unreliable way of confirming the diagnosis; too many extraneous factors can cause a false positive result. The breath hydrogen test, while more accurate, requires meticulous laboratory skills to obtain proper measurements. When an absolute diagnosis is required, a **Biopsy** of the small intestine is performed. Actually, an observed relationship between the consumption of foods containing lactose and the development of subsequent symptoms is usually sufficient; removal of lactose from the diet followed by relief of symptoms tends to confirm the diagnosis. And commercial lactase preparations (LactAid) are now available; when they relieve symptoms, they help substantiate the diagnosis.

LEAD

Lead is a trace element (only a trace is normally found in the body) that can produce a toxic reaction (plumbism) when sufficient amounts enter the body. At one time most paint had a lead base. Infants who chewed on toys or cribs painted with lead-based paint were apt to suffer lead poisoning. Today most paints are lead-free; however, old walls, furniture, and toys that have been painted over may still have lead paint underneath, posing a hazard if the paint chips or peels. Lead poisoning can also occur in people whose occupation puts them in contact with lead and people who are exposed to heavy vehicular traffic (policemen).

Whole blood, urine, and body tissues such as liver, bone, and hair may be examined. The urine may also be examined for delta aminolevulinic acid (ALA) and coproporphyrin as a screening test for those whose jobs involve contact with lead.

When performed: To aid in the diagnosis of lead poisoning; in children with pica (the regular eating of dirt and other foreign material); during pregnancy.

Normal values: Normally traces of lead up to 40 mcg per 100 ml may be found in the blood. Urine lead should not exceed 100 mcg per 24-hour sample.

Abnormal values: Levels over 40 mcg per 100 ml of whole blood or over 100 mcg in a 24-hour urine specimen are indicative of lead intoxication.

Risk factors: Negligible (see general risk factors for blood testing.)

Pain/discomfort: Minimal (see general pain/discomfort factors for blood testing).

Accuracy and significance: All tests for lead poisoning are quite accurate; lead is either present in excessive amounts or it is not. Lead testing is assuming even greater significance in the evaluation of children with learning disabilities.

LIPIDS

The total lipids test includes the measurement of the three major lipids (fats) in blood serum: cholesterol (an alcohol, not a true fat, yet still so categorized medically), triglycerides, and phospholipids. The test also includes the free fatty acids and other fats, but at present these have no diagnostic significance. Phospholipids (e.g., lecithin) also offer little diagnostic information, but a few physicians employ the phospholipid/cholesterol ratio as an experimental indication of atherosclerosis (see **Cholesterol**).

Triglycerides comprise the greatest amount (by weight) of lipids in the blood as well as in the foods we eat and are considered true fats (olive oil is made up in large part of triglycerides). While triglycerides come primarily from fats in the diet, like cholesterol they can also be manufactured by the liver. Triglycerides are the blood fats that reflect light; thus, in samples taken after a fatty meal or when there is some metabolic defect, they may be seen as a turbid layer in a test tube of serum that has been left standing. Alcohol and carbohydrates, more than fatty foods, cause a great increase in blood triglyceride levels.

The triglyceride test may be performed independently, but it is commonly measured along with cholesterol. The two tests, along with observation of the serum after refrigeration overnight in a test tube, are considered together to arrive at a classification of hyperlipidemia when an excess of serum lipids exists. Lipidemia (the normal amounts of fat in the blood) is often confused with lipoproteinemia, which is another classification of the various densities of the protein molecules that attach themselves to and carry the lipids in the blood (see **Lipoproteins**).

Blood is taken from a vein and the serum of plasma is tested. For triglycerides, the patient should follow a normal diet for at least two weeks before the test and should then eat nothing for 14 hours before the blood is taken. Certain drugs such as hormones, steroids, birth control pills, and diuretics must not be taken for a month before the tests.

When performed: Blood lipids are measured to reflect familial (inherited) disorders of fat metabolism (not necessarily disease-producing); they can point to possible liver, kidney, and thyroid diseases, and at times signify bile tract obstruction; today, however, they are tested mostly as an experimental indication of atherosclerosis.

Normal values: Total lipids usually range from 400 to 1,000 mg per 100 ml (they are normally increased after a meal containing fat). Triglycerides range from 30 to 145 mg per 100 ml; phospholipids, from 125 to 350 mg per 100 ml; the phospholipid/cholesterol ratio, from 0.7 to 1.8.

Abnormal values: There is as yet no scientific agreement on the relative merits of serum lipid measurements for the prognosis of heart and artery disease. Thus, while six varieties of hyperlipidemia (elevated serum lipid levels) have been postulated as a guide to the degree of risk for atherosclerosis, these hypothetical abnormalities are just that—hypothetical. The types are classified according to whether triglycerides, cholesterol, or both are elevated (along with the appearance of the plasma and the patient's symptoms, if any).

Type I, while very rare, shows only high triglycerides. Patients may suffer abdominal pain, but the risk of heart disease is thought to be low.

There are two kinds of type II: the most common, IIa, shows only an increased cholesterol level; IIb shows elevated cholesterol and triglycerides. Both are alleged to be indications of heart disease.

Type III, extremely rare, shows high cholesterol and triglyceride levels but also shows elevated glucose (sugar) levels. It too is alleged to be a warning sign of heart disease.

Type IV, similar to but more common than type III, shows only a marked triglyceride elevation.

Type V, rare, also shows only a triglyceride elevation and is believed to be a combination of types I and IV.

It has been postulated that the lower the phospholipid/cholesterol ratio (decreased phospholipids), the greater the possibility of atherosclerosis. Again, the reasoning behind the classification of lipids is to discover if there is a way to utilize such typing as a means of identifying those at risk for atherosclerosis.

Falsely elevated triglyceride levels are commonly found in patients taking thiazide diuretics, steroid hormones, and birth control pills.

Risk factors: Negligible (see general risk factors for blood testing).

Pain/discomfort: Minimal (see general pain/discomfort factors for blood testing).

Accuracy and significance: Most lipid tests are for purposes of research as no absolute evidence of a direct relation with heart disease has yet been scientifically proven. While the significance of the various lipid measurements is still under study, it should be remembered that wide fluctuations of the various lipid levels also occur with a number of other diseases. However, for the detection of an inherited problem of cholesterol metabolism, the tests are considered quite accurate. Whether treatment of these metabolic disabilities will be of value has yet to be determined.

LIPOPROTEINS

When **Lipids** (fat molecules) combine in the blood with protein molecules, they are called lipoproteins. Lipoproteins are classified according to their density; those with more fat and less protein have the least density (lightest weight); those with the least fat and the most protein have the highest density. Classifying the different lipoproteins is called phenotyping.

The lipoprotein containing the least amount of protein (1%) consists largely of triglycerides and is called a chylomicron. The very-low-density lipoproteins (VLDL), sometimes called pre-beta, contain more than half triglycerides as well as almost equal amounts of cholesterol and phospholipids and up to 10% proteins. The low-density lipoproteins (LDL), sometimes called beta, are nearly half cholesterol, with almost equal amounts of triglycerides and phospholipids along with 20% proteins. The high-density lipoproteins (HDL), sometimes called alpha, are composed mostly of proteins and phospholipids. The presence of increased amounts of high-density lipoproteins in the blood has been associated with a noticeable lack of heart and artery disease. Thus, in tests for **Cholesterol,** the amount of high-density lipoproteins is more important than simply total cholesterol alone. HDL levels are rarely influenced by the type of fat (saturated or polyunsaturated) a person eats; they are increased by exercise, weight loss, niacin (vitamin B_3), and moderate amounts of alcohol while decreased on a high carbohydrate diet.

The four different lipoproteins are also utilized in ascertaining the six types of hyperlipidemia (see **Lipids**). Type I shows almost all chylomicrons. Type II has two variations: IIa is mostly very-low-density lipoproteins; IIb is mostly both very-low-density lipoproteins and low-density lipoproteins. Type III shows abnormal low-density and very-low-density lipoproteins. Types IV and V show increased very-low-density lipoprotein. Type V also shows an increased amount of chylomicrons. The classifications are primarily measurements to see if predisposition to artherosclerosis (heart and artery disease) can someday be predicted. Blood is taken from a vein for testing.

When performed: To study and classify people with elevated lipids (cholesterol or triglycerides) as a possible aid in detecting patients with greater than average risk of heart and artery disease.

Normal values: There are, at this time, no definite standards; the descriptions above give an indication of the usual composition of each lipid protein.

Abnormal values: The presence of excessive amounts of very-low-density lipoproteins is tentatively assumed to be a prognostic sign of artherosclerosis. In contrast, large amounts of high-density lipoproteins are believed to be a prognostic sign of some built-in protection against atherosclerosis.

Risk factors: Negligible (see general risk factors for blood testing).

Pain/discomfort: Minimal (see general pain/discomfort factors for blood testing).

Accuracy and significance: As with lipid testing, lipoprotein measurements are primarily in the nature of research. The medical significance of all of these tests is still under study, especially their significance in relation to diet, stress, smoking, and ordinary daily activities.

LYMPHOCYTE TYPING (B and T cells)

One particular white blood cell (see **Blood Cell Differential**), the lymphocyte, is now classified into two distinct types of cells: the B cell (it is thought this form originates in the bone, hence the letter B, and in various bursa or body cavities containing lymph tissue) and the T cell (it is thought that the thymus gland, hence the letter T, controls the production and maturation of this form even though T cells are also formed in the bone). Each of the two cell types seems to have a distinct purpose; the B cells make antibodies (see **Agglutination**) found in the blood, tears, and other body fluids that fight the antigens of specific diseases, and are sometimes called "helper" cells. T cells seem to be more generalized in their control of immunity to certain diseases as well as attacking viruses. They are sometimes called "killer" cells. T cell reactions also are believed to be the way that the skin reacts to injections of disease material by showing redness and swelling (see **Skin Reaction**). Although the two lymphocytes look the same under the ordinary light microscope, they can be distinguished through an electron miscroscope, or by mixing them with sheep red blood cells (only the T cells will cling to the sheep cells and produce a distinctive rosette pattern).

By determining the quantity of the two lymphocytes in the blood (taken from a vein), in the lymph nodes, or in **Bone Marrow** (taken by aspiration or **Biopsy**), it is possible to diagnose the specific type of leukemia and assess the possible response to treatment. It is also possible to determine whether certain conditions are cancerous; the state of a patient's immunity; and the activity of some autoimmune conditions such as systemic lupus erythematosus.

When performed: To detect and differentiate between certain cancers such as the leukemias; to help detect and evaluate conditions of immunodeficiency; to help diagnose various skin diseases particularly when cancer might be the cause of a psoriasis-like rash and other common rashes; to help diagnose Hodgkin's disease (enlargement of the lymph glands and spleen); to test the possible effect of certain drugs on a patient prior to organ transplant or skin grafting; to assist in the prognosis of certain cancerous conditions.

Normal values: From 5 to 25 percent B cells and 45 to 85 percent T cells (while the range seems wide, most people average 10 percent B cells and 65 percent T cells). It is also considered normal to have approximately 20 percent null cells, or cells that appear to be either B or T.

Abnormal values: Lower than normal amounts of B cells suggest decreased immunity (a patient may have one of several serious infections such as pneumonia); an increased amount of B cells is present in certain leukemias. Decreased T cells indicate an extreme susceptibility to virus, parasitic and certain fungus diseases; an unusual sensitivity to certain drugs that can cause decreased immunity. Patients with T-cell deficiency may not react to diagnostic skin tests. An increase in T cells points to leukemia and other cancers.

Risk factors: Negligible (see general risk factors for blood testing; for bone marrow aspiration or lymph node biopsy, see general risk factors for catheter or needle insertion).

Pain/discomfort: Negligible (see general pain/discomfort factors for blood testing). The needle used to obtain a biopsy or bone marrow specimen may cause some discomfort (see general pain/discomfort factors for catheter and needle insertion).

Accuracy and significance: While the test is considered fairly accurate when used in lymph cell diseases, it is of less value in helping to distinguish other conditions. However, when other diagnostic tests are equivocal, lymphocyte typing may offer an answer. As B-and-T-cell numbers can vary from day to day, some doctors believe a patient's normal limits must be determined before an accurate evaluation can be made and appropriate drugs administered.

M

MAGNESIUM

One of the most abundant minerals in the body, magnesium is found in all cells and is active in many biochemical processes, particularly in enzyme reactions. Magnesium is important to the regulation of the body's calcium supply and usage. A normal diet (particularly nuts and vegetables) affords the body about 0.5g of magnesium every day. Blood is collected from a vein and serum is examined.

When performed: The test is performed whenever patients exhibit symptoms such as twitching and quivering muscles, irritability, and weakness. It is also used to determine whether these symptoms are caused by lowered **Calcium** levels rather than by lowered magnesium levels. Low magnesium levels seem to prevent effective potassium therapy, so the test is especially important when a patient has a low serum potassium level but shows no positive response to administration of potassium; when a heart attack is suspected but is not easily confirmed.

Normal values: Serum magnesium levels range from 1.5 to 2.5 mEq per liter (2 mg per 100 ml). Values vary with different laboratory techniques.

Abnormal values: Lower than normal values are found with parathyroid, thyroid, and adrenal gland hyperactivity, and with malnutrition, chronic alcoholism, pancreatitis, and diuretic therapy. Higher than normal values are found with dehydration and with inactive adrenal glands; after a heart attack.

Risk factors: Negligible (see general risk factors for blood testing).

Pain/discomfort: Minimal (see general pain/discomfort factors for blood testing).

Accuracy and significance: Although magnesium abnormalities are reflected in a wide variety of diseases and nutritional conditions, the test is also considered to have some significance in helping diagnose muscle irritability. It is usually performed with a **Calcium** test. Some doctors think the serum magnesium level is a more accurate measurement of heart muscle damage, especially if that damage is very small, than cardiac enzyme tests (**Creatine Phosphokinase, Lactic Dehydrogenase**).

MELANOGEN-MELANIN

Malignant melanoma is a skin condition of black spots that are believed to start from an inherited nevus (mole); it is the most dangerous of all skin cancers. Many patients with melanomas secrete colorless melanogen in the urine, which then turns to dark brown or black melanin after several hours' exposure to air. The addition of ferric chloride hastens the reaction. A single urine sample is used for testing.

When performed: When a patient has blue-black, brown-black or jet black moles or pigmentation on the skin, or when a light brown mole turns darker.

Normal values: No melanogen (turning to melanin) should be detected in urine.

Abnormal values: The presence of melanin in any quantity usually confirms the diagnosis of malignant melanoma. At times, a black-colored urine must be distinguished from alkaptonuria (see **Aminoaciduria**).

Risk factors: None.

Pain/discomfort: None.

Accuracy and significance: The test is significant if melanin is found in the urine. The absence of melanin, however, does not guarantee the absence of melanoma.

MERCURY

Mercury is a metallic element that can be toxic when taken into the body in sufficient amounts. Mercury can enter the body by inhalation if it is in the air; by contact with the skin (many skin ointments used to include mercury); by injection, as when it is used as a diuretic drug; and mostly by ingestion, as when eating fish containing even a trace of the metal. There are two different forms of mercury; the inorganic form (such as that used in thermometers), which causes vomiting, diarrhea, and kidney failure (most mercury is ultimately stored in the kidneys); and the organic form (such as that used in drugs), which causes weakness, brain damage, loss of balance, mental illness, and muscle pains.

When small amounts of mercury are taken into the body over long periods of time (years), no symptoms may appear until they build up to a toxic level. Urine is most frequently examined for mercury; blood from a vein may also be tested, as well as hair, nails, and other tissues.

When performed: On people who work with mercury (dental assistants, mirror makers, people who manufacture or use certain insecticides); with patients who seem to have mental illness, especially irritability or depression, when there is no known cause or provocation and when no psychiatric diagnosis can be made; when there is weakness, muscle tremors or cramps, brain damage, or kidney damage that cannot be diagnosed.

Normal values: There should be less than 10 mcg of mercury per 100 ml of urine and less than 2 mcg per 100 ml of blood. Hair and nails normally show a slight trace of the metal, usually less than 10 mcg per gram.

Abnormal values: While the amount of mercury varies tremendously in different individuals before it causes symptoms, in most instances a urine level greater than 20 mcg per 100 ml, a blood level greater than 20 mcg per 100 ml, or tissue amounts greater than 100 mcg per gram are indicative of mercury intoxication.

Risk factors: Negligible (see general risk factors for blood testing).

Pain/discomfort: Minimal (see general pain/discomfort factors for blood testing).

Accuracy and significance: The test is quite specific for mercury toxicity when large abnormal values are found. It is especially significant in explaining psychiatric symptoms that can come from mercury poisoning.

METHANOL

Methanol (sometimes called methyl alcohol or wood alcohol) is occasionally ingested accidentally in place of ethanol (ethyl alcohol), the basis for liquors. One ounce of ethanol is usually metabolized and excreted by the body in three hours (depending on the quantity taken in). In contrast, it takes the body more than 24 hours to eliminate each ounce of methanol. More than an ounce of methanol can cause blindness and even death. Sterno is a solid form of methanol.

Isopropyl alcohol (regular rubbing alcohol) and ethylene glycol (the primary ingredient of automobile antifreeze) are also poisonous, but to a somewhat lesser degree than methanol. (Ethylene glycol causes oxalate crystals in the urine; see **Urinary Tract Calculus.**) Blood from a vein or urine may be tested.

When performed: When a patient has a combination of breathing and vision difficulties or is in a coma and no diagnosis can be made; when the ethyl **Alcohol** test is positive, but there are no signs of drunkenness.

Normal values: There should be no trace of methanol, isopropyl alcohol, or ethylene glycol in the blood or urine.

Abnormal values: Any amount found in the blood or urine is abnormal; values greater than 50 mg per 100 ml of blood can be fatal.

Risk factors: Negligible (see general risk factors for blood testing).

Pain/discomfort: Minimal (see general pain/discomfort factors for blood testing).

Accuracy and significance: The test can be very significant, and even life-saving, when performed on a patient who appears drunk but whose breath has no alcohol odor.

MONONUCLEOSIS

The many and varied complaints of patients with infectious mononucleosis—including sore throat, headache, swollen glands (enlarged lymph nodes), abdominal pain, bleeding, and neurological problems—make diagnosis difficult. The specific cause of the disease is the Epstein-Barr virus, a member of the **Herpes** family of viruses. The disease was once thought to be spread by kissing and thus was called the "kissing disease." In infectious mononucleosis, the patient's antibody level reaction to sheep red blood cells rises. The heterophile antibody (an immunoglobulin) test is the primary aid for diagnosis. Blood is taken from a vein and the serum tested as in the **Agglutination** test. The Forssman antibody test is even more specific. There are several other "spot" tests to detect mononucleosis antibodies; most require only one drop of fingertip blood placed on a chemically treated spot on a slide (Mono-Diff, Mono-Test, Mono-Spot). A marked increase in atypical lymphocytes in a **Blood Cell Differential** also points to infectious mononucleosis.

When performed: When there is suspicion of infectious mononucleosis; to differentiate infectious mononucleosis from other diseases.

Normal values: Normally there may be very small amounts of antibody to sheep red blood cells (below a dilution of 1:112).

Abnormal values: Antibody levels are elevated to a dilution of 1:224 or more in approximately 70% of patients with mononucleosis; elevated levels may persist for weeks.

Risk factors: Negligible (see general risk factors for blood testing).

Pain/discomfort: Minimal (see general pain/discomfort factors for blood testing).

Accuracy and significance: The various "spot" and biochemical tests for mononucleosis are considered to be 85 percent accurate. The test is significant in helping the doctor differentiate mononucleosis and other diseases with similar symptoms.

N

NONSTRESS FETAL ASSESSMENT [NST]

The nonstress test for fetal assessment, sometimes called the fetal heart rate acceleration test (FHRAT), helps to evaluate potential problems of pregnancy. It is used almost routinely for those pregnant women for whom the doctor feels there is a greater-than-average risk of problems such as high blood pressure, diabetes, or previous pregnancy problems.

In the past, when a difficult pregnancy was suspected, a small amount of hormone oxytocin was administered to increase contractions of the uterus. The procedure is known as the oxytocin challenge test (OCT) or the contraction stress test (CST). No matter what the impetus, the purpose is to stimulate fetal activity (induce the baby to kick or move in the womb) and then to note if the baby's heart rate increases as it should. Usually the mother lies in a bed which elevates her head and knees. When the baby kicks or moves, the mother presses a button that records the baby's heartbeat.

When performed: On pregnant women, primarily those who are known to have, or are suspected of having, pregnancy problems; when there is doubt as to the exact location of the placenta; when there is a question about the baby's position and condition (such as the possibility that the umbilical cord is wrapped around the baby's neck, or the possibility that the baby's size is not in accord with the duration of the pregnancy); when a pregnancy exceeds the estimated delivery date; when the mother stops feeling normal movements in the womb.

Normal values: The baby's recorded heartbeat should increase at least 15 beats per minute within 20 minutes following kicking or movement. This is called reactive or positive.

Abnormal values: Failure of any acceleration of the baby's heartbeat during fetal movement. This is called nonreactive. Most often if there is a nonreactive response to the nonstress test, a stress test using oxytocin is administered before considering the response abnormal.

Risk factors: None with the use of the nonstress fetal assessment test; there is always a minor risk when the hormone is used.

Pain/discomfort: None, although some pregnant women find the test anxiety-provoking.

Accuracy and significance: Very accurate in helping to observe and predict the condition of the fetus and the course of some but not all pregnancy problems. The test can be life-saving for the infant.

NUCLEAR SCANNING [Radioactive Uptake, Scintillation, Radioisotope]

Nuclear scanning, or radionuclide organ imaging, may be performed on many parts of the body to aid in diagnosing and treating disease. Its primary function is to outline the size, shape, and exact location of an organ (liver, kidney, vein, etc.) or a chamber or duct within an organ. Nuclear scanning tests are also fairly precise in measuring organ function.

A radioactive material (radioisotope or radionuclide) is injected or ingested into the body; depending on the organ to be studied, it may be inserted into an arm vein or administered through a catheter (thin, hollow tube) that starts in an arm or leg vein or artery and is pushed through the blood vessels to the specific organ being tested. In a heart scan, for example, the catheter may start in the arm or the neck and end directly inside the heart chamber being studied. To test the thyroid, a patient drinks radioactive iodine. Various chemicals are known to select certain body organs and after being made radioactive they can be detected within the organ by rectilinear scanners or gamma cameras, both of which work on the same principle as the Geiger counter in detecting uranium. A faster modification of the process is called scintography.

The amount of radioactivity in the injected chemicals is so

small as to cause no known harmful effects to the body. Virtually all radioactivity is gone within a day or so. The scanning machines that detect the radioactivity do not give off any radiation.

In many instances, the radioactivity is visualized on a photographic plate or an X-ray plate. Sometimes a computer printout is made on paper outlining the organ being studied. The results show the size and shape of the organ as well as any part of the organ that failed to pick up radioactive material—usually indicating a defect (disease, tumor). Any excess of radioactivity in an area usually means the organ is enlarged or hyperactive. Through measurement of the flow of radioactive material through an organ, the function of that organ can be determined. When the kidneys are tested, measurement of blood flowing into and out of the kidney is called a renogram; measurement of the size, shape, and position of the kidney is called a renal scan. Usually both kidneys are measured at the same time to better detect which kidney, if only one, is affected.

Most often the nuclear scanning test is referred to by the organ being studied; examples are discussed below.

Brain scan: Radioactive chemicals (mostly technetium) are used for brain imaging; normal brain tissue will not pick up most of the tracer material. A concentration of radioactive material usually indicates an increased number of blood vessels and a disease process. The scanning is performed twice, immediately after the injection of radioactive material and then 24 hours later.

Bone scan: Usually radioactive strontium is used (since it replaces calcium) and a uniform uptake (or concentration) throughout all the bones is normal. An increased concentration in a specific area is abnormal and usually represents cancer, but arthritis and fractures can sometimes give a similar picture. Radioactive gallium is used in testing for hidden bone infections, since gallium seems to seek out inflammatory tissue. Usually a bone scan is performed a few hours after injection of the material.

Lung scan: There are two kinds of lung scanning: a perfusion scan and a ventilation scan. They may be performed separately or together to aid in diagnosis. The perfusion scan is more common. Radioactive albumin is injected into a vein and the scanning is performed immediately. The primary purpose of a perfusion scan is to diagnose pulmonary embolism. When the two different lung scans are performed together, it is also possible to evaluate pulmonary function in emphysema and other lung obstructions, to locate a growth and follow the course of that growth before and after treatment, to measure the size of the heart, and to discern areas of infection and lung collapse. The ventilation scan is performed by having the patient breathe in radioactive xenon gas and then passing the scanner over the lungs. Inhaled radioactive xenon can show normal or abnormal bronchial passageways and areas of the lung that do not receive air.

Liver scan: Nuclear scanning is probably the best way to study the liver without surgery. Radioactive gold or rose bengal (a dye) is injected into a vein. Normally the chemical is absorbed by the liver within 20 minutes and shows a uniform appearance when viewed by the scanner. If, however, there is pathology (growth, cirrhosis, or abscess), that area will not take up the chemical and the absence of radioactivity indicates disease.

Spleen scan: The same chemicals used for a liver scan are often used to visualize the spleen; however, radioactive red blood cells (erythrocytes) give an even better image (since the spleen's function is to remove ineffective erythrocytes from the blood). The test is used to help diagnose an unknown mass in the upper left portion of the abdomen, to evaluate the size and functioning of the spleen, and to diagnose spleen injury. Spleen scanning takes place about four hours after red blood cell injection.

Pancreas scan: A radioactive selenium-amino acid compound is injected in a vein. The pancreas normally takes up this amino acid immediately and the radioactive element allows imaging of the organ in about ten minutes. Pancreatic disease is difficult to diagnose, and this test helps detect cancer, cysts, and infection by the organ's failure to show absorption of the radioactive material. At times Triolein is injected as a means of diagnosing malabsorption or fat-absorption problems.

Esophagus and stomach scan: When patients have difficulty in swallowing (dysphagia) they are sometimes given a syrupy radioactive solution to swallow. This is also called a radionuclide transit (RT) test, during which the path of the radioactive material is followed by gamma camera. Many doctors prefer this test to the barium swallow (see **Radiography**) as the barium swallow can be performed only once, and interpretation of the barium's path is highly subjective. An esophageal scan can be performed several times without risk of excessive radiation exposure. **Gastroesophageal Reflux** is also evaluated in a reverse form of esophageal scan; radioactive measurements follow the reverse flow to see if the stomach's contents go back into the esophagus.

Red blood cell survival scan: To reach a precise evaluation of hemolytic anemia and other causes of red blood cell destruction or loss, some of the patient's blood is withdrawn and radioisotopes are attached to the red blood cells. The blood is then scanned weekly for a month; the loss of radioactive-tagged cells indicates the rate of hemolytic anemia.

Kidney and bladder scan: At times radioactive chemicals are injected into the bloodstream just before the blood reaches the kidney. The rate of kidney filtration (renogram scanning) and the rate of bladder filling and emptying (cystogram scanning) are measured as a means of testing the function of these organs.

Salivary gland scan: When there is a suspected blockage of the ducts that empty the salivary glands into the mouth, usually due to a stone or infection, radioisotopes can be injected into the glands to locate the blocked area.

Heart or cardiac scan: Radioactive thallium is injected into a vein and is absorbed by heart tissue, allowing visualization of the size and shape of the heart. This test is particularly valuable when pericarditis (excessive fluid around the heart) is suspected. Scanning takes place immediately after injection of the chemical. Other radioactive chemicals are used to outline the inside chambers of the heart. A blood pool scan shows heart contractions clearly and can help indicate the amount of damage after a heart attack.

In perfusion imaging, radioactive chemicals can be directed into the coronary arteries supplying oxygen to the heart muscle to reveal the blocked or narrowed arteries. This procedure is also used while a patient is exercising to detect heart muscle that has inadequate circulation only when under physical stress. "Cold Spot" imaging is another term for visualizing the heart with radioactive chemicals. "Cardiac catheterization" is yet another term used; however, it is also applied to angiology or angiography (see **Radiography**) when dye, rather than radioactive chemicals, is utilized.

Testicular or scrotal scanning, sometimes called an orchiogram, consists of an injection of radioactive material into the testicular artery, and is used to diagnose pain and/or swelling in one or both testicles. It is particularly useful in diagnosing epididymitis (an infection of the cord-like duct next to the testicle) and when an undiagnosable tumor is felt.

Vein scan: Various radioactive chemicals injected into a vein will be absorbed in blood clots if a thrombus or phlebitis is present. The clot is easily visualized. The test may also predict patients who are prone to thromboembolism.

Thyroid scan: See **Thyroid Function.**

Spinal fluid scan: Radioactive albumin is injected into the lower-back spinal fluid space (see **Cerebrospinal Fluid**) and observed as it passes around the cord into the brain spaces. The chemical takes about 24 hours to reach the brain area and remains there for two to three days. This test is especially valuable in diagnosing hydrocephalus (abnormally large head); it is also indicated when there is suspicion of a spinal fluid leak. The test is sometimes called cisternography, spinal cord scan, or intrathecal scan.

Placental scan: When there is doubt about the exact position of the fetus during pregnancy, the injection of an extremely tiny dose of radioactive albumin will help show the location of the placenta so as to place the fetus. When there is suspicion of intrauterine bleeding, usually due to a damaged placenta, this test will help diagnose the condition and can be life-saving to the patient.

In some cases, instead of a diagram or illustration of the radioactivity, a counter is placed over the organ and the amount of radioactivity is "counted" and recorded as to its intensity. This technique is often used in testing organ function, since it is easier and continuous.

(*Note:* Radioimmunoassay is a technique [not a specific test] which uses radionuclides [as used in scanning] for measuring minute quantities of hormones, certain drugs, and antigens that can cause disease [see **Agglutination; RAST**]. It is another method to verify hormone deficiency or excess, drug toxicity, allergy, and infections.)

When performed: In general, scanning is performed when it is necessary to visualize an organ and to follow the progress of certain diseases. More specific indications for nuclear scanning are noted in the descriptions of the scanning procedures above.

Normal values: Normal values are noted in the specific scanning descriptions above.

Abnormal values: Whether an organ should or should not pick up and reflect radioactivity is discussed under each organ-scanning procedure. The normality, abnormality, and degree of abnormality are determined by a physician with extensive experience in the field.

Risk factors: Depending on the organ being scanned and the particular technical process, the risk ranges from negligible (see general risk factors for blood testing) to slight when there is a single injection of radioactive material (see general risk factors for the use of radioactive material). The increase of risk parallels the number of instruments used and the complexity of the procedure (see general risk factors for catheter and needle insertion, and contrast substance use). Whenever catheters are inserted and directed to a sensitive area of the body (heart, brain, and other internal body organs) the risk increases in proportion to the distance the catheter must travel. Catheters within the heart and major arteries, particularly those to the lungs, can cause fluctuations in heart rhythm and have been known to stop the heart's beating completely (cardiac arrest). Catheters have also been known to damage the heart's valves. In summary, the more complicated a procedure; the longer it takes; or the larger the body area being scanned; the greater risks associated with nuclear scanning become.

Pain/discomfort: Pain and discomfort are minimal when the test involves only the injection of a radioactive substance (see general pain/discomfort factors for blood testing). When the test necessitates the insertion of a catheter (see general pain/discomfort factors for catheter and needle insertion) many patients complain of the manipulation of their bodies for prolonged periods of time. Unless the procedures are explained in detail before the test, patients tend to be quite apprehensive, especially when a catheter is directed to the heart. Some patients undergoing a lung scan complain of a sense of suffocation.

Accuracy and significance: In general, nuclear scanning is considered reasonably accurate, but much depends on the organ or area of the body being scanned. For example, heart scans can be extremely significant in differentiating the causes of chest pain. A number of doctors believe thallium scanning (without catheterization) is quite precise in locating damage to heart muscle and indicating its scope. When a thallium scan is performed while a patient is exercising, and the test appears normal, angiography (see **Radiography**), with its use of catheters, is not necessary. Lung scanning is not absolutely precise unless large defects exist. The majority of doctors think only incontestably normal scans are diagnostic, while abnormal scans are not always especially specific. Overall, nuclear scanning is considered to have an accuracy rate of from 50 to 80 percent.

O

OCCULT BLOOD

In medicine the word "occult" means present but invisible. Thus occult blood procedures test for blood that can be seen only through microscopic or chemical examination. Virtually all body fluids, excretions, and secretions can be tested for occult blood; most often the test is performed on feces and urine. It has been proposed that if everyone's feces were properly tested for occult blood twice a year, almost all bowel cancer could be eliminated.

A person can lose about an ounce of blood a day from the bowel (amounting to a pint in two weeks) without noticing any bleeding. In contrast, visible bleeding occurs when more than 2 ounces of blood enter the bowel (from a bleeding ulcer, from a growth in the colon or large intestine, or from hemorrhoids). When that blood mixes with the stomach acid in the bowel, it turns black and is termed melena. Thus a general assumption is that black, tarry bowel movements indicate bleeding somewhere in the upper intestinal tract, while bright red blood indicates lower-bowel and rectal bleeding.

There are three different tests for occult blood: guaiac (Hema-Chek, Hemoccult), orthotoluidine, and benzidine. The orthotoluidine test is the most sensitive but will give a false positive result when the patient's diet includes meat. The guaiac test usually does not react to dietary meat but is the least sensitive. In most instances, a patient is told not to eat any meat or even to brush his teeth for at least three days before the test, since the slightest trace of blood from meat or from irritation of the gums can give a false positive test.

When performed: Whenever gastrointestinal or kidney disease is suspected; whenever a patient has an anemia that cannot be diagnosed.

Normal values: Urine, feces, and other body secretions should show no occult blood.

Abnormal values: A positive occult blood test, after eliminating all extraneous causes (brushing the teeth, irritating the throat, blowing the nose too hard, meat diet, taking excessive amount of iron pills), is considered abnormal. Occult blood can be found in the bowel with patients taking aspirin or other drugs that irritate the stomach. Alcoholic gastritis may also cause a positive test.

False positive results can be caused by eating turnips, horseradish, and taking large doses of vitamin C just prior to being tested.

Eating beets will color the feces red but will not cause a positive test. A positive urine occult test usually indicates pathology somewhere in the urinary tract, from the kidneys to the bladder to the ducts that carry the urine.

Risk factors: None.

Pain/discomfort: None.

Accuracy and significance: Although the test is valuable, unfortunately it can show 30 to 60 percent false positive results. The manufacturers of the Hemoccult test, however, claim their method results in only one percent false positive results. When the test is positive more than once, and all the extraneous factors that could cause a false positive result have been considered, the finding is significant enough to warrant an extensive search for the cause of hidden bleeding.

(A feces specimen should not be taken from a toilet bowl in which any of the automatic cleaning compounds or devices are used.)

OSMOLALITY

Osmolality is a measure of the osmotic pressure of a liquid. In medicine osmotic pressure indicates the amount of dissolved material (minerals, hormones, etc.) in a body fluid, most commonly blood or urine. Large amounts of sodium, sugars, fats, and other substances increase the blood's osmolality; in fact, the amount of sodium alone in the blood can sometimes be used as a reasonable measure of serum osmolality. Blood osmolality regulates body water (the feeling of thirst, when water is needed, and the control of urine output), and it depends primarily on blood electrolytes (see **Chloride; Potassium; Sodium**). Blood is taken from a vein and the serum is tested. Urine is also tested for osmolality.

The osmolality test is considered more accurate than the urine specific gravity test, which offers somewhat similar measurements (specific gravity measures the presence and quantity of all the particles of varying sizes that are contained in the liquid). A common method of testing for osmolality is to measure the exact degree at which the liquid freezes, since soluble particles in a liquid affect the freezing point.

When performed: When dehydration is suspected; in alcoholism; when excessive amounts of fats are in the blood (hyperlipidemia); in uncontrolled diabetes and in unexplained instances of edema (water retention); to measure the effects of intravenous therapy.

Normal values: Normally osmolality should range from 280 to 295 mOsm per liter (about the same as normal plasma) in blood and 300 to 1,200 mOsm per liter of urine.

Abnormal values: Levels are increased (hyperosmolality) with water loss (vomiting, diarrhea, excess sweating) or inadequate water intake (300 mOsm per liter is considered moderate to severe dehydration), with brain or kidney damage, and with diabetes insipidus. Decreased levels occur when excess water is taken in or administered (such as with intravenous therapy) and when diuretic drugs are used (which cause excretion of a great deal of sodium ions, lessening the amount of blood electrolytes). Markedly decreased levels in the urine indicate failure of the kidney's concentrating ability.

Risk factors: Negligible (see general risk factors for blood testing).

Pain/discomfort: Minimal (see general pain/discomfort factors for blood testing).

Accuracy and significance: The test is most often performed in a hospital where the effects of intravenous solutions can be monitored. Osmotic pressure is considered an accurate measurement of the body's state of hydration or dehydration. When blood and urine osmolality are measured together, they help to confirm the diagnosis of diabetes insipidus (a hormone imbalance causing a patient to drink an unusually large quantity of fluid and to urinate excessively; see **Vasopressin**).

OXALATE

Eating many foods that naturally contain the chemical oxalate (sorrel, spinach, cabbage, tomatoes, rhubarb, and even chocolate) usually has no adverse effect; in some people, however, it can cause hyperoxaluria (an abnormally excessive amount of oxalate in the urine). If it then combines with calcium, oxalate can on occasion cause kidney stones. A rare inherited condition known as primary hyperoxaluria or oxalosis (as distinguished from secondary or ordinary hyperoxaluria) causes kidney infections and high blood pressure. Oxalate is measured in urine. Since oxalate levels can be lowered by altering the diet, the test aids not only in diagnosis but also in following the progress of treatment. Kidney stones of oxalate can also form when a patient has a bowel infection such as colitis or diverticulitis. Patients seem even more susceptible to oxalate stones after surgery for intestinal disease; they also occur following intestinal by-pass surgery performed to help patients lose weight.

When performed: The test is used whenever a patient has symptoms of kidney or bladder stones. It is also performed when there are certain intestinal inflammation problems that do not respond to therapy, when the intestine had been operated on for cancer or ulcers, or when, in rare instances, an intestinal bypass procedure is performed to promote weight loss. (It is believed that the presence of excessive oxalates after surgery represents a vitamin B_6 deficiency from poor intestinal absorption.) Oxalate levels are measured when there is suspicion of ethylene glycol (automobile antifreeze) or oxalic acid (bleach) poisoning.

Normal values: Oxalate levels normally range from 0 to 40 mg per 24-hour specimen of urine.

Abnormal values: Levels greater than 50 mg per 24-hour sample of urine are considered abnormal. With hyperoxaluria, the urine usually shows white, cloudy formations.

Risk factors: None.

Pain/discomfort: None.

Accuracy and significance: The test quite accurately indicates excessive oxalate levels in the urine. The significance of the test is such that when increasing oxalate levels are found, a diet can be prescribed to reduce the oxalates and help prevent the formation of kidney stones.

OXYGEN

Oxygen in the blood is measured in a variety of ways. The *oxygen content* is the amount of the gas actually present in the blood. The *oxygen capacity* is the amount of oxygen that would be found in the blood if all it could hold were present. Both measures indicate just how much oxygen is available to support life, or the percentage of oxygen saturation of the blood. And blood oxygen is measured as the *partial pressure of oxygen* (Po_2), sometimes called *oxygen tension*.

Oxygen is rarely tested alone; it is almost always measured along with the blood's **Carbon Dioxide** (CO_2) and **pH** (hydrogen ions that indicate the acidity of the blood; although the blood is in fact alkaline, "acid" is used to differentiate between the increase and decrease in the pH). Once the Po_2 and the pH are known, the amount of oxygen attached to hemoglobin (hemoglobin saturation) can be determined. These three different tests are known as the blood gas group.

Whole blood is taken from an artery for most oxygen testing; in an emergency it can be taken from a vein to measure content or saturation. The sample must be collected in a syringe that is coated inside with oil to prevent any air from reaching the blood; the needle tip must be sealed immediately and the syringe packed in ice. (A new device claims to measure Po_2 simply by touching the skin.) Elderly patients should be reclining when the blood is taken, since blood oxygen is lowest in that position and yields a truer value.

When performed: Primarily in respiratory diseases and in conditions that affect the lungs and interfere with transfer of oxygen to the blood; to determine if oxygen therapy will be effective; when there is heart failure; when there is suspected hypnotic or narcotic drug overdose; as a means of better evaluating kidney problems.

Normal values: Normal values for the different measures of oxygen are as follows:

Oxygen tension (Po_2): 85 to 105 mm Hg (after 40 years of age it may be lower).

Oxygen content: 15 to 23 volumes % for arterial blood and 10 to 16 volumes % for venous blood.

Oxygen capacity: 16 to 24 volumes % (levels depend on how much hemoglobin is present, since each gram of hemoglobin holds 1.39 ml of oxygen).

Oxygen saturation: from 94% to 100% of capacity for arterial blood and from 60% to 85% of capacity for venous blood.

Abnormal values: Oxygen values are decreased (hypoxemia) with any chronic obstructive lung disease (such as emphysema) or during an asthmatic attack. Almost any respiratory complication of disease can reduce oxygen utilization as reflected by lowered oxygen values for all the tests. Polycythemia (too many red blood cells) will also lower oxygen values. Exercise can decrease the amount of oxygen in the blood.

Risk factors: Negligible (see general risk factors for blood testing).

Pain/discomfort: Minimal (see general pain/discomfort factors for blood testing).

Accuracy and significance: Although oxygen measurements are usually performed on extremely ill and hospitalized patients, the primary purpose of the tests is to confirm the physician's judgment as to the level of blood oxygenation. Oxygen tests can provide an early warning of hypoxemia. The significance of this test lies in the constant monitoring of the patient's blood for its oxygen content, and the ability to prevent damage to tissues such as the brain from the loss of oxygen.

P

PARASITE

Although the word "parasite" literally refers to a plant or animal form that attaches itself to and exists on another living organism, in medicine the term usually refers to an infestation by some form of worm-like organism that causes disease. When doctors suspect that a patient is suffering from a parasitological invasion, they usually order an "ova and parasite" test—most often as part of a **Feces Examination.** "Ova" refers to the egg stage of a parasite's development; it is sometimes easier to detect egg forms than it is to see actual parasites. Not all parasites assume the familiar worm-like shape. Some are single cells that slither around (the amoeba that causes diarrhea, abdominal cramps and abscesses); some move quite actively and have tiny hairs called flagella protruding from their single-celled bodies (the giardia that is becoming the most common cause of gastrointestinal illness, which is usually acquired during foreign travel, and the trichomonas that cause vaginitis); and some combine both attributes (the trypanosomes that cause sleeping sickness, muscle and heart infections and many different types of difficult-to-diagnose fevers).

In actuality, malaria is really a parasitic disease, as are trichinosis (in which worms, most often acquired from eating inadequately cooked pork, lodge in muscles, causing severe pain), schistosomiasis (swimmer's itch), **Toxocariasis,** and all the many different tapeworm illnesses, which are becoming much more common thanks to the public's growing taste for raw or undercooked meat and fish.

There are many other different, and usually rare, parasitic infestations. Doctors are aided in arriving at a diagnosis through various tests such as **Complement Fixation, Agglutination, Counterimmunoelectrophoresis,** and **Skin Reaction,** as well as direct examination of the blood, urine, feces and other body tissues and secretions. The most important step in discovering that a parasite has caused a disease is to consider its possibility, something that is not always an obvious choice in today's practice of medicine. When an illness is difficult to diagnose, and especially if the patient's eating habits have recently changed, or if he or she has recently traveled to areas where these parasites are common (particularly the tropics), tests for parasites that relate to one's symptoms should be carried out.

PARATHYROID [Parahormone, Parathyrin, PTH]

Until recently, **Calcium** testing was the principal way to diagnose parathyroid disease. The parathyroid glands (usually four tiny, isolated glands buried within the thyroid gland substance but distinctly different from the thyroid) help control the body's need for and use of calcium. Calcium is necessary for muscle contraction—especially heart muscle—nerve transmission, blood clotting, and to keep the body's myriad cells alive. With hyperparathyroidism, or an excess of parathyroid hormone, calcium increases in the blood (**Phosphorus** usually decreases); when parathyroid hormone production diminishes, calcium does also. Hyperparathyroidism usually results from a parathyroid gland tumor, but it is also found with rickets (vitamin D deficiency), and abnormalities of other endocrine glands. When hyperparathyroidism is present, it is often accompanied by a stomach ulcer, kidney stones, high blood pressure, heart rhythm abnormalities, bone pain, or even psychosis. For testing, blood is taken from a vein; when a more precise diagnosis is needed the hormone is also tested for its two components, C-terminal and N-terminal. Decreased parathyroid hormone (hypoparathyroidism) commonly occurs following the surgical removal of the thyroid glands as a treatment of thyroid disease. It can also occur after X-ray treatments to the neck for thyroid disease and after treatment for parathyroid tumors. And for some as yet unknown reason, it has been found in patients suffering from candidiasis (a fungus infection of the mouth called "thrush"; the fungus can also infect the lungs and vagina).

With hypoparathyroidism, there is often an extreme sensitivity of the muscles which can tighten and twitch involuntarily. There can be muscle pains, particularly in the abdomen, frequent urination, and abnormal mental manifestations such as depression and delirium. With severe cases, there is hair loss, loose teeth, brittle nails, and eye cataracts.

There is also an inherited condition known as pseudohypoparathyroidism, in which parathyroid hormone may be present but does not act on the kidneys as it should. Lastly, there is pseudopseudohypoparathyroidism, a condition that imitates pseudoparathyroidism but one in which the blood's calcium remains normal (unlike the other hypoparathyroid disorders).

Occasionally the Ellsworth-Howard test is used to help eliminate pseudohypoparathyroidism; by injecting the patient with parathyroid hormone its effect on the kidney's ability to handle calcium and phosphorus can be observed.

When performed: Primarily when blood calcium tests are abnormal; when there are repeated episodes of muscle pains and tetany (muscle twitching); when there are repeated episodes of kidney stones; when abnormal bone X-rays cannot be explained; when personality changes cannot be diagnosed.

Normal values: Total parathyroid hormone should be from 100 to 600 pg per ml; however, as laboratory procedures differ, each laboratory may have its own standard; C-terminal and N-terminal measurements also vary but range between 200 to 1,200 pg per ml. Calcium measurements must be made simultaneously with and correlated with parathyroid hormone values.

Abnormal values: With hypoparathyroidism, parathyroid hormone levels are generally lower than normal; with pseudohypoparathyroidism and hyperparathyroidism the levels are elevated. They are normal with pseudopseudohypoparathyroidism. Hormone levels must always be evaluated with blood calcium values to help arrive at a specific diagnosis.

Risk factors: Negligible (see general risk factors for blood testing).

Pain/discomfort: Minimal (see general pain/discomfort factors for blood testing).

Accuracy and significance: Parathyroid hormone measurements are rather imprecise as all of the hormone is not always detected. The significance of the test is in its differentiation among the many causes of calcium disorders and the various parathyroid syndromes.

PARTIAL THROMBOPLASTIN TIME [PTT]

Thromboplastin is one of the 12 factors in the body that cause the blood to clot. The partial thromboplastin time (PTT) test measures the efficacy of eight of those factors, primarily Factors VIII and IX (the antihemophilia factors). It is gradually replacing the older **Bleeding and Clotting Time** tests. Blood is drawn from a vein and plasma is examined. The test serves the same function as the blood clotting time which must be measured immediately after the blood is taken; the advantage of the PTT is that the blood sample may be measured later in a laboratory.

When performed: In diagnosing hemophilia; to monitor therapy of hemophilia; when heparin is prescribed.

Normal values: Normal partial thromboplastin time averages 35 to 50 seconds, depending on the laboratory.

Abnormal values: Elevated PTT levels (more than 50 seconds) occur with hemophilia and with patients taking heparin.

Risk factors: Negligible (see general risk factors for blood testing).

Pain/discomfort: Minimal (see general pain/discomfort factors for blood testing).

Accuracy and significance: The test is far more accurate than the routine bleeding and clotting time tests, and is particularly significant when following the progress of a patient receiving heparin. To insure the efficacy of partial thromboplastin time measurements, the test must be performed before heparin is administered to establish a baseline measurement.

PEPSINOGEN

Pepsinogen is a substance secreted by certain stomach cells and converted by stomach acid to the digestive enzyme pepsin. Normally it is present in blood serum. Recent research studies of men with stomach cancer, who had blood samples collected for other reasons years before they showed any evidence of cancer, revealed that a great many of these men had lower than normal pepsinogen levels prior to the onset of their cancer. It has since been observed that changes in the stomach lining cells, which may or may not be precancerous, decrease the blood's pepsinogen levels. Yet longtime smokers, many with symptoms of gastritis (an inflammation of the stomach wall) and a tendency to ulcers rather than cancer, have higher blood levels of pepsinogen. The blood for testing is usually taken from an arm vein.

When performed: As a screening test to evaluate the risk of stomach cancer; as a confirmatory test in the diagnosis of stomach cancer; to help differentiate among the causes of stomach pain and bleeding.

Normal values: 30–45 ng per ml for men; 20–40 ng per ml for women. If reported by mcg, both sexes average 45–150 mcg per ml for a 24-hour period.

Abnormal values: Less than 40 ng per ml is reason to suspect the presence of stomach cancer; greater than 60 ng per ml is reason to suspect the presence of gastritis. Smokers have higher than normal levels (greater than 75 ng per ml) without signs or symptoms of gastritis.

Risk factors: Negligible (see general risk factors for blood testing).

Pain/discomfort: Minimal (see general pain/discomfort factors for blood testing).

Accuracy and significance: It has been postulated that men with a low pepsinogen level have seven times the risk of having stomach cancer than do men with normal or elevated pepsinogen levels. Whether women show the same risk factor has not been determined as yet. The test is considered 35 to 50 percent accurate in helping to diagnose stomach cancer, gastritis, and ulcers.

pH

pH is a measure of how much hydrogen gas is in the blood; it reflects the number of hydrogen ions that are present per liter. A pH of 7, which is neutral (neither acid nor alkaline), means there are 100 nanoequivalents of hydrogen ions per liter of blood. The body functions best when the blood pH is 7.40—that is, when it contains about 40 nanoequivalents of hydrogen ions per liter. Therefore, the blood is normally very slightly alkaline (on the base side when considered on an acid-base relationship).

The balance is so delicate that when the pH goes below 7.38 (a difference of only 2 nanoequivalents of hydrogen: far less than a billionth of a gram), normal body functions are disrupted and the pathological condition of acidemia (acidosis) exists. The body immediately struggles to correct the condition, which can be fatal if allowed to persist. A drop in pH also causes severe constriction of arteries and a lack of oxygen to tissues. Should hydrogen ions be lost from the body (or neutralized) and the blood pH rise above 7.44, the opposite pathology occurs—a condition known as alkalemia (alkalosis). If the alteration is caused primarily by bicarbonate, it is called metabolic; if the change is caused by carbon dioxide, it is called respiratory. Either condition reflects an acid-base balance disturbance.

Since most normal metabolic reactions in the body tend to create acids, the blood is always slightly alkaline (to neutralize the acids). Breathing out carbon dioxide (which is acid) also helps keep the pH properly balanced. Preferably, blood from an artery is tested; properly collected venous blood can be measured in emergency situations. The blood must not be exposed to air. The pH is also measured in urine, spinal fluid, lung fluid, semen, and many other body secretions.

When performed: Almost always in conjunction with **Carbon Dioxide** and **Bicarbonate** tests and frequently with **Oxygen** testing; whenever there are respiratory or kidney problems that cannot be positively diagnosed; when a patient is in a coma or very confused; following vomiting or diarrhea; with severe muscle cramps; when certain drug poisoning is suspected.

Normal values: Normal pH in the blood ranges from 7.38 to 7.44. The body will not survive a pH lower than 6.8 or higher than 7.8.

Abnormal values: Levels below 7.35 indicate acidosis: either respiratory (from a lung condition that prevents the normal exchange of oxygen and carbon dioxide from the blood to the air, such as asthma, emphysema, an injury that causes a blood clot in the lung, or fractured ribs) or metabolic (from drug poisoning such as aspirin or from diabetes, diarrhea, or kidney disease). A pH above 7.45 indicates alkalosis: either respiratory (from deliberate fast breathing, certain drugs, or liver disease) or metabolic (from taking diuretics, steroids, or alkaline antacids for ulcers or burning stomach, or from vomiting or adrenal disease).

Urine pH is normally acid, especially on arising, but it becomes more acid (sometimes abnormally so) with kidney disease or lung disease, and after taking certain drugs or eating a great deal of meat. Urine becomes less acid (and sometimes alkaline) with various drugs and when the diet is high in vegetables and fruits. Spinal fluid is normally alkaline but becomes acid when excessive drugs are administered and in certain lung diseases. Most other body fluids are alkaline; when they become acid, pathology is usually indicated (an acid semen means decreased fertility).

Risk factors: Negligible (see general risk factors for blood testing).

Pain/discomfort: Minimal (see general pain/discomfort factors for blood testing).

Accuracy and significance: When pH is measured with carbon dioxide and bicarbonates, it can help differentiate between the various causes of acidosis and alkalosis. Knowledge of serial pH measurements can lead to the precise treatment of acidosis and alkalosis conditions which can be life-saving. Measurements of pH in the urine are not critical; simple paper dipstick tests are usually sufficient.

PHENYLKETONURIA [PKU]

Phenylketonuria (PKU) is an inherited amino acid enzyme deficiency that can cause mental retardation because of the body's inability to metabolize a protein amino acid, phenylalanine, which is then abnormally found in the urine. It occurs once in every 10,000 births and is most common among people from northern Ireland and western Scotland. Early treatment of this metabolic disorder—by a diet low in phenylalanine (using synthetic proteins in place of plant and animal proteins)—can prevent mental retardation; thus the testing of newborn infants is essential to early diagnosis and treatment. A very small amount of phenylalanine is necessary for normal growth, and children differ markedly in how much they can eat without showing symptoms.

The primary test for phenylketonuria is the blood Guthrie Bacterial Inhibition Assay (GBIA). A small amount of blood is usually drawn from the infant's heel for testing. The test cannot be performed until at least 24 hours after the infant has had its first milk meal. (Breast-fed infants must be tested again after one month.) Urine can also be tested for PKU, but blood will show a positive reaction much sooner than urine. If the Guthrie test is positive, a blood phenylalanine analysis is performed to confirm the diagnosis.

The dinitrophenylhydrazine (DNPH) test and ferric chloride urine test help detect PKU as well as other inherited metabolic defects. There are also special plastic strips coated with chemicals that turn color when dipped into the urine (or even placed on a wet diaper) of a child with phenylketonuria, but occasionally they give a false positive reaction.

When performed: Testing of newborn infants for PKU is now mandatory throughout most of the United States; the exceptions are Delaware, North Carolina and Vermont, although many states will not test children when the parents object. In other situations, the test is utilized when mental retardation is suspected.

Normal values: Normally there are less than 4 mg per 100 ml of demonstrable phenylalanine in the blood.

Abnormal values: When a child has PKU, the blood concentration of phenylalanine is kept between 3 and 7 mg per 100 ml. A concentration greater than 20 mg per 100 ml indicates a metabolic disorder. The urine will show 100 mcg per ml or more with PKU.

Risk factors: Negligible (see general risk factors for blood testing).

Pain/discomfort: Minimal (see general pain/discomfort factors for blood testing).

Accuracy and significance: The test is extremely accurate when properly performed and is significant in the mental retardation it has already prevented. (The chemicals used in manufacturing certain brands of disposable diapers can prevent any reaction when testing for PKU while other brands can give a false positive reaction. Disposable diapers should not be used for this test.)

PHOSPHORUS

Phosphorus metabolism is directly related to calcium metabolism and is associated with many body functions, most controlled by the parathyroid glands. Ninety percent of the phosphorus in the body is stored in the skeleton. Approximately 1 g of phosphorus is ingested daily by the average adult; primarily from dairy foods, meat, nuts and vegetables. Although the test is reported as phosphorus, usually phosphate ions (phosphorus combined with something else such as oxygen phosphates) are measured. It is possible to be poisoned by inorganic phosphorus as opposed to organic phosphorus (see **Cholinesterase**). Matches, fireworks, and some rodent poisons contain phosphorus, which may cause symptoms imitating liver disease. Blood is collected from an arm vein and the serum is examined. Phosphorus is also tested in urine and feces.

When performed: In kidney disease, hypoparathyroidism, suspected vitamin D deficiency (rickets), and undiagnosed nerve and muscle disease, when phosphorus poisoning is suspected.

Normal values: Normal phosphorus levels range from 2.5 to 4.5 mg per 100 ml of serum (higher in children).

Abnormal values: Phosphorus levels may be increased in kidney disease, hypoparathyroidism, conditions of bone destruction and repair (healing fractures, certain bone diseases), and hypervitaminosis D (excess vitamin D), and sometimes in patients taking Dilantin, pituitrin, or heparin. Phosphorus levels may be decreased in certain rare diseases of the kidney tubules, alcoholism, hyperparathyroidism, and vitamin deficiency. Increased urine and feces phosphorus usually reflects a decrease in the serum.

Risk factors: Negligible (see general risk factors for blood testing).

Pain/discomfort: Minimal (see general pain/discomfort factors for blood testing).

Accuracy and significance: Although the test is a fairly accurate measure of phosphorus levels in the blood, abnormal values exist in so many conditions that the test is not useful for a specific diagnosis unless it is used in conjunction with other tests. To avoid false results, the glassware employed in the test must be kept free of cleaning solutions containing phosphorus. Patients who suddenly stop using alcohol a day or two before the test, or who are surreptitiously taking diuretic drugs, can also cause the test to yield abnormal values.

PLACENTAL LACTOGEN

Human placental lactogen (HPL), also known as human chorionic somatomammotrophin (HCS), is a hormone produced by the placenta (the blood supply around the fetus during pregnancy). It first appears in the blood after about the fifth week of pregnancy and gradually increases in amount until the baby is born, after which it disappears. Its appearance and gradual increase are an indication of normal pregnancy. Blood is taken from a vein and the serum is tested.

When performed: The HPL test is used whenever there is suspicion of trouble during pregnancy, especially if the patient has a sudden onset of vaginal bleeding. It has been suggested that the test be routinely performed during all pregnancies as a means of detecting potential miscarriage.

Normal values: No HPL is usually found until after the fifth week of pregnancy. At that time about 0.5 mcg per ml can be detected. The level then rises to between 7 and 10 mcg per ml just before delivery.

Abnormal values: Slightly increased values may be found with a large placenta (multiple births), but the test is not a positive indicator. A sudden decrease in HPL during pregnancy is considered a warning sign that a miscarriage is about to occur, usually because the fetus either is abnormal or is having some difficulty (such as insufficient oxygen or separation of the placenta from the uterus). Certain rare tumors may cause an increased amount of HPL in the blood.

Risk factors: Negligible (see general risk factors for blood testing).

Pain/Discomfort: Minimal (see general pain/discomfort factors for blood testing).

Accuracy and significance: Although the test may have to be performed several days in succession, it is a particularly significant guide for an obstetrician managing a high-risk pregnancy. Many obstetricians consider it an accurate forecast of complications in the placenta and an abnormal pregnancy.

PLATELET COUNT

Platelets, or thrombocytes, are minuscule bodies (less than half the size of red blood cells) that are essential to the blood-clotting process. They are manufactured in bone marrow at the rate of about 100,000 each day. When bleeding occurs, platelets group or clump together (aggregate), swell up, stick to the injured area, and attempt to act as plugs to stop the bleeding. The normal life span of platelets is about eight days. Only one drop of blood is necessary for examination and may be taken from the fingertip, heel, or earlobe or from a tube of blood drawn for other tests. Platelets are usually counted manually under the microscope; electronic counting is also performed. Platelets are also examined for size (young, larger platelets are more effective for clotting).

Note: The newly developed platelet aggregation test (Aggregometer) helps distinguish between inherited (hemophilia, Von Willebrand's disease) and acquired bleeding problems. Drugs such as aspirin and aspirin-like products used for arthritis and generalized pain can keep platelets from aggregating and thus cause bleeding. This new test is also used as an indication of susceptibility to stroke in older people.

When performed: When there are obvious bleeding tendencies; before surgical procedures or tooth extractions; with fractures; to check liver function; when polycythemia or certain kinds of anemia are suspected; when leukemia is being treated.

Normal values: There should be between 150,000 and 500,000 platelets per cu mm (lower for children). Normal values vary with different laboratory methods.

Abnormal values: Platelets are usually increased (more than 500,000 per cu mm) in rheumatoid arthritis, most cancers, trauma (hemorrhage), polycythemia, and some anemias (iron deficiency). They are decreased in bleeding tendencies (usually less than 20,000 per cu mm before bleeding occurs), purpura (a condition in which even the slightest bruise causes a black-and-blue mark from bleeding under the skin), some anemias, certain leukemias, and infectious mononucleosis.

Risk factors: Negligible (see general risk factors for blood testing).

Pain/discomfort: Minimal (see general pain/discomfort factors for blood testing).

Accuracy and significance: Platelet counts are quite accurate and very significant in reaching a diagnosis of bleeding tendencies. They are especially important when following patients receiving chemical treatment for leukemia which tends to destroy body platelets.

PLETHYSMOGRAPHY

Venous thrombosis (a clot attached to the wall of a vein), usually in a deep vein of the leg (and far more common in the left leg than in the right, for reasons as yet unknown), is becoming a common illness. Deep-vein thrombosis (and its potential consequence, pulmonary embolism or lung clot) frequently follows surgical procedures when patients must lie quietly for long periods after the operation. Phlebography (see **Radiography**) is the best way to diagnose deep-vein thrombosis (thrombophlebitis); however, when X-ray is difficult or when it is impossible to locate a vein in the foot for injection of a radio-opaque dye (because of excessive swelling, low pain threshold, etc.) venous impedence plethysmography is used. This is a noninvasive technique (the skin is not broken with injections) and is a safe, fairly reliable way to test for thrombosis.

In venous impedence plethysmography, a standard blood pressure cuff with measuring wires is connected to an impedence analyzer, which records the blood flow through the vein around the area of the leg where the clot is suspected. The blood pressure cuff is inflated to create pressure around the upper leg and thus slow or stop the flow of blood in the veins below the cuff. The pressure is released suddenly and the rate of venous blood flow is recorded. The test can be performed at home, in a doctor's office, or at the bedside of a hospitalized patient.

Ocular plethysmography is a test to detect and evaluate blood flow through the carotid arteries to the brain. With the patient sitting in a chair, special eye cups are placed over the eyes while the pulsations behind the eyes are recorded. The eyes are tested simultaneously to determine if one carotid artery pulse is slower than the other, which indicates blockage.

Penile plethysmography, using similar equipment, is used to differentiate psychological from physical **Impotence.**

When performed: Whenever there is swelling of the leg (usually but not always painful) that cannot be specifically diagnosed; prior to and following extensive surgical procedures, especially when the patient has been forced to lie on the operating table for a long period of time; whenever patients are bed-ridden for more than several days at a time; as a screening test for the prevention of thrombosis and pulmonary embolism and occasionally to follow the progress of the treatment of a clot; in cases of impotence.

Normal values: After the pressure in the blood pressure cuff is applied, the impedence analyzer should show a slow steady rise as the lower veins fill up but are unable to empty; as soon as the pressure is released, a sudden surge of blood into all the leg veins should be recorded.

Abnormal values: When a thrombus (clot) is present a vein will show very slow filling, and when the pressure above the vein is released the sudden surge of blood will not be recorded. Abnormal values for other uses of plethysmography depend on the physician's experience and interpretation.

Risk factors: None.

Pain/discomfort: There may be some embarrassment when penile plethysmography is performed. When ocular plethysmography is performed a few patients find the eye cups uncomfortable but not painful.

Accuracy and significance: Plethysmography is a relatively new test procedure and its overall accuracy has not been definitively established. While a number of doctors believe venous impedence plethysmography is probably the most significant way to identify thrombosis, other doctors will not accept a diagnosis of a leg vein clot unless it can be seen on an X-ray. Today, penile plethysmography is being replaced by the penile tumescence monitor. Ocular plethysmography is a significant non-invasive way to measure blood flow to the brain without risk to the patient. If contact lenses are left in place while ocular plethysmography is performed, inaccurate values can result.

PORPHYRINS

Porphyrins are pigments that come from red blood cells and from the liver; when present in the urine they indicate disease (porphyria). Erythropoietic (red blood cell) porphyria is a rare, inherited condition characterized by the excretion of red-tinted urine shortly after birth. Hepatic (liver) porphyria may be inherited or acquired after birth as a consequence of drug use, alcoholism, or exposure to certain chemicals such as lead and fungicides. Virtually all people who have excessive porphyrins in their system are hypersensitive to sunlight. Exposure to sun results in edema, blisters, and other skin lesions, mostly ulcers and scarring. Other symptoms that occur with porphyria include generalized body pains (most commonly in the stomach), confusion, and convulsions. During an acute attack, a patient may have high blood pressure, an extremely rapid pulse, and fever.

The porphyrin test measures a number of different types of porphyrins (such as coproporphyrins, protoporphyrins, and uroporphyrins); it is usually not necessary to distinguish the type of porphyrin to establish a diagnosis. Two specific products that immediately precede the formation of porphyrins are porphobilinogen and delta aminolevulinic acid, called ALA (see **Lead**). Determination of these specific products helps pinpoint the diagnosis by showing whether the porphyria is erythropoietic or hepatic, inherited or acquired. A 24-hour sample of urine is the most common test. Porphyrins may also be measured in the feces, in the blood serum taken from a vein, and in red blood cells alone.

When performed: Primarily when a patient complains of reddish or reddish purple urine; when there is photosensitivity, hyperpigmentation, ulceration of the skin, excessive hair growth, undiagnosable stomach pains, unexplained convulsions, and other nervous disease manifestations that cannot be otherwise diagnosed; as an indication of a possible acute attack of porphyria and as a measure of progress while treating the disease; as an aid in testing for lead poisoning.

Normal values: Normally there are no porphyrins in the urine and no more than 1,000 mcg in a 24-hour feces specimen. There may be up to 100 mcg per 100 ml in red blood cells and up to 60 mcg per 100 ml of blood serum.

Abnormal values: Porphyrins are increased in the urine in porphyria, liver disease, certain cancers, and lead poisoning. They may also be increased with alcoholism, the use of estrogens (including birth control pills), psychic trauma, menstruation, and pregnancy. Eating beets or blackberries or taking certain laxatives containing phenolsulfonphthalein (Ex-Lax), danthron, or cascara may give a false porphyrin-like color to the urine, as will certain azo-dye urinary anesthetics (Pyridium) and rifampin, an antibiotic. Patients who are malingering have been known to add ketchup or tomato juice to their urine in order to simulate illness.

Risk factors: Negligible (see general risk factors for blood testing).

Pain/discomfort: Minimal (see general pain/discomfort factors for blood testing).

Accuracy and significance: Porphyrin measurements are quite accurate and are very significant in helping to diagnose and differentiate between the various types of porphyrias. They are of significant aid in determining why some patients cannot tolerate sunlight, whether hyperpigmentation of the skin is present, and to women who have excessive hair on the face, the cause of which has not been diagnosed.

POTASSIUM

Potassium is a blood electrolyte (see **Sodium**) that is essential to maintaining the proper balance of fluids within body cells. (Sodium acts in the same manner but is responsible for the water *surrounding* the body cells.) Potassium is particularly important to help carry out enzyme reactions throughout the body and to regulate heart muscle action. The typical daily diet contains about 3 g of potassium (less than half as much as sodium), but the body excretes almost all of it. Foods richest in potassium include dates, apricots, bananas, oranges, and tomatoes. Most problems come from too little potassium in the body, a condition caused more by reactions to drugs than by disease or lack of the mineral in the diet. Very little potassium is lost in sweat (which contains large amounts of sodium).

Blood is taken from a vein and the serum is examined. In this test particularly, but also in many others, the common practice of asking the patient to clench and open the fist (to help find a vein in the arm) or leaving the tourniquet on too long can cause great errors in measurement. Potassium is also measured in the urine, the spinal fluid, sweat, and saliva.

The most accurate measurement of potassium is total body potassium. The patient lies inside a steel walled room; a nuclear counter is passed over the entire body for 30 minutes and detects the amount of radioactive potassium present (see **Nuclear Scanning**).

Once serum or total body potassium has been determined, a physician can reasonably estimate potassium changes by alterations in the **Electrocardiogram**.

When performed: When there are symptoms of muscle weakness, lethargy, heart rhythm abnormalities, or hormone problems; when patients are taking diuretic drugs; to help determine the source of acidosis, which can cause coma.

Normal values: Potassium levels should range from 4 to 5.5 mEq per liter in serum and 25 to 100 mEq per liter in a 24-hour urine sample.

Abnormal values: Elevated amounts of potassium (hyperkalemia) are found with kidney failure, liver disease, and adrenal cortical hormone deficiency. A large amount of potassium in the blood, usually secondary to kidney failure, can cause the heart to stop beating. Urine levels are most often the opposite of serum levels (high blood potassium with low urine amounts). A few exceptions, however, exist with malabsorption (the potassium is not taken into the bloodstream through the intestines) and with diarrhea.

Serum potassium levels may be decreased in diabetes, vomiting, and diarrhea; from taking laxatives, diuretic drugs, and certain forms of penicillin; with heart rhythm irregularities; and when there is a body magnesium deficiency.

Salivary changes in potassium occur with adrenal disease, and sweat changes occur with certain inherited conditions.

Risk factors: Negligible (see general risk factors for blood testing).

Pain/discomfort: Minimal (see general pain/discomfort factors for blood testing).

Accuracy and significance: The test is reasonably accurate but it is important that the collection of blood for testing be precise. Should a quantity of red or white blood cells and platelets be present and break down during the collection process, abnormally false elevations will result. The test is significant as a confirmation of a doctor's suspicions rather than as a tool to reach a specific diagnosis.

PREGNANCY

Although pregnancy is not really a disease, the bodily changes caused by pregnancy are sufficiently complex to be considered a deviation from normal. After fertilization occurs and the fertilized ovum is implanted in the uterus, the newly formed tissue material that attaches the fertilized egg to the uterus produces a hormone substance called human chorionic gonadotropin (HCG). Most pregnancy tests ascertain the presence of HCG in the serum or urine. Formerly, the blood or urine from the patient with suspected pregnancy was injected into a rabbit (A-Z test). If the rabbit's ovaries showed signs of pregnancy, the test was considered positive. The rabbit test is rarely used today; rats, which are easier to obtain than rabbits, have been substituted should this particular version of the test be requested (Friedman).

The newer tests for pregnancy depend on **Agglutination.** Either HCG-sensitized red cells or latex particles (which are treated to act like red blood cells) are added to a patient's serum or urine in a test tube. The pregnant patient has antibodies to chorionic gonadotropin that will react (agglutinate) by clumping together and settling at the bottom of the test tube. The same test may be performed on a slide. When a drop of urine is placed on the slide with sensitizing chemicals, agglutinizing can be seen if pregnancy exists. A slide test takes only two to three minutes and is accurate 96% of the time. These tests are called DAP, Neocept, Pregnosticon Dri-Dot (or Slide), UCG, and Pregnate, to name a few. Do-it-yourself early pregnancy tests (EPT) are usually tube tests that are very accurate when pregnancy is at least four weeks along but not very accurate when pregnancy is in its very early stage.

When performed: When there is suspicion, or fear, of pregnancy. Pregnancy tests should be routinely performed on all women of child-bearing age (at least from age 12 to age 50) when hospitalized, prior to any X-ray test or treatment or before embarking on any course of drug therapy.

Normal values: A positive test in the presence of pregnancy is normal.

Abnormal values: False positive pregnancy tests may occur when certain hormones are temporarily increased (such as after the menopause); when red blood cells or excessive protein are found in the urine; when certain tranquilizing drugs such as barbiturates, Compazine, Phenergan, Stelazine or Thorazine are present. Even penicillin and methadone can cause false-positive results. In addition to urinary infections, hepatitis and some rare uterine and ovarian tumors can produce false-positive reactions. Menstrual irregularities can also cause abnormal values.

Lower-than-normal HCG levels can indicate an ectopic pregnancy (in which the fetus grows outside the uterus). A sudden drop in HCG levels has been interpreted as signalling the possibility of a spontaneous abortion.

Risk factors: Negligible (see general risk factors for blood testing).

Pain/discomfort: Minimal (see general pain/discomfort factors for blood testing).

Accuracy and significance: When properly performed, urine and blood tests for pregnancy are considered to be 92 to 98 percent accurate. Levels of HCG are detectable within three weeks after one's last menstrual period, or about a week after pregnancy begins. The more sensitive the test, the earlier pregnancy may be detected. When the test is negative, but the possibility of pregnancy is still suspected, the test must be repeated in seven days. When the amount of HCG is measured and followed, the test is considered to be 60 to 80 percent accurate in helping diagnose ectopic pregnancy and predicting spontaneous abortion.

PROLACTIN [HPRL, hPRL]

Prolactin (sometimes called lactogenic hormone) is a pituitary hormone that causes the breasts to enlarge and secrete milk. It must be present in order for a mother to nurse her child. In addition, prolactin has been reported to act as a **Growth Hormone** under certain conditions. Blood is taken from a vein and the serum or plasma is tested.

When performed: When a mother who has just given birth is unable to nurse; when certain brain tumors are suspected; when women have menstrual problems; during pregnancy when fetal difficulties are suspected.

Normal values: Prolactin levels range from 5 to 25 ng per ml in both men and women but are normally increased in women during pregnancy and while nursing.

Abnormal values: Increased prolactin is found in both men and women during stressful (anxiety-producing) situations; when brain tumors involve the hypothalamus portion of the brain; in certain pituitary tumors (although if the pituitary is destroyed, prolactin levels may be reduced); and in women taking certain drugs—especially those for high blood pressure and some tranquilizers—that may, in turn, cause the breasts to secrete milk without any relation to pregnancy. Prolactin is usually absent when a mother of a newborn is unable to nurse her child.

Risk factors: Negligible (see general risk factors for blood testing).

Pain/discomfort: Minimal (see general pain/discomfort factors for blood testing).

Accuracy and significance: Basically, the test's only significance is in helping to determine the reason a mother is unable to nurse her child following pregnancy. However, it is also used to help evaluate a high-risk pregnancy, and it is considered approximately 65 percent accurate in predicting fetal problems. Unfortunately, this predictive value is accompanied by a high false-positive rate. The test helps to diagnose brain tumors in the pituitary-hypothalamic areas of the brain, lung tumors, other hormone disorders, and kidney problems. When evaluating prolactin levels, the doctor must consider the patient's use of tranquilizers, antidepressants, some high blood pressure drugs, and procainamide, all of which tend to lower prolactin values.

PROTHROMBIN TIME [Quick Test]

Prothrombin (Factor II) is one of the 12 known factors necessary to stop bleeding (normal body coagulants). Like four other clotting factors, it is manufactured in the liver from vitamin K, which is obtained in the diet primarily from green leafy vegetables, fish, and liver. It is important to know a patient's diet when testing for prothrombin time, since an excess of such foods will alter the test. Coumarin anticoagulant drugs such as warfarin (Coumadin) and dicumarol are often prescribed to prevent thrombophlebitis subsequent to surgery or after an injury. Anticoagulants have, on occasion, also been prescribed after heart attacks and to prevent eye problems in diabetes. They interfere with the liver's ability to make clotting factors.

Although the prothrombin time test indicates the level of prothrombin in the blood, it is more a measure of the overall blood coagulation response to the taking of coumarin anticoagulant drugs. When anticoagulants are given, it may take from three to seven days before the prothrombin time test reflects the drug activity. It is important to know what drugs a patient is taking in addition to anticoagulants before evaluating the prothrombin time. Blood is taken from a vein and the plasma is tested. The test must be performed within an hour after the sample is taken for accurate results, unless the blood sample is immediately frozen.

When performed: Primarily as an indication of the activity of certain anticoagulant drugs (but not heparin); as an indication of how the liver is functioning; as a measure of a patient's dietary intake of vitamin K.

Normal values: Normally it takes 12 to 14 seconds for a fibrin strand (first sign of clotting) to be seen. The test is always run with control plasma that is known to be normal. The result is sometimes reported as the number of seconds it takes a patient's blood to clot compared with the control; more often it is reported as a percentage of the control's plasma prothrombin time compared to patient's prothrombin time, called percentage concentration or percentage of patient's prothrombin activity.

Abnormal values: Any amount of time greater than the control is considered an abnormal value; the longer the patient's prothrombin time in seconds, the lower the percentage of prothrombin activity. When anticoagulants are prescribed, an abnormal value is indicative of the effectiveness of the drug. Ideally, a patient taking a coumarin product should have a prothrombin time two to two and a half times longer than the control, or show between 12% and 20% prothrombin activity.

The prothrombin time is affected when anticoagulants are taken with other drugs. Barbiturates, oral contraceptives, mineral oil, and antacids will shorten the prothrombin time, while aspirin, thyroid hormone, insulin, and oral antidiabetic drugs will lengthen it. It is also prolonged with liver disease; when used for this condition, the test is usually repeated after the patient is given a large amount of vitamin K. Eating large quantities of food containing vitamin K (salads, fish) will shorten the prothrombin time and require additional anticoagulant drug for effectiveness. Eating commercial French-fried potatoes made with methylpolysiloxane for crispness (the chemical is listed on the label if bought packaged for home use; it is impossible to know about this when dining out) will cause an abnormally decreased prothrombin time for at least a week afterward and could cause a patient to take a dangerous overdose of an anticoagulant drug.

Risk factors: Negligible (see general risk factors for blood testing).

Pain/discomfort: Minimal (see general pain/discomfort factors for blood testing).

Accuracy and significance: The test is sufficiently accurate for monitoring the blood level of a patient taking warfarin-type drugs. The more frequently the test is performed, the less the chance of bleeding or clotting problems.

PULMONARY FUNCTION

Measurements of how well the lungs take in the air, how much they can hold, how well they utilize air, and how well they can expel it are important in diagnosing the many different kinds of breathing problems. (The amount of **Oxygen** and **Carbon Dioxide** in the blood are also important measures of the lung's effectiveness.) There are two main types of lung disease. The first type can be caused by loss of lung tissue, inability of the lungs to expand properly, or inability to transfer oxygen to the blood. The second type results from obstruction or narrowing of the main passageways of air (the trachea and bronchial tubes) in the lung.

Most lung function tests are performed by having the patient breathe into a spirometer, an instrument that records the amount of air put through it and the rate of air passage for a specified time. The various tests for pulmonary function are listed and explained below.

Vital capacity (VC), sometimes called forced vital capacity, is probably the most common test of lung volume. It measures how much air the patient can forcefully exhale after inhaling as much air as possible. Usually the body's surface area is calculated and the number is multiplied by 2.5 to obtain the number of liters (a liter approximates a quart) of air that a patient should be able to expel at one time. An average-size 150-pound man should be able to take in and breathe out about 5 liters (5,000 ml) with one forced breath; any amount from 4,000 ml to 6,000 ml is considered within normal limits for men of that size.

Forced expiratory volume (FEV), sometimes called timed vital capacity, is the same as vital capacity with the addition of a time element: the patient is asked to take as deep a breath as possible and then force out the air as hard and as quickly as possible. The amount of air exhaled during the first second of time (FEV_1) is measured. Sometimes measurements of exhalation last for two or three seconds (FEV_2, FEV_3). Normally a person will exhale at least 80% of his vital capacity in the first second and 95% by the third second.

Maximal voluntary ventilation (MVV), sometimes called maximum breathing capacity (MBC), measures the greatest amount of air a person can breathe each minute. The patient is asked to breathe as rapidly and deeply as possible for 15 seconds. The total amount of air exhaled is then multiplied by four, giving the result in liters per minute. The normal amount, like that for the vital capacity, is determined by the individual's body surface area. Someone in good physical condition should have an MVV of almost 20 times the VC.

Several other measurements may be made of amounts of air the lungs hold. A few of these include the *residual volume* (the air that remains in the lung after the vital capacity is exhaled), the *tidal volume* (how much air is expired with each normal breath), and the *functional residual capacity* (the sum of the last bit of air that can be exhaled during the vital capacity test and the residual volume). These tests are performed by having the patient inhale known amounts of certain gases such as nitrogen and helium and noting which of those gases are absorbed and which are exhaled; they can also be performed with the plethysmograph (a special machine that measures changes in the body's overall volume during breathing; the patient sits in an enclosed controlled-air chamber that resembles a diving bell).

Pulmonary compliance measures how well the lungs can be stretched or distended and then how well they recoil after a full breath; normal is determined by body surface area.

Diffusing capacity shows how well the lungs can transfer oxygen to the blood and eliminate carbon dioxide from the blood at the end points of air passage in the lung (tiny sacs called alveoli). A small amount of carbon monoxide is inhaled and the amount the blood absorbs is measured; normally it should absorb all of it.

Maximum expiratory flow rate (the rate during the middle half of forced vital capacity) and *maximum midexpiratory flow* (the average flow during the middle half of the total expired volume) are two additional measurements used to confirm the results obtained by other tests.

Bronchial inhalation challenge, sometimes called methacholine inhalational challenge because the drug methacholine is commonly used, helps differentiate between asthma and other lung conditions which appear similar. After vital capacity measurements are established, the patient inhales methacholine, or some histamine preparation, and vital capacity volumes are again observed. When the patient has asthma rather than a problem of deliberate hyperventilation or a non-allergic disease that affects normal breathing, the drug causes bronchial constriction and a reduction of vital capacity. Patients who wheeze but otherwise have normal pulmonary function measurements are usually given this test. It also helps to diagnose breathing difficulties that can come from heart failure rather than lung disease, a chronic cough produced by a sinus infection rather than lung irritation, and difficulty in breathing that can come from chest tumors rather than allergies.

When performed: Whenever there are breathing difficulties such as wheezing, persistent coughing, shortness of breath, repeated episodes of fainting or coma, or difficulties due to exposure to environmental contaminants such as coal dust, asbestos, moldy hay, moldy sugar cane, or compost; when a patient has been working with birds or poultry; following use of certain drugs (especially heroin, methadone, and some antibiotics); with heart failure, chest injuries, and certain nervous system diseases; when there is suspicion of a growth in the lungs; when anxiety causes breathing difficulties; to measure progress in treating lung diseases; to determine when a patient can breathe on his own after being in a mechanical respirator.

Normal values: Most normal values for breathing tests must take into account the age, height and weight (body surface area) and sex of the individual (obviously, the smaller the person, the smaller the lung capacity). After the normal or expected values for a person's size are determined, the measurements are obtained and compared against the standard. A deviation of up to 20% from expected values is considered within normal limits.

Abnormal values: In almost all of the pulmonary function tests, results showing a person's breathing or lung capacity to be less than 80% of the expected value (as determined by the person's body surface area) are considered a sign of disease. In general, the tests, when used together, help diagnose restrictive types of lung disease from obstructive types. If the tests show abnormal results, the normal procedure is to administer a bronchodilator drug such as isoetharine (usually by inhalation) and then repeat the measurements; if the drug produces bronchodilatation and causes marked improvement, the lung disease is usually considered reversible. For example, with asthma the vital capacity will increase after a bronchodilator drug; with emphysema there will be no improvement. The vital capacity measurement is reduced with nerve diseases that affect respiratory muscles (Guillain-Barré disease, myasthenia gravis), edema of the lungs, and conditions that take up space in the lung area such as tumors.

The other lung function tests will give less than predicted results depending on the specific cause of the disease and the extent of the disease process. In chronic bronchitis (an obstructive type of disease) the vital capacity and the FEV_1 are reduced. In sarcoidosis (where the lung alveoli, which transfer oxygen to the bloodstream, are thickened), the FEV_1 is usually normal because there is no obstruction to the bronchial tubes. The lungs will not recoil normally with emphysema.

Sudden changes in forced expiratory volume measurements may be one of the earliest indications of heart disease.

Risk factors: If an undiagnosed pulmonary disease exists such as weakness in the lung's air sacs, there is a slight risk of collapsing the lung during the performance of the test.

Pain/discomfort: Wearing a nose-closing piece and having to breathe through a special tight-fitting mouthpiece can be quite uncomfortable, especially for prolonged periods of time. Sitting in the sealed, controlled-air chamber causes anxiety in a number of patients.

Accuracy and significance: Pulmonary function studies, when performed in their entirety, are considered 90 percent accurate in helping to diagnose the specific cause of lung disease. The tests are particularly significant in that there are very few false positive results.

PULSE ANALYSIS

The word "pulse" refers to the sudden expansion of the walls of a blood vessel, usually a medium-to-large-sized artery, as blood is forced through the artery by each heartbeat. Most people are familiar with "taking the pulse" when the doctor feels for the artery on the inside of the wrist (see **Blood Pressure**). But there are other pulse test measurements that can be made, depending on the blood vessel's location in the body. The pulse of the carotid artery is tested by placing two fingers on either side of the neck, a bit toward the front, and noting the artery's force or pulsations. At times, a stethoscope is used to listen to the sound of the surging blood, and it is not unusual to place a sensitive recording instrument over the carotid area to visualize graphically the carotid pulse—which, in fact, also reflects the action of the heart valves between the heart's left ventricle and the aorta (the body's largest artery). Occasionally, the pulse of the carotid vein, which is adjacent and parallel to the carotid artery, is measured to test the efficacy of the heart's right side (there are no heart valves between the vena cava, the body's largest vein, and the right atrium, the heart's upper right chamber, which first receives venous blood). The right side of the heart directs blood into the lungs.

The brachial pulse is felt for just above or below the collarbone; the femoral pulse is located on either side of the groin; the popliteal pulse is located behind the knees; there are also pulses along the ankle and on the back of the foot that are routinely tested during a physical examination. When pulsations are felt over veins, other than the carotid, they usually signify an arteriovenous fistula, a direct opening between an artery and its adjacent vein. Such abnormalities cause the heart to work harder than it should, and the result can be heart failure.

The pulses on both sides of the body are tested and they should be of equal force; the same pulses are tested while taking deep breaths.

When performed: To help confirm heart and heart valve disease; to detect circulation blockages often caused by another organ compressing the artery (and usually the adjacent nerve as well); to help diagnose an aneurysm (a ballooning out of a major artery frequently as a consequence of a weakened arterial wall); to help evaluate decreased circulation to the body, especially to the brain; to help diagnose a coarctation (a constriction of severe narrowing and almost always of the aorta); to help distinguish among a variety of lung conditions such as asthma and emphysema; to help confirm the diagnosis of pericardial disease (the pericardium is the sac around the heart; it can become filled with fluid or tighten from an infection and impair heart function).

Normal values: The pulse should be firm and forceful and equal on both sides of the body; it is normal for the pulse rate to increase slightly when a breath is inhaled and to decrease as air is exhaled.

Abnormal values: The most common abnormality is a diminished pulse beat, usually on one side of the body but at times on both sides. This almost always indicates decreased circulation which can mean an inadequate supply of oxygen and nutrients in reaching the body tissues. The causes can be atherosclerosis, blood vessel defects, injuries, or congenital malformations. Pulsus paradoxus is an abnormality in which the pulse can disappear when a deep breath is inhaled; it usually signals an obstructive lung problem.

Risk factors: None.

Pain/discomfort: None.

Accuracy and significance: In many instances, the measurement of pulsations is subjective and depends primarily on a doctor's training and experience. Graphic records, on the other hand, can provide significant characteristic patterns that quite accurately indicate disease. Most often, pulse analysis is a supportive test used in conjunction with more definitive tests for heart and blood vessel pathology.

(**Note**: Pulse analysis is not the same as the "pulse test," once proposed as a detect-it-yourself allergy test. In the "pulse test," it was purported that the pulse would increase to a specific rate when an offending substance was eaten or inhaled.)

PUPILLARY REFLEX

The pupils of the eye (the openings in the center surrounded by the colored iris) open and close (widen and narrow) when exposed to different amounts of light and when focusing on near or far objects. The smaller the opening, the more clearly objects can be seen at different distances (in photography this is called "depth of field"). To test pupillary reflexes, first, a strong light is directed into the eye to note the pupil's reaction; second, the patient is asked to look at objects both close up and far away and the pupil is observed.

When performed: Whenever brain, nerve, or eye disease is suspected; whenever certain drug abuse or overdose is suspected.

Normal values: Normally, when a bright light is directed toward the eye (or when a person is in bright sunlight), the pupils contract and become very small (miosis). As the amount of light diminishes, the pupils widen. When a person looks at an object close up, the pupils usually contract (accommodation). If light is directed to one eye only, normally the pupil of the other eye also becomes smaller, even if it is blocked off from the light source. As people become older, pupil size normally becomes smaller. Both pupils should be round and of the same size.

Abnormal values: In patients with Argyll-Robertson pupil, light will not diminish pupil size, but looking at a close object will.

The condition is most often a result of syphilis. In patients who are blind in one eye, the pupil may still respond to light in the other eye, but not to direct light. When the pupil does not react at all, it is usually indicative of nerve-brain disease. Various drugs can cause either sustained dilatation or contraction of the pupil. Narcotic drugs usually cause fixed "pinpoint" pupils.

Risk factors: None.

Pain/discomfort: None.

Accuracy and significance: The test is highly accurate and significant because the measurements are totally objective. Observation of pupil abnormalities, however, cannot necessarily distinguish the particular cause of an abnormal pupillary reflex, nor can it differentiate between the various drugs that cause pupillary changes.

R

RADIOGRAPHY

Radiography, or the use of X-rays, is an intergral part of many different testing procedures. A chest X-ray for a cough, for instance, is no different from a specific screening blood test for anemia or infection; it may not always reveal a specific disease, but it offers clues toward a diagnosis. Much depends on the type of X-ray. There are X-rays of specific parts of the body or specific organs taken from different angles. There are X-rays using a contrast dye (usually an iodine solution) that cannot be penetrated and that causes great contrast on the X-ray film, silhouetting or imaging whatever tissue the dye fills; the dye reveals organs that normally would not be seen by X-ray alone. The dye may also be used to show concentration in an organ or to follow how efficiently and rapidly an organ eliminates that dye (excretion test).

An X-ray of a bone will show if that bone is broken (or has a slight crack) and thus is essentially a test for fracture. The chest X-ray will show any pathology in the lung as well as the size, shape, and position of the heart and, like the standard electrocardiogram, will help diagnose suspected heart problems; in this sense it is a "test" for coronary disease. A fluoroscopic examination will show heart movement (using X-rays) and, with the use of contrast dye, will delineate just what happens when a person swallows; the contrast dye outlines the stomach, the intestines, and the large bowel. The gall bladder, joint cavities, the spinal canal, the uterus and tubes, the lungs, and even arteries and veins are also outlined by contrast dye.

Angiography is the particular study of the arterial blood vessels by X-rays and contrast media. In cerebral angiography, the dye is injected into the neck arteries and X-ray pictures are taken of the circulation of the brain. (The dye fills and outlines arteries that normally cannot be visualized by X-ray.) Coronary angiography is similar, except that the dye is injected into the coronary arteries (those that feed heart muscle) via a catheter (thin tube) from the arm or neck through the heart into the aorta; the dye is specifically placed to fill the tiny arteries that supply the heart, the plugging of which seems to cause most heart attacks. Angiography is also performed on the pulmonary arteries leading to the lungs.

Because angiography involves the positioning of cardiac catheters through X-rays, other heart observations can be made without dye, or after the dye is administered. Various pressure measurements are recorded from inside the heart's chambers, and in the large arteries leaving the heart (the pulmonary artery which leads to the lungs and the aorta which leads to the rest of the body). The amount of oxygen in the blood can also be recorded. Then, too, intraatrial pacing studies can be done. For these studies, a special sensory electrode placed inside the heart's atrial or upper chamber records the origin, direction, and time of the nerve impulse that establishes the pace of the heartbeat. At times the electrocardiogram is recorded from inside the heart rather than from outside it.

Digital subtraction angiography (DSA) is a form of angiography that does not use catheters and, hence, avoids their risks. A computer is employed in this technique to enhance the X-ray images on a TV screen. This test is easily performed, and does not require hospitalization. Furthermore, it offers excellent results when surveying the body's major arteries—especially those in the abdomen, extremities, and heart chambers.

Electrokymography, also called radarkymography, is a means of observing the heart in action. The image of the moving heart is shown on a fluoroscope, permitting observation of the heart's borders, measurement of the size of the heart's contraction, and evaluation of the elasticity of those arteries leading to the lungs and of the aorta, which carries blood to the rest of the body. At times the beating heart is photographed in motion for a permanent record. This form of radiography is particularly valuable when a heart wall aneurysm (a weakened area of the muscle wall that balloons out) is suspected.

Venography is similar to angiography except that the dye is injected into a vein instead of an artery. This test is especially valuable for detecting thrombophlebitis (a clot blocking the passage of blood in a vein, usually—but not always—existing along with an infectious process). There are many newer tests to detect thrombosis (using sound waves or air pressure measurements); however, phlebography (X-rays of dye in the vein) is still considered the most accurate for blood clots in veins. Normally no clot or blockage is seen in veins.

Pyelography (intravenous pyelography, or IVP) is the study of the kidney, ureters, and bladder by X-rays and contrast media. When the contrast dye is injected into the bloodstream (usually through an arm vein), it will almost immediately concentrate in the kidneys and then pass down into the bladder. Normally the dye shows in the kidney within minutes and assumes an expected silhouette. If cysts, tumors, or other diseases are present, the dye will take longer to appear and abnormal filling defects will be seen. In special circumstances, the dye is injected directly into the kidney arteries (usually by catheters inserted into leg arteries and pushed up to kidney level) to determine if both kidney arteries are of normal size and shape and are not narrowed or blocked. This is called a renal arteriography test and is particularly useful in cases of undiagnosed high blood pressure.

The same test can be performed by inserting a contrast dye through a cystoscope into the urethra and then via tiny tubes into the ureters and watching the dye fill up in the kidneys; it is called retrograde pyelography. This form of the test is usually used when there is some doubt about kidney function and when the cause of the problem is thought to be below the kidneys.

Oral cholecystography, using X-rays and contrast media, will detect gallstones (a plain X-ray of the liver and gallbladder area usually will not). The patient follows his usual diet for several days prior to the test; at dinner the night before and breakfast just prior to the test no fat is ingested. The patient takes special dye tablets the night before. If the bile ducts and gallbladder are normal, the X-ray (taken the next morning) will show the gallbladder filled with the dye. The patient is then given a fatty meal to eat; X-rays are taken every 15 minutes afterward to determine if emptying of the gallbladder is normal. If stones are present, they usually are seen in contrast to the dye. If the gallbladder does not fill up with the dye the next morning, the test is usually repeated with a double dose of the dye tablets before the results are considered abnormal. An abnormal test can mean gallstones, but it can also mean a sluggish or infected gallbladder or liver disease.

Cholangiography, sometimes called intravenous cholangiography (IVC), is another test of the functioning of the ducts that carry bile from the liver to the gallbladder and then to the intestine. It is usually employed when two oral cholecystography tests fail to show the gallbladder, or after a patient has had gallbladder surgery and still has symptoms. The dye is injected into an arm vein; X-ray pictures are taken every 15 minutes (usually for an hour) until the bile ducts and the gallbladder can be visualized. It is especially valuable when a gallstone is suspected in a bile duct rather than in the gallbladder. Occasionally this test too must be performed a second time in order to find the gallstone or to ascertain that the gallbladder is not functioning.

Transhepatic cholangiography may be performed when it is impossible to tell whether jaundice is caused by bile stones or by liver damage. A needle is inserted into the liver and after a bile duct is located, dye is injected directly into the duct. If the liver is not outlined by the dye, bile stone blockage is indicated and surgery is usually performed immediately to remove the obstruction.

A *gastrointestinal (GI) series,* or contrast radiography of the gastrointestinal tract, can consist of many different tests. The patient may swallow a mouthful of barium (a compound that resists X-rays and shows up in marked contrast on the X-ray film). As the barium passes down the esophagus into the stomach, the size, shape, and activity of the esophagus can be observed through fluoroscopic examination. When sufficient barium is ingested to fill the stomach, it can be seen both by fluoroscopic examination and by X-ray pictures. Any filling "defect" (a place where the normal outline of barium should be seen but is not) is usually an indication of disease (ulcer, growth, or infection). When barium is in the stomach, it is common to tilt the patient so that his head is lower than his feet; the procedure helps to diagnose a hiatal hernia (a weakness of the lower end of the esophagus and the diaphragm around the esophagus), which can cause consistent heartburn. The barium is then followed into the upper (small) intestines where the physician searches for other defects. Sufficient barium is usually given to outline the entire small intestine.

To test for disease in the large intestine (the colon and rectum), barium is usually instilled by enema until the lower bowel is filled. Again, defects in places where barium should normally be seen can indicate disease. In contrast, visible pouches of barium can indicate polyps or diverticuli. After the barium is expelled, X-rays are again taken to see if any residual barium has been captured by the bowel; this can also indicate a disease process (at times additional air is introduced to exaggerate the contrast). If a complete gastrointestinal series is to be performed, the barium enema is given first. A barium enema can also help prevent unnecessary surgery for appendicitis by revealing the cause of abdominal pain.

Amniography utilizes X-rays to help outline the fetus within the mother's uterus. A contrast dye is injected into the amniotic sac which surrounds the developing infant; the resultant shadows can reveal an abnormal physical development such as a tumor or some organ growing outside the infant's body rather than inside. The fetus may swallow the dye and show an abnormality in its digestive tract. (See **Amniocentesis**.)

Arthrography refers to X-rays of the joints using a contrast media (dye) or air to outline the joint spaces. Arthrography may be performed on almost any joint. Most frequently the knee is examined, in order to diagnose meniscal injury. (Menisci are the small cartilage cushions in the knee joint that separate the bones of the upper and lower leg.) Fluoroscopy is used after the dye is injected to help locate the area to be studied; then X-ray films are taken.

In *myelography*, sometimes called a myelogram test, contrast dye is injected into the spinal canal (using the **Cerebrospinal Fluid** test technique), in order to study the bones of the spinal column (almost always the lower, or lumbar, spinal column) and especially the spaces, or discs, between the bones. Usually the patient is placed on a special table so that his position can be changed to distribute the dye better and, of even greater importance, so that as much of the dye as possible can be withdrawn at the end of the test. If it is not possible to withdraw all the dye, the removal technique is repeated the following day.

In *bronchography* contrast media are dropped into the lungs through a catheter (tiny tube) inserted into the trachea in order to examine the bronchial tubes—their size (opening), location, and number. The technique, though not in frequent use, is still a fairly definitive test for bronchiectasis (abnormally dilated passages of the bronchial tubes).

Hysterosalpingography is a test to discover whether the fallopian tubes are open to allow passage of the egg or ovum from the ovary to the uterus. It is one of many fertility tests conducted when a couple is unable to have children (see **Rubin**). The tubes may be closed as a result of infection (appendicitis, gonorrhea) or other disease or abnormally located uterine tissue.

Pneumoencephalography (PEG) is a test to outline the cerebrospinal fluid spaces within the brain. Sterile air or a gas is injected into the spinal column (using the **Cerebrospinal Fluid** test technique) and rises up the brain area, replacing the fluid normally present and giving a clear outline of the spaces, called ventricles. Should defects be seen (such as a suspected tumor or loss of brain substance), the patient may be moved about to provide better visualization. At times a cisternal puncture is used instead of the usual cerebrospinal fluid tap in the lower spine, usually when the patient has a vertebral defect. With the cisternal puncture, the needle is inserted at the base of the skull just above the first vertebra. **Computerized Tomography** is being used as a less dangerous substitute for this particular test.

Lymphangiography is a test to determine the effectiveness of the lymph vessels and lymph glands (lymph is a transparent fatty fluid that goes from body tissues back into the bloodstream). When lymph vessels become obstructed or inoperative, edema (water retention) usually results; cancer tends to be spread via the lymph system. Dye is slowly injected into the lymph vessels to be studied, and the patient is X-rayed at that time and then again in 24 hours.

Mammography is the use of X-rays to visualize breast tissue (mammary glands), primarily to detect a growth and secondarily to distinguish, when possible, a malignant from a benign growth. The test is usually performed prior to any breast surgery and especially on women over the age of 30 who have a family history of breast cancer. Usually, the breast is X-rayed from the top and from the side. Xeromammography is a special X-ray technique that is said to provide greater detail with less X-ray exposure.

Many physicians feel the danger of too much X-ray makes this test unsatisfactory. While breast X-rays have some advocates, it is a fact that many "masses" detected through these processes are not always cancer and that one out of five "lumps" is not detected. Mammography is also used to detect early adult-onset diabetes; should calcification of the breast arteries be observed in the course of the procedure, diabetes diagnostic studies are warranted.

The newest form of radiography is the Dynamic Spatial Reconstructor (DSR) that utilizes a great many X-ray tubes in a half circle around the patient; each X-ray is detected by a television receiver opposite it. This device allows three-dimensional images of organs in motion, such as the heart beating or the lung breathing.

When performed: In general, radiography is performed to detect any disease process that cannot be diagnosed by other means. Specific indications are discussed in the descriptions of the procedures above.

Normal values: Each area of the body has a standard photographic pattern. Through training and experience the physician can determine whether the patterns seen on an X-ray (including minor variations for individual patients) are normal.

Abnormal values: The finding of suggested pathology or the absence of an X-ray shadow that should be visible is considered abnormal, as described in the various procedures.

Risk factors: With the ordinary X-ray picture there is always a slight risk. As more X-ray pictures are taken that risk increases due to the accumulation of radioactive damage. Any radiography test using a contrast dye can cause a reaction in a patient—from minor itching and a rash to a fatality (see general risk factors for contrast substance use). The patient must always be screened for any allergy to the dye to be used; patients with allergic diseases such as hay fever or asthma must be tested with extreme caution for an allergy to the dye. The dye used in intravenous pyelography has been known to lead to kidney failure; the odds of this occurring are highest in patients with diabetes. When contrast medium (the dye injected to enhance the X-ray image) is used it also appears to cause a ten-fold increase in radiation damage to the body's cells, especially to the cells' chromosomes. Manipulative procedures that are part of radiological examinations, such as the use of catheters, greatly increase the risks (see general risk factors for catheter and needle insertion). Whenever catheters are inserted and directed to particularly sensitive parts of the body (heart, brain, and other internal body organs), the risk increases in proportion to the distance the catheter must travel. Catheters in the heart and major arteries, and especially in the lungs, can cause fluctuations in heart rhythm. They have been known to cause cardiac arrest, in which the heart stops beating completely, and to damage the heart valves directly. It has been reported that some of the catheters used in angiography cause hemoptysis (spitting-up of blood). The more complicated the procedure, the longer it takes, and the greater the body area being X-rayed, the greater the risks associated with radiography.

With angiography and its related tests, much depends on the training and experience of the medical team performing the catheterization. Deaths resulting from the test reportedly range from one in every 100 tests to one in every 1,000 tests. The more times a patient has the test, the greater the risk seems to be. If angiography is performed in an institution doing fewer than 100 of the procedures a year, the risks are some eight times greater than they are when the test is performed in a hospital doing a minimum of 400 of the procedures a year.

As with many medical decisions, the risks in testing must be weighed against the benefits. Too much X-ray exposure, the possibility of sensitivity to dyes, and the use and manipulation of medical instruments such as catheters may well cause problems far worse than the suspected disease for which the patient is being tested. Whether the benefits of the testing outweigh the hazards is something that must be decided solely by the patient and/or his or her family after a full and frank discussion with the physician.

One indirect risk factor in radiography can come from the technicians who take the X-ray pictures. At the present time, only 11 states require X-ray technicians to be licensed or to demonstrate evidence of their knowledge and ability to operate the radiographic machines properly and safely. In California, even doctors may not take X-ray pictures until they show proof of their skills; only one out of six doctors in California is legally permitted to operate X-ray equipment. Although it is estimated that nearly 200,000 technicians perform X-ray services, fewer than half are known to have had any formal training or to hold proper credentials. The Food and Drug Administration states that "it's reasonable to assume incompetence by some technicians" is partly responsible for the 2,000 to 4,000 annual deaths from cancer attributable to the use of X-ray equipment.

Pain/discomfort: When the test involves only a simple X-ray picture, there is no pain or discomfort. When radiography requires multiple pictures over a period of time, the patient can experience some discomfort lying on a hard table. Some patients, too, find unusual positioning uncomfortable (when the search is for a hiatus hernia the patient must be almost upside down). Many patients find swallowing barium distasteful and not a few patients are embarrassed by the ordeal of a barium enema. (See general pain and discomfort factors for catheter and needle insertion.) When air is inserted through the uterus to test the patency of the fallopian tubes a number of women complain of abdominal pain for several hours after the test. The prolonged use of the catheter in angiography can make patients apprehensive and lead them to complain of discomfort, although the catheter itself rarely causes pain.

Accuracy and significance: It should be remembered that the results of almost all radiographic tests are in large measure subjective, and depend primarily on a doctor's interpretation of the shadows, or in some instances the absence of shadows, on the X-ray picture, fluoroscopic, or television screen. Despite the impressiveness of all the equipment and procedures used in radiography, it is not as accurate as most people imagine. Unless the pathology is obvious, it is all too easy for the radiologist to miss seeing a fracture, an ulcer, a gallstone, a kidney stone, or a cancerous growth. Many doctors believe **Ultrasound** is far more accurate than intravenous cholangiography in diagnosing gallbladder problems; cholangiography usually reveals specific gallbladder problems in fewer than one out of every five patients. Pyelography is not considered very accurate in evaluating urinary tract infections. Mammography has only a fair degree of accuracy. More than one out of 10 suspected cancer patients examined by the best trained mammographers did not have cancer, while one out of five known cancers was missed. Only one out of three existing breast cancers is detected by mammography alone. Although radiologists specializing in angiology working with heart surgeons might feel cardiac angiography is the best method of diagnosing heart disease, most non-surgical cardiologists are not too impressed with such diagnostic techniques; they feel there are many non-invasive, far less risky, diagnostic tests that are at least as good, if not better, than angiography.

One particular study seems to reflect the accuracy of X-ray diagnosis. When highly experienced radiologists were asked to review the chest X-rays of 143 patients known to have lung cancer, 78 of whose X-rays displayed clear-cut evidence of cancer, the doctors missed the obvious diagnosis in 27 cases. The conclusion was reached from this and other published studies that there is an error rate of 20 to 50 percent in the detection of cancers that are visible on X-rays. The chances of accuracy can be increased by having more than one radiologist "read" the X-rays.

RAST

Although skin tests (see **Skin Reaction**) are still the most common way to test for allergy, the newest technique for measuring a potential allergic reaction is called the RAST test (sometimes called radioimmunosorbent assay test or radioallergosorbent test). It begins as a generalized measurement of a patient's serum immunoglobulin E, or IgE (see **Immunoglobulin**), which will react to known allergy-causing substances (the many varieties of grasses, foods, animal danders, molds, house dust and house dust mites, insect stings, trees, weeds, and cosmetics). The test is a form of Coombs' test reaction (see **Agglutination**). If a patient's blood contains antibodies to certain allergy-provoking substances, these antibodies will combine with known nuclear-radiolabeled allergens and can be so detected.

A positive RAST test (one that shows a reaction) is really a qualitative measure of IgE in the body; the test not only detects the allergens but can also show how much of an allergen it takes to cause an allergic manifestation (asthma, hay fever, eczema). The RAST test is much less time-consuming (one day versus several months), less painful (one needleprick versus scores), and less dangerous (no chance of severe allergic reactions) for a patient than skin-scratch tests for allergy.

Blood is taken from a vein and the serum is examined. Usually the serum is tested against specific groups of known allergy-causing antigens (such as all the grasses and trees and various weeds, animals, and house dust mites). When a grouping shows a positive reaction, further tests are performed on individual items in that group if known antibodies are available (not all known antibodies have been processed into allergens for testing).

When performed: To help find the specific cause of an allergy; as a means of measuring progress in the treatment of allergies.

Normal values: A RAST negative reaction indicates that no allergenic antibodies are present.

Abnormal values: A RAST positive reaction, especially in the presence of high serum IgE levels, indicates the presence of allergenic antibodies. Sometimes a positive test is reported as from class I to class IV, the latter indicating a very large amount of antibodies. Because different laboratories may show different results (some will report a positive reaction where others report negative), it is usual to have RAST tests repeated by more than one laboratory.

Risk factors: Negligible (see general risk factors for blood testing).

Pain/discomfort: Minimal (see general pain/discomfort factors for blood testing).

Accuracy and significance: Many doctors consider the RAST test more accurate than traditional skin testing. In patients with true allergic disease the RAST test is approximately 80 percent accurate in detecting the allergic substance. It reaches its highest level of accuracy when used to uncover food allergies; its level of accuracy decreases when used for pollens and other environmental irritants.

RED BLOOD CELL

The red blood cells (erythrocytes) contain hemoglobin (about 60% of the body's iron), which is the essential carrier of oxygen in the blood. Besides carrying oxygen to all parts of the body, red blood cells pick up certain waste products (such as carbon dioxide) that are given off later by the lungs. In testing, the red blood cells are counted as well as stained to reveal the size, shape, and hemoglobin content. Sickle cells are seen directly this way, as are certain anemias (see **Blood Cell Differential**). Blood taken from a vein is most commonly used; a drop of blood, usually from the fingertip or earlobe, can also be collected. The blood is viewed through the microscope and counted manually or by automated machines.

When performed: When there is suspicion of one of the anemias or polycythemia (a disease where the bone marrow makes too many red blood cells); in certain parasitic diseases; to verify certain poisonings; to help determine blood loss after hemorrhage. Some states require the testing of newborn babies for sickle cell anemia; they are Arizona, Colorado, Georgia, Louisiana, New Mexico, North Carolina, and Wyoming unless there is parental objection.

Normal values: Normal levels for men range from 4 to 6 million red cells per cubic millimeter (cu mm) of blood. Women may have a slightly lower count, and newborn babies a higher count.

Abnormal values: Higher than normal values are usually found with polycythemia, dehydration, certain kidney diseases, and lung conditions where there is difficulty in breathing and the body needs more oxygen. Lower than normal values are usually found with anemias, severe infections, certain cancers, **Malaria**, lead poisoning, and after prolonged bleeding.

Risk factors: Negligible (see general risk factors for blood testing).

Pain/discomfort: Minimal (see general pain/discomfort factors for blood testing).

Accuracy and significance: Although blood cell counting is fairly accurate, there is recent evidence that when blood cells are counted by automatic machines the results can show false lower-than-normal amounts. It is important, therefore, to know whether or not a blood cell count was performed by an automatic machine.

RED BLOOD CELL INDICES (Red Blood Cell Profile)

New electronic equipment has made determination of the red blood cell (erythrocyte) indices a valuable aid not only in classifying anemia but in determining the basic cause of the anemia and in helping to decide the specific therapy. The three indices are (1) mean corpuscular volume (MCV), a ratio of the hematocrit to the red blood cell count, expressed as the area of cubic microns (cu μ) per cell; (2) mean corpuscular hemoglobin (MCH), a ratio of the hemoglobin to the red blood cell count, expressed as picograms (pg) of hemoglobin per cell; and (3) mean corpuscular hemoglobin concentration (MCHC), a ratio of hemoglobin to hematocrit, expressed as a percentage. (See **Hematocrit; Hemoglobin; Red Blood Cell.**) Blood is taken from a vein (or from a fingertip, earlobe, or heel) and placed in a special indices chamber.

When performed: When the cause or type of anemia cannot be determined; after the cause of an anemia is determined, to follow the progress of therapy; in certain cases of liver disease and suspected vitamin deficiencies.

Normal values: Normal levels for MCV range from 83 to 103 cu μ; for MCH, from 27 to 35 pg; for MCHC, from 32% to 36%.

Abnormal values: The MCH and MCV are lowered with some genetically caused anemias and with iron deficiency, liver disease, and blood loss. The MCHC is increased with anemias due to inadequate blood formation. The MCV and MCHC are increased with pernicious anemia, tapeworm infestation, and when taking certain medicines.

Risk factors: Negligible (see general risk factors for blood testing).

Pain/discomfort: Minimal (see general pain/discomfort factors for blood testing).

Accuracy and significance: The test is of value in helping to differentiate among the various types of anemia and is a significant aid to the doctor in diagnosing hemolytic anemias and anemias from **Folates** deficiency.

REFLEX

A reflex test is a measure of the reaction of the body to stimulation. Most commonly muscles are measured for their reflex reaction. Testing for the reflex reaction of the eyelid, the cornea (surface of the eye over the iris and lens), the pupils (see **Pupillary Reflex**), and the skin surface can help in the diagnosis of disease. (See **Caloric** test for ear reflex responses.)

In general, a muscle is tested by applying sufficient pressure to cause stretching of its fibers. In the knee-jerk reflex test, for example, the tapping of the patellar tendon (usually with a rubber hammer) just below the kneecap stretches the attached thigh muscle that lifts the lower leg. The muscle reacts by contracting (shortening) and the lower leg lifts suddenly and involuntarily.

Arm and leg muscle reflex tests are called "deep" reflex tests because of the force of the tap necessary to elicit a response. When a reflex is tested by gentle stroking motion over or near the muscle, it is called a "superficial" reflex test. For example, when the upper abdomen is stroked, the stomach muscles contract and pull the umbilicus (navel) upward. If a gentle stroke is applied just inside the upper thigh, adjacent to the testicle, the scrotum (the sac that holds the testicle) will suddenly rise upward on the same side that is stroked because of contraction of the cremasteric muscle.

Virtually every muscle can be tested this way, but only about a dozen reflex tests are routinely performed. Each muscle reflex represents an area of the spinal cord where the nerves to that muscle arise and, of course, the nerve itself. Thus testing for a specific muscle reflex can determine the exact area of the nervous system involved. For example, the bicep (the usually large, bulging muscle of the upper arm) is activated by nerves that come from between the fifth and sixth cervical vertebrae (the neck bones of the spine).

Failure to elicit the reflex, or an extremely exaggerated reflex, indicates disease of the nerve from the muscle to the spinal cord, disease of the spinal cord itself, or disease of the nerves from the spinal cord. The knee-jerk reflex is indicative of nerves that come from the lumbar (lower back) portion of the spine. Superficial reflexes also indicate nervous system locations. Pathology in certain nerves that come directly from the brain can be determined by the corneal reflex. When the colored part of the eye is touched with a piece of cotton, both eyes should immediately close as a reflex action. Failure of the eyes to close, or only one eye closing (either the same side or the opposite), indicates disease inside the brain.

The usual instrument for testing reflexes is the rubber hammer, but the edge of the hand will do as well. When it seems impossible to obtain a positive reflex reaction, the patient may be asked to perform some other muscular act to draw attention away from the area being tested. This will relax the muscle and allow a normal reflex. To obtain a knee-jerk reaction, for example, the physician may ask the patient to interlock his fingers and pull hard with both hands.

The Bender-Purdue reflex test, sometimes called the symmetric tonic neck reflex test, is performed primarily to determine whether an infant will hold his head up high and look forward and up when creeping. The position and use of the arms, hands, knees, and feet are also recorded. The manner of the child's movements is said to be indicative of the child's ability to learn (to be educated).

For pupil reflex tests see **Pupillary Reflex**. The eyelids should close when touched and at the sight of any approaching object; unless the patient is requested to do otherwise, both eyelids should close simultaneously. Blinking should also be simultaneous.

Another specific reflex test is the cold face test (CFT). Some doctors ask patients to hold their breath and then immerse their faces in cold water for 15 seconds. Others cover the patient's face with a large ice bag. The cold face test, while somewhat similar to the **Cold Pressor** test, is a measure of the heart rate's reflex response. Normally the application of cold slows the heart, but in patients who have had a stroke, or have multiple sclerosis or severe diabetes, the heart rate does not slow as it should. If the heart slows as expected, the possibility of brain disease can usually be eliminated.

When performed: As part of a routine physical examination to ascertain the functioning of nerves, muscles, and spinal cord; whenever nerve, muscle, or brain damage is suspected; after any injury.

Normal values: Pressure or stimulus on any relaxed muscle should cause a contraction of that muscle, or at least a reaction indicating that the pressure or stimulus was acknowledged by the body. Experience has taught doctors the expected responses so that weak or overly strong reactions can be noted. The reflexes on exact opposite sides or parts of the body should be about the same.

Reflex reactions are usually recorded on a "plus" scale from 1 to 4: 4-plus means hyperactive; 1-plus means weak or inadequate; 2-plus and 3-plus are average.

Abnormal values: Total absence of a reflex or extreme hyperactivity is considered abnormal. Specific pathological reflexes include the Babinski, in which stroking the sole of the foot causes the toes to point up and separate (normally the toes turn down as a response). The reaction is indicative of brain disease. The abnormal doll's-eye reflex occurs when the head is rotated from side to side and the eyes follow the movement to each side (normally they continue to look straight ahead). This is indicative of severe brain disease, but it can also occur with a large overdose of barbiturate drugs.

Risk factors: Negligible, with the exception of the doll's eye reflex, performing this test on a patient with a neck injury is extremely hazardous.

Pain/discomfort: Minimal, although there are those who find it uncomfortable to immerse their faces in cold water.

Accuracy and significance: Reflex responses are quite accurate and assist the doctor in diagnosing nerve, brain, and muscle diseases. They are especially significant in identifying malingerers. The cold face test is valuable because an ice pack can be placed over the face of an unconscious or comatose patient to help determine if brain damage is present.

RENIN

Renin is an enzyme produced by the kidney. (A renin-type substance that acts exactly like renin is also produced by the liver as an adverse reaction when oral contraceptive drugs or other female hormones are taken.) Renin regulates the production of the hormone aldosterone, which in turn controls the salt and water balance in the body. It also metabolizes to form other compounds that cause the muscles around the arteries to tighten and become smaller in size, thus raising the blood pressure.

The test is really a renin activity measurement, since an angiotensin compound made from renin is actually measured. It is important to know how much salt the patient has been eating for at least three days prior to the test (the less salt, the higher the renin values). The patient should be lying down for several hours before the test (standing and even sitting increases renin activity).

Usually blood is taken from a vein and the plasma is tested. It is now becoming common to measure renin activity separately in each of the kidney veins, since the comparative values are important in evaluating the potential success of kidney surgery as a treatment for high blood pressure.

When performed: To diagnose one cause of high blood pressure and to help ascertain the type of therapy and whether that therapy will be effective; when adrenal disease is suspected.

Normal values: Plasma renin activity (PRA) measures from 0.2 to 4 ng per ml per hour, depending on the amount of salt in the diet and for how long the patient was in an upright position before the test. Normal values are higher in the early morning hours. When renin activity is measured in each of the kidney veins, there should be no significant difference between the left and right vein.

Abnormal values: PRA is increased with high blood pressure caused by kidney disease, sometimes with chronic kidney disease alone, following kidney injury, with certain adrenal tumors, and with chronic liver disease. Increased values can also occur with pregnancy, with certain diuretic drugs, and with a salt-free diet. Values are usually decreased when patients are eating large amounts of salt or foods containing salt, when patients are taking certain steroid hormone drugs, when the adrenal glands secrete excessive aldosterone, and when high blood pressure comes from eating large amounts of licorice.

Risk factors: Negligible (see general risk factors for blood testing).

Pain/discomfort: Minimal (see general pain/discomfort factors for blood testing).

Accuracy and significance: The test is significant for those few patients with high blood pressure resulting from kidney disease as it helps to pinpoint this particular diagnosis. The test is also useful if there is a suspicion that only one kidney is involved; renin activity can indicate the specific kidney. Because of the many factors that can interfere with renin evaluations, the test is accurate only when it is performed with precision.

RHEUMATOID FACTOR (RF, RA, RAF, Rheumatoid Arthritis Factor)

The majority of patients suffering with rheumatoid arthritis have an **Immunoglobulin** antibody called rheumatoid factor. The more rheumatoid factor detected in the blood, the greater the possibility that rheumatoid arthritis exists. Unfortunately, a number of other diseases can also elevate RF levels (liver, lung and heart conditions, syphilis, and some worm infestations). Blood is taken from a vein and tested through various **Agglutination** techniques.

When performed: Primarily on patients with arthritic symptoms to help confirm the diagnosis.

Normal values: No rheumatoid factor or very low levels of it (a low titer, or detection of the substance before any substantial dilution of the blood). The older one gets, the greater the possibility the blood will reveal some rheumatoid factor without evidence of arthritis.

Abnormal values: Titers greater than a dilution of 1:160 (RF present in very diluted serum).

Risk factors: Negligible (see general risk factors for blood testing).

Pain/discomfort: Minimal (see general pain/discomfort factors for blood testing).

Accuracy and significance: It is reported that 80 to 90 percent of patients with rheumatoid arthritis have a high titer of RF. However, failure to have any RF in the blood does not indicate the patient is free of rheumatoid arthritis. Thus, elevated levels of RF only help confirm the doctor's diagnosis. There is some disagreement among doctors as to whether the sheep cell or latex agglutination technique is the most accurate; most prefer the sheep cell method.

RUBELLA (German Measles)

German measles was once considered a mild childhood disease. It is now known that if a pregnant woman is exposed to this virus infection and contracts the disease, especially during the first three months of pregnancy, she has a 50 percent chance of giving birth to a child with a congenital defect (deafness, cataracts, heart problems, abnormal growth of various organs, blood disorders). The test for rubella, therefore, is primarily one of determining an individual's susceptibility to the disease by measuring the amount of German measle antibodies in the blood. Usually an attack of rubella causes a lifelong immunity, which can be measured. If no rubella antibodies are detected, however, there is a vaccine that can help bring about immunity and prevent birth defects. Prior to the use of the vaccine, the results of a German measles epidemic could be tragic; in the United States, in 1964 and 1965, in the wake of such an epidemic, more than 20,000 infants were born with congenital malformations; there were in addition 30,000 stillbirths. Blood is taken from a vein for testing.

When performed: Whenever there is some question whether a woman is immune or susceptible to the disease. Four states require women obtaining a marriage license to be so tested; they are California, Colorado, New Jersey, and Rhode Island. The law does not usually require immunization, however, if susceptibility is found. Some states may require rubella testing as a condition of employment; in New York, for example, a woman employee of the State Health Department may be fired if she is found to lack immunity and refuses rubella immunization. Every woman should be tested prior to pregnancy so that proper immunization can be performed where indicated; many doctors suggest routine testing of all young girls at puberty. The test is also administered to help distinguish German measles from other, similar diseases such as regular measles (rubeola), exanthem subitum, or other infections that produce a rash and drug eruptions. All 50 states now have laws requiring that children be vaccinated for rubella before attending kindergarten, but this alone will not insure that all women of child-bearing age are protected; thus the screening tests are of vital importance.

Normal values: In this test, a "normal" value is evidence of immunity to the disease; that is, that the disease once had infected the individual.

Abnormal values: Evidence of susceptibility, or no immunity.

Risk factors: Negligible (see general risk factors for blood testing).

Pain/discomfort: Minimal (see general pain/discomfort factors for blood testing).

Accuracy and significance: The test is quite accurate in detecting immunity, or the lack of it, to German measles; it can sometimes indicate when the infection occurred. Usually, evidence of immunity appears within a week after exposure to, and contraction of, the disease. Its significance in helping prevent birth defects is obvious.

RUBIN

The Rubin test is one of several tests performed in cases of infertility. Specifically, it determines whether the fallopian tubes (which carry the ovum, or egg, from the ovary to the uterus) are open or blocked. Carbon dioxide gas is forced into the uterus under pressure; if the tubes are normal (open), the gas is detected in the abdomen. Occasionally the test procedure itself acts therapeutically to open blocked tubes.

When performed: When disease of the fallopian tubes is suspected; in cases of sterility.

Normal values: Normally the carbon dioxide passes easily through the tubes into the abdomen.

Abnormal values: Obstruction of the fallopian tubes may occur in endometriosis and infections (particularly following previous delivery or abortion) or following peritoneal inflammation (appendicitis). Occasionally the patient may have a spasm of the tubes during the test, giving a false negative result. Therefore, if the test is negative (tubes blocked), a second test should be performed for verification.

Risk factors: Although it is possible to force an excess of air into the abdominal cavity and cause trauma, this happens very rarely.

Pain/discomfort: After the air is inserted there is an uncomfortable feeling of fullness in the abdomen and occasionally discomfort around the liver. Once the test is completed, there is almost always an aching sensation in the shoulder resulting from the pressure of gas pushing up against the diaphragm. Actually, this discomfort indicates the fallopian tubes are open.

Accuracy and significance: The test is quite significant in revealing whether a woman's fallopian tubes are open or blocked. Should air escape from the apparatus during the test there could be a false negative result, giving the impression of blockage.

S

SCABIES INFESTATION

Scabies is a dermatological condition caused by a biting, burrowing mite. The incidence of scabies is increasing greatly, even among people who keep themselves fastidiously clean. A skin test in which extracts of the mite are injected is the primary method of differentiating between scabies and other dermatological conditions. Another test is to paint the skin with fluorescein dye and then shine ultraviolet light over the area; the burrowing tunnels then fluoresce. Serum immunoglobulin A is reduced in patients with scabies (see **Immunoglobulin**).

When performed: To differentiate certain rash-causing itching patterns from syphilis or lice infestations; whenever venereal disease is suspected; when a woman has a dermatitis of the nipples or a man has a rash over his scrotum; when a patient has a localized rash over the buttocks.

Normal values: There should be no evidence of the mite on direct examination and no reaction to the skin test.

Abnormal values: A positive skin test reaction (a hard, red nodule forms) confirms the diagnosis of scabies.

Risk factors: Negligible.

Pain/discomfort: Children often find the injection of the solution under the skin uncomfortable.

Accuracy and significance: The test is reasonably accurate, but direct examination of the skin showing the tunneling is generally sufficient.

SCHILLER

In gynecological examinations, many doctors "paint" the cervix (entrance to the uterus) with an iodine solution in order to isolate any suspected area of disease. Normal cells contain glycogen (starch), which iodine will stain. Although the Schiller test is not a specific diagnostic tool, it does point out suspicious areas for further study. Before the cervix is stained, the cervical mucus (discharge) is also examined for threadiness (called spinnbarkeit). The time it takes for the thready components of the mucus to be stretched indicates the phase of the menstrual cycle.

When performed: During a routine gynecological examination; whenever the patient has a persistent vaginal discharge or bleeding or a vaginal infection that is not easily cured.

Normal values: After being painted with iodine, the cervix should show a uniform brown (sometimes slightly bluish brown) color.

Abnormal values: Any area of the cervix that does not take the stain and remains white or pink indicates a lack of normal starch-containing cells (most commonly from infection, cancer, or injury) and a bit of the unstained tissue should then be taken for **Biopsy**. False positive tests (lack of staining without subsequent disease) occur in one out of three patients often due to infected or unestrogenated cells.

Risk factors: Negligible, unless the patient is allergic to iodine in which case there can be irritation.

Pain/discomfort: Usually minimal, if the doctor exercises care. Should the iodine solution touch the vagina's outer edge or other sensitive parts, there can be severe stinging or burning.

Accuracy and significance: The Schiller treatment of the cervix is not a specific test, yet it is highly significant as it directs a doctor's attention to potential disease conditions.

SEDIMENTATION RATE (ESR)

The erythrocyte sedimentation rate (ESR), called "sed rate" by most physicians, is a measure in millimeters (mm) of how far the red blood cells (erythrocytes) cling together, fall, and settle toward the bottom of a specially marked test tube in an hour's time. The cells group together and then form a sediment, as mud does in still water. Essentially it is an indication of any infectious process going on in the body. The various methods of performing the ESR are labeled according to the different sizes and shapes of tubes (Cutler, Westergren, Wintrobe) in which whole blood, usually taken from a vein, is placed.

When performed: With any suspected infection or tissue damage; to detect if an unsuspected disease is present; to follow the progress of disease (an increased ESR that begins to return to normal is a good prognostic sign).

Normal values: Normal values differ slightly depending on the tube used: Cutler, 2 to 10 mm fall in one hour; Wintrobe, 0 to 20 mm fall in one hour; Westergren, 1 to 12 mm fall in one hour. In general, a fall of up to 10 mm in one hour in men is considered normal; in women and elderly people, rates of up to 20 mm in one hour are still within normal range.

Abnormal values: The ESR is increased (falls faster) with certain infections (not with typhoid fever or with most virus diseases), tissue damage as with heart attack (not with angina), rheumatic fever, rheumatoid arthritis (not degenerative arthritis), kidney disease, thyroid disease, and some other hormone disorders, some cancers, and many connective tissue diseases or autoimmune conditions. It is also increased after poisoning, during menstruation, and in pregnancy.

Risk factors: Negligible (see general risk factors for blood testing).

Pain/discomfort: Minimal (see general pain/discomfort factors for blood testing).

Accuracy and significance: Because the test shows abnormal values in such a wide range of conditions, it is basically a screening device which suggests the possibility of illness when it is elevated. Although the test is still performed in doctors' offices, it has been replaced in most laboratories by various enzyme measurements (SGOT, SGPT, CPK, LDH) as part of **Comprehensive Multiple Test Screening** panels.

SEMEN

The semen, seminal fluid, or ejaculate is the single most important test of testicle function and fertility. (Fertility has nothing to do with potency.) In barren marriages, 30% of the husbands are infertile; more than half of these men can be helped to become fertile. Besides sperm (spermatozoa), normal semen contains spermatocytes, Sertoli cells, sperm nutrients, red and white blood cells, macrophages, lecithin crystals, and secretions from the prostrate as well as other glands (fructose, citric acid, proteins, prostaglandins, and hormones).

Semen is usually examined for volume, viscosity (thickness), **pH** (acidity), motility (movement: whether sluggish or quick), morphology (form and structure of sperm), amount of sperm (sperm count) and fructose level (deficient fructose levels in semen seem to parallel testicular hormone, or androgen deficiency).

It takes approximately ten weeks for sperm to form, so that the sperm sample analyzed is actually indicative of bodily functioning over the preceding ten weeks. Thus a single examination that indicates irregularities cannot be considered valid. If any abnormality is noted, at least three more specimens should be examined for verification.

After sexual abstinence for four to six days, the patient collects a specimen either by masturbation or by coitus interruptus. Masturbation is perferable so that none of the sample is lost. Semen should be examined immediately, but no later than two hours after collection. The one exception is the postcoital (after-intercourse) test where, because of religious convictions or extreme embarrassment, the woman reports to her doctor as soon as possible after normal intercourse and the specimen is removed from the vagina.

The Huhner test is an examination of the sperm in the semen, which is taken from the vagina after intercourse to determine if the sperm can penetrate the cervical mucus to fertilize the egg.

When performed: As a test of gonadal function; in suspected infertility; after vasectomy to measure success of the surgery; when rape is suspected.

Normal values: Volume: the normal ejaculation is 2.5 to 5 ml of seminal fluid (about one teaspoon). A low-volume ejaculation (1 ml) may still be normal and may contain a high sperm count.

Viscosity: Semen seems to gel just after ejection but normally liquefies in 15 to 30 minutes. It should not be examined until it has liquefied.

pH: Normally the pH level ranges between 7.2 and 8.0 (slightly alkaline).

Motility: At least 70% to 90% of normal sperm are motile (active) in the first hour after ejection, and 50% should still be motile up to ten hours after ejection.

Morphology: In a sample, 80% to 90% of sperm should appear to have a normal form. The normal sperm has head, neck, and tail. Slight variations in the size and shape of the head (tiny, large, round, elongated and double heads) may be normal.

Sperm count: The normal semen sample contains 60 to 120 million sperm per ml. Patients who have more are not considered more fertile than others.

Fructose level: Normal fructose is 315 mg per 100 ml.

Abnormal values: Volume: A low volume of semen (less than 2.5 ml) may be, but is not always, associated with fertility problems unless accompanied by a low sperm count. An exceptionally high volume (more than 5 ml) can also be an indication of infertility.

Viscosity: Failure of the semen to liquefy from its gel form after 15 to 30 minutes may be associated with infertility.

Motility: Immobile or sluggish sperm are abnormal, and usually indicate infertility.

Morphology: Variation from the normal size and shape in more than 20% of sperm is indicative of infertility problems. The different ways the sperm takes up stain are significant. Frequency of senile or juvenile forms, diffuse staining, or lack of staining are abnormal variations. Usually the fewer the sperm, the more abnormal forms that are seen.

Sperm count: A sperm count below 60 million per ml is considered abnormal. Organic disease of the genitals (mumps, prostatitis, occlusion of ducts), endocrine or other systemic disease, spinal cord injury, hypopituitarism, and even a form of anxiety (anorexia nervosa) can cause low or no sperm count.

Rape test: When there is a question of sexual intercourse, an examination for semen (especially sperm) may be performed. The presence and activity of sperm taken from the vagina may indicate the approximate time intercourse took place. If no sperm are found, suspected semen and/or vaginal fluid are sometimes examined for prostatic **Acid Phosphatase**, the presence of which usually indicates intercourse. Sperm can live for up to six days after intercourse within the cervix portion of the uterus, but evidence of sperm has been found as long as four months after a rape-murder.

Abnormal sperm have been found in men who are heavy cigarette smokers with no evidence of other testicle dysfunction.

Risk factors: None.

Pain/discomfort: The collection of sperm can embarrass some patients.

Accuracy and significance: The test is totally objective and hence quite accurate. However, men with completely normal values can still be infertile, and men with some abnormal values can still father a child. The significance of the test, after several examinations at different times, is that when a cause for infertility is found, it can be corrected in at least half the men with testicle dysfunction.

SENSORY

Many different tests measure a patient's ability to perceive various sensations (pain, a light touch, temperature differences, vibrations, etc.). Discovering the exact locations where sensations are decreased (or at times increased) can help indicate the area in the nerves or spinal cord where disease originates. In addition, when patients complain of unusual sensations (burning, tingling, pins and needles), tests must be performed to isolate the area involved.

In most sensory tests, the patient is asked to keep his eyes closed so that the sensitivity of the skin area being tested can be measured directly. Various objects (cotton, pins, tubes) are touched to or pressed on the skin to elicit a response. Sensory ability is affected by a great many conditions (injuries, tumors, drugs, poor nutrition, infection, and inherited diseases).

When performed: Whenever nerve, muscle, spinal cord, or brain disease is suspected; when patients complain of an inability to feel normal sensations or experience unusual sensations.

Normal values: A patient should be able to locate and discriminate between a pin prick on the skin, a touch with a piece of cotton, pressure from the doctor's hand, tubes containing warm and cold water applied to the skin, and a vibrating tuning fork touched to any bone area. The patient should be able to tell if a toe is being pushed up or bent down as well as which fingers and toes are being touched. These feelings should be equal on both sides of the body.

More discriminating types of sensory tests measure the ability of the brain to interpret sensation. For example, the skin may be touched at two points at the same time; normally a patient can describe the touching and how far apart the points are. Normal patients can also distinguish different materials that touch them (cotton versus silk), specific shapes, and letters or numbers that the doctor outlines with a finger on the palm of their hand or other skin area.

Abnormal values: Although any absence or diminution of sensory ability usually indicates disease, the area affected must always correspond to a specific nerve distribution, called a dermatome. For example, if the patient complains of loss of feeling in the knee area, a definite area above, below, and alongside the knee should also be affected. If the loss of feeling does not correspond to the anatomical distribution of the nerve, other causes for the complaint (hysteria, attempting to mislead the physician, etc.) must be considered.

Risk factors: None.

Pain/discomfort: None.

Accuracy and significance: The tests are of value in diagnosing the existence of nerve and spinal cord disease, but they are not sufficiently precise to distinguish between the possible causes of an illness. They are particularly significant in detecting malingerers.

SEROTONIN (5-HIAA, HIAA)

Serotonin (hydroxytryptamine) is manufactured in the blood from tryptophan (one of the amino acids in the protein we eat) and is then metabolized into 5-hydroxyindolacetic acid (HIAA), a compound that can be tested for in the urine. Serotonin acts to transmit nerve impulses and also constricts blood vessels. An excess of serotonin seems to be implicated in both flushing and blueness of the skin, rapid heartbeat, diarrhea, precipitation of asthma, and increased blood clotting (it is also found in the platelets). Exposure to the sun seems to increase serotonin production. Blood from a vein may be tested for serotonin, but it is more common to test a 24-hour urine sample for HIAA. Recently the test has been performed on mentally retarded patients (usually from inherited developmental disabilities) and on patients with **Depression**.

When performed: Primarily when a carcinoid tumor (usually in the intestinal tract) is suspected; when there is unexplained cyanosis (bluish color to the skin) and an enlarged liver; on patients with inherited metabolic deficiencies; on mentally ill patients.

Normal values: Serotonin in whole blood ranges from 0.05 to 0.20 mcg per ml. HIAA in urine ranges from 2 to 8 mg per 24-hour sample.

Abnormal values: With a carcinoid tumor (called an argentaffinoma), values of HIAA may go up to 1,000 mg per 24-hour urine specimen. Certain tranquilizers, antidepressant drugs, and foods that contain serotonin (such as avocados, bananas, pineapples, and eggplants) may cause elevated levels. Decreased serotonin levels are found in patients with Down's syndrome and in those with depression who are not being treated with lithium.

Risk factors: Negligible (see general risk factors for blood testing).

Pain/discomfort: Minimal (see general pain/discomfort factors for blood testing).

Accuracy and significance: The test is particularly significant in helping to diagnose a carcinoid tumor and is equally important in helping to eliminate this tumor from diagnostic considerations. The accuracy of the test in mental retardation and mental illness is still under study.

SKIN REACTION

Many diagnostic tests measure the allergic sensitivity of the skin as an indication of either susceptibility to or previous contact with disease-producing substances. Common skin reaction tests (also called intracutaneous, intradermal, or subcutaneous tests) include the tuberculin or Mantoux test, the Tine test (application of tuberculin sensitive substance to the surface of the skin), and the purified protein derivative (PPD) which is similar to the tuberculin test. A new modification of the tuberculin test uses the

Tine surface application with PPD rather than the traditional tuberculin substance. There is the Schick test for susceptibility to diphtheria; the Dick test for sensitivity to the Streptococcus toxin (scarlet fever); specific tests for tularemia, mumps, aspergillus, candida, tricophyton, coccidioidomycosis, histoplasmosis, and trichinosis; and the various tests that measure allergic sensitivity to foods and pollens. Skin tests may also be used to detect immune reactions.

About 0.1 ml (much less than a drop) of the testing material is injected just under the top layer of the skin, producing a small, whitish bump. (If no bump is raised, the material has been injected too deeply.) The usual sites are the inner hairless portion of the lower arm and the back, but the injection can be made anywhere on the body. If the testing substance is mixed in a solution that in itself could cause an allergy, the mixing solution alone—without the testing element—is injected in the opposite arm as a control measure. Sometimes a tiny bandage soaked in the testing solution is placed on the arm and covered with adhesive tape; this is called a patch test. The newest test for allergies is called the radioimmunosorbent assay test (see **RAST**).

It should be noted that the Food and Drug Administration considers a number of commonly performed skin tests to be ineffective—specifically, those to test for trichinosis, histoplasmosis, lymphogranuloma, diphtheria, and the "old tuberculin" test for tuberculosis (the PPD is accepted by the FDA). The federal government is trying to remove the substances used in these tests from the market.

When performed: When allergy is suspected; to diagnose certain specific infections; in dermatological conditions that are difficult to diagnose; to measure immunological sensitivity.

Normal values: There are really no normal values for skin tests since positive responses do not always indicate the presence of disease. For example, a person who was once exposed to tuberculosis but who has no infectious activity whatsoever may still have a positive skin reaction. A person who has had diphtheria may have lost his immunity and thus have a positive reaction. With allergy tests, it is not unusual for the skin to react positively to certain substances that have no direct effect on the nose or lungs and that therefore may not be causing allergic disease in other parts of the body.

Abnormal values: Since a positive test may not necessarily be abnormal, any positive reaction must be interpreted in light of a patient's medical history and physical findings. A reaction is positive when the site of the injected material turns red and/or a raised bump (wheal) at least ¼ inch in diameter can be felt. The reaction generally appears 24 to 72 hours after the injection but may last for several days.

Risk factors: Negligible (see general risk factors for catheter and needle insertion).

Pain/discomfort: Minimal (see general pain/discomfort factors for catheter and needle insertion).

Accuracy and significance: Although the efficacy of many skin tests is questionable, they can help to eliminate certain disease possibilities. The Tine test is probably the most commonly used screening test for tuberculosis, but it gives false negative as well as false positive results. The PPD test, given by injection just under the skin, is the most accurate. Once a patient has been adequately treated for tuberculosis a positive tuberculin skin test may become negative. However, it should be remembered that a positive tuberculin skin test does not necessarily mean the existence of active tuberculosis. Many doctors do not consider the skin reaction tests for food allergies of value; too often the tests cannot be judged significant as there are many false positive reactions to food testing. Allergy specialists acknowledge that there are many variables that can affect the accuracy of skin testing for hay fever, asthma, and other sensitivity illnesses. For instance, the particular area of the body on which the test is performed can affect the results; different parts of the arm react to the testing material in different degrees, and the skin on certain parts of the back can prove twice as reactive as the skin on the arms. Then too, the time of day can alter a skin test result; for some people tests performed in the morning are three times as reactive as those performed in the afternoon; others have a totally opposite reaction response. If skin reaction tests are placed too near one another on the body, a positive reaction in one site may trigger a false positive reaction in the adjacent site. False positive reactions also occur when the same needle is used to inject different test materials without being adequately cleaned between tests. A false negative, or lack of reaction, may occur if a patient has been taking an antihistamine drug for up to three days prior to testing (antihistamine drugs do not seem to interfere with **RAST** testing), and there are many false negative results, or lack of a response, when the testing material is more than one month old.

SLEEP MONITORING

Insomnia or hypersomnia (too much sleeping, as opposed to not enough) are well known symptoms of many different illnesses, but it is only recently that sleep laboratories have been established to observe patients during their usual sleeping hours. Direct observation of the individual, along with mechanical measurements such as the **Electrocardiogram,** the **Electroencephalogram,** and **Electromyography** along with tests of **Pulmonary Function** and **Blood Gases** (when several of these tests are utilized, they may be referred to as polysomnography), can help in diagnosing many sleep disorders, such as nighttime breathing difficulties. An annoying problem such as loud snoring can be the key to an underlying severe heart or lung disease that was previously undetected. Measurements of various hormone levels, especially those related to blood pressure, kidney function, and the **Catecholamines,** may also be performed while the patient is sleeping.

Severe breathing difficulties during sleep are called sleep apnea syndromes. Some doctors feel that they are the cause of, or at least reflect, a great variety of illnesses. Anatomical deformations, such as a deviated septum in the nose, abnormally large tonsils, tongue malformations and tumors in the upper respiratory tract have been found to cause sleep apnea. Brain and nerve disease may also be responsible for the temporary cessation of breathing during sleep. Sudden death as a consequence of sleep apnea is being reported in medical journals with increasing frequency.

Most sleep monitoring takes place at sleep disorder centers; these clinics are almost always associated with hospital or university medical centers. As of October 1981, there were 27 sleep disorder centers certified by the Association of Sleep Disorder Centers that test patients for difficulties in sleeping, staying awake, and even for troublesome behavior during sleep. Some of these centers will only test patients when referred by a doctor but others will accept self-referral.

An up-to-date list of fully accredited sleep disorder centers can be obtained from a doctor or from the Association of Sleep Disorder Centers, P.O. Box YY, East Setauket, NY 11733.

When performed: When repeated episodes of snoring cannot be diagnosed; when unexplained chest pains occur during the night; when the cause of high blood pressure cannot be determined; when there are breathing difficulties during sleep; when patients sleep too much during the day or cannot keep themselves from dropping off to sleep at inappropriate times.

Normal values: Each of the various monitoring devices that can be utilized at a sleep center shows normal or usual patterns during sleep (the heart rate decreases, blood pressure falls, some hormone activity increases while other hormones decrease in amount, brain waves change their pattern, etc.); specialists in sleep disorders know what to expect and can distinguish normal from abnormal findings.

Abnormal values: Deviations from normal or expected body activities and responses.

Risk factors: Negligible (see general risk factors for blood testing).

Pain/discomfort: Minimal (see general pain/discomfort factors for blood testing).

Accuracy and significance: Many doctors feel that sleep monitoring is still in an experimental stage but that it can help uncover some previously unsuspected diseases. The true significance of sleep monitoring has yet to be established.

SODIUM

Sodium is one of the blood electrolytes. (Atoms or ions of **Bicarbonate, Chloride,** and **Potassium** are the other major electrolytes.) It is essential to maintaining the body's normal water metabolism and acid-base balance, and to keep the proper amount of fluids in the bloodstream and in the tissues *around* the cells (potassium holds the water *in* each cell). On a typical diet, the average adult takes in about 6 g (about 0.2 ounce) of sodium a day. The ingestion of excess sodium from salt (sodium chloride), monosodium glutamate (MSG), and the many heavily sodium-based flavor enhancers (such as disodium inosinate and disodium guanylate) found in processed foods can cause water retention (edema), headache, and several other symptoms. A loss of body sodium (from excessive sweating, vomiting, or fever) produces dehydration. Blood is taken from a vein and the serum is tested. Sodium is also measured in the urine, in **Sweat,** occasionally in the spinal fluid, and in saliva.

When performed: When there is a persistent water retention; to help diagnose various hormone disorders; to determine the cause of coma; to confirm suspected cystic fibrosis of the pancreas (it has been suggested that all patients with chronic lung disease be sodium tested for cystic fibrosis).

Normal values: Normal sodium levels range from 135 to 150 mEq per liter in serum and 40 to 200 mEq per liter in a 24-hour urine sample.

Abnormal values: Increased sodium levels (hypernatremia) are found in some endocrine disorders, especially those of the adrenal glands (Addison's disease); in dehydration; and in patients taking certain hormones and drugs such as steroids, contraceptive pills, and sodium-formulated medicines. Kidney disease, heart disease, and high blood pressure can also cause increased amounts of sodium in the blood. Decreased serum sodium is found in diabetes, inadequate adrenal function, and patients taking diuretic drugs.

Urine sodium usually parallels serum sodium, except with dehydration or with certain hormones or drugs that cause the kidney to excrete excessive amounts in the urine.

Sodium is greatly increased in sweat and saliva (as are chlorides) with cystic fibrosis of the pancreas (mucoviscidosis), a congenital condition that usually expresses itself through repeated lung infections.

Risk factors: Negligible (see general risk factors for blood testing).

Pain/discomfort: Minimal (see general pain/discomfort factors for blood testing).

Accuracy and significance: While sodium measurements are quite accurate, a deviation from normal occurs in such a variety of conditions that basically the test serves only to confirm a doctor's suspicions.

SPUTUM

Sputum is the mucous secretion (phlegm) from the lower respiratory system (the lungs, the bronchi, the trachea, and the larynx). The sputum examination usually does not include the nose or sinus secretions, which are part of the upper respiratory tract. In infections and other inflammatory conditions, sputum volume and viscosity (thickness) increase.

Sputum is collected for microbiologic **Culture** or **Cytology** examination. Some is placed on culture plates to check for bacterial growth, some is placed on slides for microscopic study, and some is examined by the Papanicolaou stain for tumor study. Most clinicians request a specimen of all the sputum a patient produces in a 24-hour period; a few find a single specimen sufficient for diagnostic study. Usually sputum is obtained by coughing. It can also be aspirated (suctioned) through a bronchoscope. See **Endoscopy.**

When performed: With suspected respiratory tract disease, when there is a persistent cough that cannot be explained, or with an undiagnosed general infection.

Normal values: Unless there is a disease process (infection, irritation, allergy, or cancer) very little sputum is produced. Any minute amounts of sputum produced should be clear, colorless, and odorless and should reveal no bacteria and very few cells or crystals under the microscope.

Abnormal values: An increased amount of yellow to greenish sputum indicates a lung infection. Reddish or brown sputum accompanies lung congestion with or without infection (pinkish, watery, foamy sputum is considered diagnostic of pulmonary edema).

In lung infections, there is a great increase in the white blood cells and fat crystals. With coliform bacteria and anaerobic infections, the sputum has an unpleasant odor. With allergy such as asthma, there is an increase in one particular white blood cell, the eosinophil, along with Curschmann's spirals and Charcot-Leyden crystals, which are quite different from the crystals seen in infection. With irritation (from dust, smog, etc.) an increase in the cells that line the bronchial passageways of the lung is seen. Elastic fibers found in the sputum on microscopic examination suggest a destructive process such as pneumonia, tuberculosis, cancer, or lung abscess.

Risk factors: None when obtained while a patient has a productive cough. If a bronchoscope is used to obtain the specimen, see **Endoscopy.**

Pain/discomfort: None, unless the specimen is obtained by bronchoscopy.

Accuracy and significance: Sputum examinations can be extremely valuable in the diagnosis of lung disease, particularly in identifying the cause of infection. If cancer cells are detected the test can be very significant when it leads to early treatment.

STRABISMUS

Strabismus is a condition in which the two eyes do not see the identical image simultaneously; usually one eye is directed in a slightly different direction from the other. Most often this condition is the result of an eye muscle weakness (eye movement is controlled by six different muscles); it can also come from brain and nerve involvement. By having the patient look at fixed points in certain directions, the physician can determine the specific external ocular muscle at fault. Forms of strabismus include heterotropia (squinting); esotropia (cross-eyes), where one or both eyes look inward; exotropia (walleyes), where one eye always looks outward; and diplopia (double vision).

Diplopia is detected when a red glass is placed over one eye and the patient, looking at a light with both eyes, sees both a red and a white dot. In the Worth four-dot test, a red glass is placed over one eye and a green glass over the other; the patient looks at a special light that shows one red, one white, and two green dots. Depending on what the patient sees, the doctor can determine which eye is affected and whether the two eyes can work together.

In the Wirt stereopsis test, polarized-lens glasses are used to ascertain the degree and possibility of fusion (the ability to use both eyes together for three-dimensional viewing). In the cover-uncover test, a patient looks at an object 20 feet away first with one eye covered and then with the cover removed. The Hirschberg test, similar in technique, is used on young children who do not easily cooperate; movement of corneal light reflex is noted. The Maddox rod test uses cylinders to measure eye deviations. All the tests help confirm the specific cause of strabismus and help determine prognosis. About one in 20 children has a form of strabismus.

When performed: Whenever patients have cross-eyes, wall-eyes, squinting, or double vision; following head or eye injury; with all cranial nerve diseases; in patients with diabetes or vascular diseases.

Normal values: When both eyes look at the identical spot or object, they should see it as one rather than two distinct spots or objects, without blurring (in this instance blurring would be due to double vision rather than loss of **Visual Acuity**). The patient should be able to control each of the six muscles of the eye so that they move in perfect harmony.

Abnormal values: Deviations are measured in units of prisms. With strabismus, a prism lens must be placed in front of the eye to correct muscular weakness or nerve defect. One prism diopter (diopter is a unit of measurement in ophthalmology) means that at a distance of one meter (a bit more than three feet) the eye sees an image one centimeter away from its true location. In the Worth four-dot test, a patient with double vision will see five dots instead of four; whether the extra dot is red or green determines which eye is affected. In the cover-uncover test, when the cover is removed the weak eye will suddenly move instead of focusing in the direction in which the uncovered eye is looking.

Risk factors: None.

Pain/discomfort: None.

Accuracy and significance: The tests are quite accurate as an aid to determining the cause of strabismus; if the cause is muscle imbalance, the tests help to identify the specific muscle. The significance of the tests lies in their ability to indicate which strabismus conditions can be corrected and to what degree.

STRING

At times a patient may present vague symptoms of bleeding from the esophagus, stomach, or first part of the small intestine, usually indicative of an irritation, an ulcer, or a parasitic infestation. A simple test to detect such bleeding, and to help justify subsequent expensive and complicated examinations, is the string test. It is so named because all the patient must do is swallow a string (usually of the same material as that used to tie the umbilical cord at birth). At times, the string is weighted at the end with a small capsule that may or may not dissolve. The distance the string travels is noted and it is then pulled back up and the stains from blood, bile, or mucus are observed. In addition, material adhering to the string can be examined microscopically to observe the types of cells that make up the linings of various organs (see **Cytology**). The presence of crystals of cholesterol, bilirubin from bile, or segments of parasites or their eggs can also be noted (parasitic infestation can exist so high up in the intestinal tract that it is difficult to diagnose through a feces examination). Finally, certain fungus overgrowths that can interfere with the effectiveness of antibiotics can be detected by the string test. Today there are commercial products which are much-improved versions of the traditional string; some use nylon and have fast-dissolving capsules and color markers in the string to make diagnosis easier and quicker.

When performed: As a screening test when there is a suspicion of bleeding or other pathology in the upper digestive tract; when a patient's **Feces Examination** is normal, but there is a suspicion of worms or other parasites; in cases of anemia when the source of bleeding has not been isolated; in malabsorption syndrome (food is not properly digested); when particular medications are not properly absorbed; when pernicious anemia is suspected; to note the presence or absence of bile.

Normal values: No evidence of blood, parasites, fungi, abnormal cells or bile crystals. Normal acid in the stomach.

Abnormal values: Evidence of bleeding, irritation, parasites, abnormal bacteria (such as those that cause typhoid), abnormal pH (acid) values in inappropriate locations (see **Gastroesophageal Reflux**), and any abnormal (cancerous) cells. Lack of stomach acid.

Risk factors: Virtually none; swallowing the string will cause no real complications.

Pain/discomfort: Some patients find it difficult to swallow the string, while others tend to vomit when swallowing the string or when it is retrieved.

Accuracy and significance: The test is considered 90 percent accurate in detecting bleeding in the esophagus, stomach, or first portion of the small intestine; approximately 85 percent accurate in detecting parasites in the upper intestine; approximately 50 percent accurate in noting malabsorption problems; quite accurate in measuring the presence or absence of stomach acid and its pH. Although this test is simple and relatively painless, the use of a gastroscope (see **Endoscopy**) is far more accurate (endoscopy can necessitate hospitalization). When testing for stomach acid in the esophagus, the gastroesophageal reflux test is more precise.

SWEAT

Testing for the chemicals in sweat (see **Sodium**) helps to detect many different diseases. Measuring the ability to sweat is a particular test for physical as well as mental disease. A very weak iodine solution (in alcohol) is painted on the skin area under study and allowed to dry; the area is dusted with starch powder. The patient is then made to sweat (by administration of direct heat, hot liquids, or certain drugs). If the sweat glands are functioning properly, the white starch powder will turn dark blue. Vapor pressure osmometry is a new sweat collection procedure that uses a heated cup to help eliminate false results. One simple sweat test is to kiss a baby to find out if the skin seems particularly salty. Many pediatricians urge parents to use this test to detect early signs of cystic fibrosis in their infants.

There is also a sweat patch test for **Alcoholism.** The patient wears a sweat patch from two to eight days; the concentration of alcohol in the sweat collected by the patch determines alcohol consumption.

When performed: Most often the test is performed to ascertain excessive sweating such as with "night sweats" (which occur only during sleep and suggest chronic infections); to differentiate malnutrition from certain specific diseases such as lupus erythematosus; to measure a spontaneous sweating reaction to anxiety; to collect sweat for cystic fibrosis screening; to distinguish alcohol drinkers from non-drinkers.

Normal values: It is normal for sweat glands to function when exposed to direct heat, exercise, or excessive alcohol, or when the body is excessively warmed by clothes or blankets. Sweat may have a color if the body is exposed to certain chemicals (as in certain occupations) or if the sweat is accompanied by color-producing bacteria. Excessive bacteria can normally cause bromidrosis, or unpleasantly scented sweat, but this is usually limited to areas with skin folds.

Abnormal values: Hyperhidrosis, or excessive sweating under inappropriate conditions (as in a cool room), may be caused by vitamin deficiencies, hyperthyroidism, brain and spinal cord disease, blood vessel disease, and following surgery where certain nerves have been severed. Psychological problems usually cause excessive sweating on the palms of the hands and the soles of the feet. The inability to sweat is usually an inherited condition. Patients with cystic fibrosis have increased sodium and chloride concentrations in their sweat. Patients who drink alcohol but deny it can be identified with this test.

Risk factors: None.

Pain/discomfort: None.

Accuracy and significance: Sweat measurements are not considered precise tests. They are reasonably significant as a confirmation of cystic fibrosis; however, false positive results occur with enough frequency to warrant blood **Sodium** testing. The inaccuracies found in sweat tests are, in large measure, due to carelessness in performing them.

SYNOVIAL FLUID

All body joints contain a small amount of straw-colored syrupy liquid called synovial fluid that helps lubricate the bone or cartilage surfaces. Three dozen different tests can be performed on joint fluid. The usual examination consists of measuring sugar levels and white blood cells, as well as searching for crystals, immunoglobulins, antigamma globulins, various forms of complement, and lupus erythematosus cells (see **Antinuclear Antibodies**). In the ropes test, the fluid is mixed with a mild acid to see if it forms a good mucin clot (a small, ropy-looking mass that stays together even with shaking).

In most instances, the patient is asked to fast the night before and the morning of the test so as not to abnormally alter the sugar level. The synovial fluid is obtained by inserting a small needle into the joint cavity (a process called arthrocentesis). Absolute sterile precautions must be observed to make sure that infection is not introduced into the cavity when the fluid is withdrawn. A joint cavity can contain up to half an ounce of fluid, but only one drop is needed to arrive at certain diagnoses.

A new test, the limulus assay (limulus is a special chemical), is now being performed whenever synovial fluid is suspected of being infected with Gram-negative bacteria (see **Gram Stain**); it can give a fairly reliable indication of infection within an hour as opposed to the several days needed to culture bacteria. The limulus test can also be used on blood to indicate the presence of small amounts of endotoxin (poisons from certain bacteria that can cause blood poisoning, sometimes called toxemia or sepsis).

When performed: Primarily when there is a swollen joint, whether hot and inflamed or not; to differentiate the different types of arthritis (from infectious to traumatic); to aid in the diagnosis of systemic lupus erythematosus; to follow the progress of any joint disease; when certain bleeding disorders are suspected.

Normal values: Normal synovial fluid is slightly yellow and clear with very few white blood cells (less than 200 per ml), no crystals, and a good mucin clot. Sugar levels and other chemical test values should approximate those found in normal plasma.

Abnormal values: With arthritis, synovial fluid tends to become more yellow or yellowish green and turns somewhat cloudy. The white blood cells increase markedly (over 10,000 per ml), and with certain diseases various types of crystals appear: uric acid crystals with gout, calcium crystals with pseudogout. With arthritis, the mucin clot is "poor"—that is, fragile and easily breakable on shaking; with gout, it is even more fragile. With infectious arthritis, synovial fluid sugar levels are reduced and the fluid is given a **Culture** test.

Risk factors: An ever-present risk in extracting joint fluid is the subsequent possibility of osteomyelitis or prolonged bone infection. When sterile conditions are meticulously observed this risk is reduced. When the test itself is correctly performed, the remaining risks are negligible (see general risk factors for catheter and needle insertion).

Pain/discomfort: Minimal (see general pain/ discomfort factors for catheter and needle insertion).

Accuracy and significance: Synovial fluid tests are significant in their ability to differentiate between joint infection and other non-infectious conditions (arthritis, gout, pathology secondary to an injury). Synovial fluid examinations are done routinely in conjunction with **Radiography.** It is these two tests, supporting the doctor's physical findings, that can help make a diagnosis of joint disease.

SYPHILIS

Many tests help to determine if syphilis is present in the body. These tests may be of the treponemal variety (looking for Treponema pallidum, the corkscrew-shaped organisms that cause the disease) or the nontreponemal variety of serological (blood) tests (see **Agglutination; Complement Fixation**) that give passive evidence of the disease if antibodies are present. The nontreponemal antigen tests include the Hinton, Kolner, Kahn, Kline, Mazzini, Wassermann, rapid plasma reagin (RPR), automated reagin (ART) and Venereal Disease Research Laboratory (VDRL). The VDRL is the most common test, but it is not completely accurate: one patient out of four with early syphilis will have a false negative reaction. These tests are not as expensive and are more easily performed than the treponemal tests, but they all may give false positive results in conditions other than syphilis (lupus erythematosus, malaria, leprosy, acute infections, and after smallpox vaccination).

The treponemal organisms are so narrow that they cannot be seen by ordinary microscopic light and need a "darkfield"; that is, they must be illuminated by reflected light in order to be observed. The darkfield examination is performed during the primary stage of syphilis; fluid from the lesion is placed on a glass slide and examined under the microscope for direct, living evidence of Treponema pallidum.

The Treponema pallidum immobilization test (TPI) takes serum from a suspected syphilis patient and adds it to complement (special serum antibodies); when both are then added to a virulent strain of live Treponema pallidum, the organisms become immobilized.

The Fluorescent Treponemal Antibody Absorption (FTA-ABS) test has been found to be more sensitive for syphilis than the TPI. It is easier to perform and therefore used more often, but one patient out of ten with early syphilis will still be missed (have a false negative reaction). False positive reactions may occur when the patient's serum contains antinuclear factor, rheumatoid factor, or increased globulins. Blood from a vein is tested. Spinal fluid is also tested to detect latent syphilis and to follow the progress of treatment.

When performed: Whenever there is a mystifying infection (syphilis is known as the great masquerader, since it imitates many illnesses); when a skin disease does not heal; with other symptoms that cause suspicion of syphilis; when certain tropical diseases are suspected; when pregnancy is diagnosed.

In most states a syphilis test is required by law before a marriage license can be issued. (The exceptions are Idaho, Maine, Maryland, Minnesota, Nevada, South Carolina, and Washington; in

Colorado men are exempt.) In Alabama, Alaska, Colorado, Kansas, Louisiana, New Mexico, North Carolina, North Dakota, Oklahoma, Utah, Wisconsin, and the territory of Puerto Rico, applicants for a marriage license must also present a certificate certifying they are free of *all* known sexually transmitted diseases.

In all states, other than Alabama, Minnesota, Mississippi, Tennessee, Wisconsin, and the territory of Puerto Rico, the law requires a pregnant woman to be tested for syphilis on her first visit to a doctor or clinic; in California a woman can be excused from the test if she objects for any reason.

Normal values: Normally there is no evidence (reaction) of syphilis in the body.

Abnormal values: The test is positive when there is active or even inactive (old) syphilis. Other conditions that can cause a positive reaction include malaria, Hansen's disease, rat-bite fever, pellagra, infectious mononucleosis, pneumonia, tuberculosis, and lupus erythematosus.

Risk factors: Negligible (see general risk factors for blood testing). Also see **Biopsy.**

Pain/discomfort: Minimal (see general pain/discomfort factors for blood testing). Also see **Biopsy.**

Accuracy and significance: Nontreponemal tests are used primarily for premarital and prenatal screening; while they serve this purpose adequately they are not of sufficient accuracy to confirm a diagnosis. Such a variety of conditions other than syphilis produce a positive nontreponemal test that the finding of an abnormal value requires extensive follow-up. Positive treponemal and microscopic tests are necessary before a specific diagnosis can be made.

SYSTOLIC TIME INTERVALS (STI)

The word "systole" refers to the time during which the heart contracts and pumps blood into the aorta and the rest of the vascular system ("diastole" is the time the heart relaxes between contractions). An electronic instrument is placed on the side of the neck so that the carotid artery pulse can be felt. The device records the pulse waves (pressure from the heart's contraction and forcible outflow of blood) in the form of specific waves that can be measured and timed.

Many cardiologists consider the STI to be the most accurate of all tests of heart muscle and vascular system functioning. It is usually performed along with a standard **Electrocardiogram** (ECG) and a phonocardiogram (PCG). The first part of the STI measures the left ventricular ejection time, or how long it takes the left side of the heart to empty itself. The second part of the test measures the pre-ejection period (PEP), or the exact time the heart muscle is activated to the time the blood begins to leave the heart. The two parts of the STI can reveal heart disease that is not detected by other tests.

The most recent innovation for measuring systolic time intervals is the Spodick-Haffty-Kotilainen ear pulse wave recording (performed as a part of the 24-hour Holter-type **Electrocardiogram**).

When performed: When suspected heart disease patients have a normal stress electrocardiogram; to check the effectiveness of certain drugs on the heart as well as to uncover toxic effects of other drugs; to follow the progress of patients who have heart attacks.

***Normal values*:** The left side of the heart should empty completely in less than 0.35 second; the pre-ejection period is even less.

***Abnormal values*:** Prolonged systolic time intervals are seen with heart valve disease, with damaged heart muscle (usually after a heart attack), and with heart damage caused by certain cancer-treating drugs.

***Risk factors*:** None.

***Pain/discomfort*:** None.

***Accuracy and significance*:** There is no unanimity of opinion about the most effective technique for measuring the heart's performance through systolic time intervals. Most radiologists prefer a form of **Nuclear Scanning,** while some cardiologists think the **Echocardiogram** is best. All agree, however, that systolic time intervals are a significant measurement of the heart's function, especially when the standard electrocardiogram is unrevealing and inconsistent with the doctor's suspicions.

T

TAY-SACHS DISEASE (Gangliosidosis)

Tay-Sachs disease is an inherited disorder that seems to occur primarily in Jewish people from Eastern Europe. (Its occurrence in those of non-Jewish origin is rare.) Children born with the disease have little or no active hexosaminidase enzyme, the lack of which causes fat to accumulate in the brain's ganglions (bundles of nerves). The consequences are mental retardation, paralysis, blindness, and cherry-red spots on the retina of the eye; the disorder is usually fatal before the child reaches the age of four. There are two tests for the disease. The first is a blood test, performed prior to pregnancy (on both parents), that helps detect carriers of the disease. The second, performed during pregnancy, is **Amniocentesis,** which can identify a fetus with the disease.

When performed: As a screening test for parents-to-be, especially among Central and Eastern European Jewish people (also known as Ashkenazi), who have a one-out-of-thirty chance of carrying the disease genes. Before or during pregnancy when there is even the remotest possibility that some distant forebear might have come from Eastern Europe or when a family member, no matter how remote the relationship, once had a child with a genetic defect.

Normal values: Evidence of the presence and activity of the enzyme hexosaminidase.

Abnormal values: Lack of any hexosaminidase enzyme, or decreased activity of the enzyme in a carrier.

Risk factors: Negligible for blood testing (see general risk factors for blood testing). See **Amniocentesis** if applicable.

Pain/discomfort: Minimal (see general pain/ discomfort factors for blood testing). See **Amniocentesis** if applicable.

Accuracy and significance: The test is considered extremely accurate in detecting carriers of the disease. A patient must inform the doctor or laboratory of the presence of diabetes, and diseases of the liver or pancreas, as these conditions, along with pregnancy and the use of birth control pills, require a modification of the test procedure for accuracy. The obvious significance is to identify those couples who run the risk of bearing a child with the disease.

TESTIS FUNCTION

There are several different tests to determine if the testicles (male gonads) are functioning normally (also see **Semen**). Two tests in particular indicate whether the tests are performing their two basic functions: producing the male hormone testosterone and producing sperm. One is the direct measurement of testosterone in blood plasma or in the urine; the other is measurement of gonadotropin (chorionic gonadotropin) in both the blood and the urine.

Testosterone is also manufactured in small amounts in the liver and by the adrenal glands (women normally produce a very small amount of testosterone in their ovaries and adrenals). Thus testosterone testing is not an absolute measurement of testicle function; however, it is a reasonable approximation. Testosterone is the hormone responsible for secondary sex characteristics such as hair distribution, voice pitch, hip configuration, and muscle development (primary sex characteristics are the sex organs themselves).

In the past, the 17-ketosteroid (17-KS) test was used to evaluate testis function. It has since been learned that almost all 17 ketosteroids come from the adrenal glands and not the testicles, as was once believed; thus the test is no longer a measure of male organ activity.

Human chorionic gonadotropin (HCG) measurements in the urine seem to be the most significant indicator of testicular activity. Gonadotropin measured in blood taken from a vein is a confirmatory test. The measurement of human chorionic gonadotropin is also used to determine if a woman is pregnant (see **Pregnancy**).

When performed: Whenever a tumor of the reproductive glands (testis or ovaries), adrenal glands, pituitary gland, or hypothalamus is suspected; whenever congenital (inherited) sex defects are being considered; with hypogonadism (testicles that do not function adequately or failure of the testicles to descend), a condition that is usually not detectable until after puberty and at times until 21 years of age; with suspected prostate trouble; with **Impotence;** as a possible indication of heart disease. Increased testosterone levels in women may explain hirsutism (excessive body hair) from ovarian tumors.

Normal values: Serum or plasma testosterone averages from 500 to 1,200 ng per 100 ml in men and from 25 to 50 ng per 100 ml in women. Men usually excrete up to 200 mcg in the urine every 24 hours; women and children excrete no more than 10 mcg per 24 hours. There should be no measureable gonadotropins in the blood or urine of men or women (except during pregnancy). At times, a 24-hour specimen of urine may contain from 5 to 50 mouse-uterine units of pituitary gonadotropins. (The test is measured by an increase in the weight of the mouse uterus after the mouse has been injected with the human specimen; pituitary gonadotropins are slightly different from chorionic gonadotropins.)

Abnormal values: Testosterone levels are decreased in hypogonadism and indicate inadequate or absent testis function such as can be caused by alcohol and many other drugs. Urine and blood pituitary gonadotropin levels are increased when hypogonadism originates in the testicle rather than the pituitary gland or hypothalamus. They are usually decreased when hypogonadism is caused by pituitary problems. Chorionic gonadotropins are increased with testicular tumors. Low testosterone levels, only in conjunction with elevated estradiol (female hormone) levels, have been implicated in susceptibility to heart disease (see **Estrogen**). Severe dieting can elevate testosterone levels.

Risk factors: Negligible (see general risk factors for blood testing).

Pain/discomfort: Minimal (see general pain/discomfort factors for blood testing).

Accuracy and significance: Although measurements of testosterone and HCG are fairly precise, abnormal values are not significant for specific diseases. However, they help to narrow the diagnostic possibilities to abnormal endocrine gland dysfunction.

THERMOGRAPHY

Thermography measures the slightest variations in temperature of soft tissue in the body using infrared heat sensors. The technique is often used in mammography (breast examination) to detect any growth in the breast (the mass will have a different temperature from other breast tissue). Today there is a specially constructed bra connected to a measuring device that, when it is worn for 10 to 15 minutes, can reveal differences in temperature on a graph. Thermography may also be used on an extremity, particularly the leg, to help diagnose a thrombus (clot) in a vein. The inflammation usually associated with the thrombus raises the temperature in the area of the clot. Measuring temperature changes of the penis, especially after showing a patient sexually stimulating illustrations, can help differentiate physical from psychological **Impotence.** The area of the body to be tested is usually placed on a heat-detection device that reacts to specific temperatures, either by color changes or a direct display of temperatures.

When performed: To aid in diagnosing breast masses; when thrombus is suspected; when other vascular conditions exist such as arterial circulation deficiencies, either from a nerve problem or as a direct defect (blood clot); to ascertain skin and adjacent tissue status (as in instances of possible gangrene).

Normal values: There are no strict normal values except in relation to other tissue; temperature response should reflect the type of tissue and the blood supply of the tissue being tested.

Abnormal values: Any unexpected change in tissue temperature in relation to surrounding tissue is considered abnormal.

Risk factors: None.

Pain/discomfort: None.

Accuracy and significance: Many doctors believe breast thermography is more accurate than X-ray mammography for the diagnosis of breast cancers. Up to 70 percent of breast cancers will show an abnormal heat pattern. When used on other parts of the body the test's chief value is as a support to other examinations.

THORACENTESIS

Thoracentesis is the removal of fluid from the space around the lungs. Normally no fluid is present. When evidence of fluid is found, usually after **Radiography** (X-ray) or **Ultrasound** testing of the chest, a small needle is inserted between the ribs (the X-ray shows exactly where) and the liquid is removed for further study to isolate bacteria, to look for blood cells, to perform a **Cytology** test and to perform various chemical tests for enzymes, glucose, and proteins. Because coughing can cause difficulty, a cough-suppressant medicine is usually given to the patient just prior to the test. At times, thoracentesis is also performed to remove large amounts of fluid and thus make breathing easier. Afterward, another chest X-ray is taken to make sure the lung did not collapse as a result of the test.

Paracentesis is the removal of fluid from the peritoneal cavity (the sac in the abdomen that holds the intestines). Normally, an accumulation of fluid does not exist in the peritoneal cavity, but when it does (called ascites), it indicates disease. A needle is inserted through the abdominal wall and the fluid withdrawn. Studies similar to thoracentesis are performed; ascites usually results from cancer, liver disease, and infections.

When performed: Whenever a patient has breathing difficulties; when a chest X-ray shows fluid around the lungs; when chest infection, fungus, or cancer is suspected; with heart or kidney failure causing edema; in certain forms of arthritis and rheumatoid disease; in certain bleeding-tendency diseases.

Normal values: There should be no measurable amount of fluid in the lung area.

Abnormal values: Any amount of fluid, called an effusion, is abnormal. Very low glucose levels in pleural (lung) fluid indicate rheumatoid diseases. Increased white blood cells in the fluid are found with cancer and infections. Increased **Lactic Dehydrogenase** (LDH) is almost always found with lung cancer. Increased **Amylase** suggests disease of the pancreas. Increased protein usually signifies an infectious or hemorrhagic process. Decreased protein usually indicates heart, kidney, or liver failure.

Risk factors: See general risk factors for catheter and needle insertion. When performing thoracentesis, especially when testing for fluid around the heart, the needle must be connected to an electrocardiograph in order to observe that the needle does not touch the heart.

Pain/discomfort: See general pain/discomfort factors for catheter and needle insertion.

Accuracy and significance: The test is quite accurate as the presence of any fluid is a positive indication of disease. It is not always significant enough, however, to diagnose a specific disease condition.

THYROID FUNCTION

There are a great many ways to assess how the thyroid gland is functioning. The primary tests consist of measuring the amounts of triiodothyronine (T_3) and thyroxine (T_4), both of which comprise the thyroid hormone. The hormone is made by the thyroid gland from tyrosine (an amino acid from protein) and iodine (which can enter the body through the skin and lungs as well as by diet). T_3 is four times as powerful as T_4, and only about half as much T_3 as T_4 is made each day. It is believed that T_3 is the "true" thyroid hormone, while T_4 may be a precursor of it.

Thyroid hormone is essential for normal growth and development, control of oxygen metabolism (energy), and production of other hormones such as the sex hormones and insulin. Thyroid hormone components are usually bound to serum proteins but unbound, or free T_4, is sometimes measured; free T_4 parallels T_4 except when certain drugs (oral contraceptives) are taken. T_3 and T_4 concentrations are measured directly in the serum. T_3 is also measured by its "uptake" (T_3U), which also shows how much thyroxine is already bound to serum proteins. A reverse T_3 test (rT_3) to detect a third thyroid hormone can be performed to determine if an abnormal thyroid function finding might come from drugs or a serious illness unrelated to thyroid function. Another commonly performed test of thyroid function is thyroxine-binding globulin (TBG), a measure of the major serum proteins to which T_3 and T_4 attach themselves. At least two different tests must be performed to understand the specific cause of thyroid disease so that appropriate treatment may be prescribed.

Other thyroid function tests that may be performed, usually when the tests described above are not conclusive, include the long-acting thyroid stimulator test (LATS), performed on babies whose mothers have thyroid disease, and various tests to detect thyroid autoantibodies (antithyroglobulin antibody, or ATA, and thyroid microsomal antibody, or TMA), which are produced when the thyroid gland acts as if it were infected and the body's immune protection system turns against itself in response. When cancer or nodules are suspected, a radioactive iodine screening test is performed (see **Nuclear Scanning**).

In the thyroid stimulation test (TSH), the patient is given pituitary gland thyroid-stimulating hormone; by observing its effect on the thyroid, the physician can determine if thyroid problems are coming from the pituitary gland rather than the thyroid itself. An older test, rarely used today, is the protein-bound iodine (PBI), which essentially measures thyroxine (T_4) amounts (but not as accurately as the newer direct T_4 measurements). The simplest routine chemical confirmation test of thyroid function is **Cholesterol.**

The Basal Metabolic Rate (BMR), one of the first tests devised for thyroid function, is based on a different measurement principle from the usual thyroid function tests (oxygen consumption rather than measurement of chemicals in the blood). The BMR is used when the more sophisticated thyroid function tests cannot be performed (for example, when laboratory facilities are not available or when the patient has taken, or been in contact with, too much iodine to allow proper chemical measurement).

In the Achilles reflex (ankle-jerk) test, or photomotography, the heel tendon that moves the foot downward is struck with a rubber hammer. The force of the reflex activity of the foot and the time it takes the tendon to react are considered measures of thyroid gland activity.

The neonatal hypothyroidism test measures the amount of thyroid hormone in the newborn infant. Diagnosis of cretinism at birth allows treatment to prevent one form of mental retardation.

Blood is taken from a vein for the chemical tests and the serum is tested. Certain tests may be performed by using a drop of blood from the fingertip or earlobe. The tests can give false values if the patient has had any sort of iodine test in the six previous months (gallbladder X-rays, kidney X-rays; bronchograms, etc., using contrast dye) or has had excessive iodine in the diet for the previous month. Previous radioactive tracer tests can also cause erroneous results. Some thyroid function tests (PBI, radioactive iodine) may be performed on urine, saliva, and feces.

When performed: Whenever there is a suspicion of a thyroid disorder; when other hormone disease is suspected; in all cases of depression; to follow the progress of treatment of thyroid disease; to screen newborn children for cretinism or congenital hypothyroidism that can cause mental retardation, nerve problems, and growth inhibition. Almost all states require such testing at birth; the exceptions are: Arkansas, Delaware, Hawaii, Iowa, Michigan, New Hampshire, North Carolina, South Carolina, South Dakota and Vermont. Many states do not enforce the law when parents object.

Normal values:

Free T_3: 100 to 250 ng per 100 ml
rT_3: 30 to 60 ng per 100 ml
T_3U: 25% to 35%
T_4: 2.8 to 6.4 mcg per 100 ml
Free T_4: 3 to 5 ng per 100 ml
TBG: 10 to 26 mcg of T_4 per 100 ml
PBI: 3.5 to 8.5 mcg per 100 ml

LATS and thyroid antibodies are not normally present in the serum. Radioactive iodine uptake should range from 10% to 20% in the first hour and no more than 50% in 24 hours.

Abnormal values: Hyperthyroidism (Graves' disease, thyrotoxicosis, toxic goiter) usually shows increased T_3, T_4, radioactive iodine, and PBI, low cholesterol values, a normal amount of TBG, and low TSH. Hypothyroidism (goiter, cretinism, pituitary disorder) usually shows decreased T_3, T_4, radioactive iodine, and PBI, and high cholesterol values, an increased amount of TBG, and an elevated TSH. Thyroiditis (inflammation of the gland) may exist with hyperthyroidism or hypothyroidism, and the tests reflect the way the thyroid is (or is not) functioning. Tumors of the thyroid (cancers, cysts) may also alter the tests, depending on how the growth affects function. Certain drugs such as estrogens and contraceptive pills will increase T_4, TBG, and PBI. Male hormones and other steroid drugs, as well as Dilantin, will cause low T_4, TBG, and PBI. While T_4 changes with some drug use, free T_4 stays normal. Pregnancy can cause false abnormal values such as elevated T_3, T_4, and TBG. Chronic kidney disease causes low T_3, T_4, and TBG along with an elevated T_3U. Excessive exposure to iodine increases PBI and decreases the radioactive iodine uptake. The taking of thyroid preparations usually increases all values. Large doses of aspirin, antiarthritic drugs, and anticoagulant drugs can alter thyroid function tests.

Risk factors: Negligible (see general risk factors for blood testing).

Pain/discomfort: Minimal (see general pain/discomfort factors for blood testing).

Accuracy and significance: Most doctors believe more than one abnormal thyroid function test must be made to help diagnose thyroid dysfunction. They also find the most accurate single screening test for overall thyroid function is the serum free thyroxin (T_4); the most sensitive test for hyperthyroidism (over-active thyroid gland) is the triiodothyronine (T_3); and, the most sensitive test for hypothyroidism (underactive thyroid gland) is the thyroid-stimulating hormone test (TSH). Furthermore, the majority of doctors believe that thyroid function tests have no real significance in patients without two or more clinical signs of thyroid disease (heart intolerance, tremor, dry skin, hair loss, changes in heart rhythm). Thyroid function tests are positive in less than half of one percent of those patients without signs and symptoms. The remaining thyroid function tests are merely more sophisticated measurements to confirm or support a diagnosis.

TONOMETRY

Tonometry is the specific measurement of the intraocular pressure (pressure of the fluid within the eyeball). It is used primarily to test for glaucoma, although there are rare instances of intraocular hypertension without glaucoma. Most glaucoma is of the chronic open-angle type, which does not occur until late in life and can usually be treated medically. The usual symptoms of glaucoma are poor vision (blurring), usually in only one eye at first, followed by gradual restriction of the **Visual Field.**

A Schiotz tonometer is placed on the pupil after a drop of anesthetic has been applied to the eye, and a gauge records the resistance of the eye to the slight pressure applied. The tonometer translates the resistance into millimeters (mm) of mercury (Hg). The procedure is similar to applying a contact lens to the eye. In another technique, called applanation, a drop of dye is placed on the eye and the slight pressure is applied and measured while the eye is observed through a special microscope. Tonometry should always be performed in a cool, dark room or false negative values will be recorded, missing the patient with glaucoma.

When the routine test result is equivocal, procedures to increase eye pressure are performed. In the water provocative test, the patient drinks a full quart of water at one time; the intraocular pressure is measured 30, 45, and 60 minutes later. If the pressure rises more than 8 mm Hg during that time, glaucoma is a reasonable diagnosis. In tonography, constant, gentle pressure is applied to the eye (using a special tonometer) for four minutes; the pressure should cause a decrease in the measured tension in normal individuals. If it does not decrease, glaucoma is the most likely diagnosis.

The Seidel test places the patient in a dark room for one hour. An increase in eye pressure during that time means that the ocular fluid does not escape when the pupils are dilated, as it normally should. A somewhat similar test is performed by dropping the drug homatropine into the eye. Homatropine causes the pupil to dilate. After an hour the eye is checked for any increase in pressure; an increase indicates glaucoma.

When performed: Tonometry is routinely performed on individuals over 40 years of age and on younger people whenever there is any vision difficulty (especially blurring) or any history of glaucoma in the family. It is also performed after any eye infection, after eye injury, with diabetes, and when there are thyroid problems.

Normal values: Normally the intraocular pressure measures between 10 and 20 mm Hg. Many physicians, through experience, can place fingers over the closed eye and the bony ridge above the eye and accurately detect normal intraocular pressure (less than 20 mm Hg).

Abnormal values: Lower than normal intraocular pressure (less than 10 mm/Hg) is rare and is usually due to an infection or sometimes follows surgery. A false lower value may occur in patients taking diuretics. Repeated pressure readings between 20 and 30 mm Hg (these readings must be taken several times; one or two tests are insufficient for diagnosis) indicate ocular hypertension and a presumption of glaucoma. Readings greater than 30 mm/Hg are almost always diagnostic of glaucoma, especially when accompanied by certain changes in visual field. Many drugs can cause increased intraocular pressure, which can then lead to glaucoma. Drugs that dilate the pupils, steroids, anticholinergics (such as used for bowel and bladder relaxation), antidepressants, antihistamines, muscle relaxants, and oral contraceptives are particularly dangerous, especially with patients who have a family history of glaucoma.

Risk factors: There is the possibility of scratching the surface of the eye should the test be performed carelessly but this happens very rarely. There is also the remote possibility of an eye infection should the instrument not be absolutely sterile.

Pain/discomfort: Although the eye is usually anesthetized prior to testing, many patients find the touching of the eyeball quite uncomfortable.

Accuracy and significance: Any one of the tonometry tests is sufficiently accurate to help detect glaucoma. The tests, when performed at regular intervals, are particularly significant as they can detect glaucoma before it seriously affects vision.

TORCH

TORCH is not a specific test but an acronym for a group of blood tests performed on a pregnant woman and/or a newborn child to ascertain the presence of antibodies to five conditions: **Toxoplasmosis, Rubella** (German measles), **Cytomegalovirus,** and **Herpes** Simplex virus I and II. These infections are known to cause a variety of physical and mental impairments in babies—blindness, blood abnormalities, deafness, enlargement of the spleen, hepatitis, mental retardation and other birth defects. The principle of the tests is related to **Agglutination, Complement Fixation,** and fluorescent antibody studies.

TOURNIQUET TEST FOR VARICOSE VEINS

The varicose vein incompetency tests are performed to determine if leg varicosities are caused by diseases of the deep veins as opposed to problems of the superficial veins (which can be seen on the surface). The patient's leg is elevated to empty the veins, and a tourniquet is applied in various areas (above and below the knee, thigh, and calf). The patient stands (Trendelenburg test) and/or walks (Perthes test), and the leg is observed to ascertain how long it takes for the superficial veins to fill.

When performed: When varicose veins cause fatigue and discomfort; when there is lower-leg dermatitis or ulcer; to discover whether the varicosities are from some condition other than vein disease (such as pregnancy or abdominal tumor); when surgery is anticipated on the surface veins (to ascertain that after surgery the deep veins will be competent, or able to carry blood).

Normal values: When the deep veins are normal, the superficial veins fill 30 seconds after the leg is lowered (with the tourniquet still in place).

Abnormal values: If, when the leg is lowered and the veins fill immediately, the connecting veins between the deep and superficial systems are not adequate, surgery will be deemed to be of no help. If, while the tourniquet is on, there is cramping or immediate filling while walking, there will probably be no benefit from surgery.

Risk factors: None.

Pain/discomfort: None.

Accuracy and significance: The tests are quite accurate in helping a doctor diagnose the cause of varicose veins; they are particularly significant in predicting the success of surgery.

TOXOCARIASIS

The larvae of the common roundworm of the dog, whose scientific name is Toxocara canis, produces the disease called toxocariasis, also called visceral larva migrans (VLM) because the worm larvae migrate throughout the body (to the brain, eyes, heart, kidneys, liver, lungs, intestines). Generally the infestation is found in young children who play on the ground, in grass, or in dirt where dogs, especially puppies, defecate. The animals' feces can contain the eggs of the worms, which contaminate the ground. When the child plays in the area and puts his fingers in his mouth the eggs enter the digestive system, become larvae, and subsequently infect the child's organs. The most common symptoms are a pneumonia-like illness, sometimes imitating asthma, an enlarged liver, and an extremely elevated number of white blood cells called eosinophiles (see **Blood Cell Differential**). The symtoms can last for years before being diagnosed; the disease can cause nerve damage, blindness, and even death. Until recently, it was extremely difficult to diagnose toxocariasis; at the very least it required a liver **Biopsy.** Now there is an ELISA, a test similar to **Agglutination,** which can prove the diagnosis when the untoward symptoms appear. Blood from a vein is tested.

When performed: Whenever a patient, particularly a very young child, has a chronic cough, recurrent fever, and the neurological signs associated with an enlarged liver. In patients with an extremely high eosinophile-type white blood cell count that cannot be explained. In children whose symptoms imitate asthma but do not respond to the asthma treatment.

Normal values: No antigen-antibody reaction to the worm eggs should be noted.

Abnormal values: Evidence of antibody reaction with a titer greater than 1,000 (a positive reaction in a very weak, dilute solution).

Risk factors: Negligible (see general risk factors for blood testing).

Pain/discomfort: Minimal (see general pain/discomfort factors for blood testing).

Accuracy and significance: The test has been shown to be at least 90 percent accurate when tested on those suspected of having the disease. It is particularly significant now that the infestation is known to be more prevalent than once believed. It is also valuable as an aid in identifying other eye problems that imitate toxocariasis. Furthermore, it can help to differentiate among other worm infestations, such as those from dog hookworms, which enter the body through the feet and migrate to the lungs and intestines.

TOXOPLASMOSIS

Toxoplasmosis is an infection caused by a parasite. A number of doctors consider it the most common infectious disease, although another parasitic infestation, *Giardiosis,* is as common. For unexplained reasons the domestic cat is the primary source of the microorganism, and infected cats, while showing no symptoms of the condition, will still excrete the parasite in their feces. Should people or animals have contact with contaminated ground, they too can become infected. Raw or partially cooked meat from infected animals—steak tartare for example—can also transmit the disease. (Sufficient cooking kills the parasite.) Symptoms and signs include nerve and muscle damage, lymph gland swelling, eye problems, and heart muscle damage. The most serious complication comes when a pregnant woman contracts the disease, shows no symptoms, and passes it on to her fetus. The consequences include spontaneous abortion, stillbirth, or a child born with the disease and all its complications, including encephalitis or physical birth defects. Tests to detect the disease include **Complement Fixation,** fluorescent antibody (see **Agglutination**), and the Sabin-Feldman Dye test performed on blood taken from a vein.

When performed: As part of the **TORCH** screening panel for pregnant women and newborn infants; when the disease is suspected because of specific unexplainable symptoms (especially those pertaining to the eye, brain, or heart); when a condition resembling infectious mononucleosis (persistent lymph gland swelling) remains undiagnosed.

Normal values: Ideally no antibodies should be detected; however, because hundreds of millions of people have had some contact with the parasite, small amounts of antibodies can be considered "normal." Therefore, a low antibody titer can be considered within normal limits. It is also considered normal when the measurable antibodies do not increase over a period of time.

Abnormal values: Usually a titer of 1:256 or more (the higher the titer value, the more antibodies present); titers greater than 1:1,000 are believed to signify active disease. A rise in antibody titers over a period of months, especially in the newborn.

Risk factors: Negligible (see general risk factors for blood testing).

Pain/discomfort: Minimal (see general pain/discomfort factors for blood testing),

Accuracy and significance: Extremely accurate in the detection of antibodies. The significance of the test is not quite as high because of the variation in titers found in numbers of people, and because different manifestations of the disease produce a broad range of titer levels. The most significant observation is of a child or pregnant woman whose negative titer is suddenly positive; a negative test (a failure to detect any antibodies) usually indicates a lack of the toxoplasma parasite. The Sabin-Feldman test, considered the most accurate, is rarely performed today except in special laboratories because of the dangers to laboratory personnel of working with a live antigen—which is what makes that test so precise.

TUNING FORK

Tuning forks are metal instruments that vibrate when struck, giving off a pure tone of a predetermined number of cycles per second (cps). They are commonly used to tune pianos or other musical instruments. In medicine, tuning forks are used primarily to measure the ability to hear sounds by both air and bone conduction (see **Hearing Function**); they are also used to measure bone conduction sensitivity in other parts of the body as part of a neurological examination. The base of the vibrating tuning fork is placed against a bone area (elbows, knees, ankles) and the sensation is noted by the patient as well as the equalness of the sensation on opposite sides of the body. There are five basic tuning fork tests for hearing.

Weber: The base of the vibrating tuning fork is placed in the center of the forehead at the hairline, and the patient is asked if he hears the tone better in one ear than the other. Normally the tone is heard equally in both ears.

Rinné: The tuning fork is vibrated and placed next to each ear opening (for air conduction) and then against the mastoid bone behind the ear (for bone conduction) to see which tone is heard longer. Normally the tone will be heard much longer via air conduction (through the ear canal).

Schwabach: The physician vibrates the tuning fork and compares his perception of the tone with that of the patient. Assuming the doctor has normal hearing, the perceptions should be about the same.

Stenger: With the patient blindfolded, two tuning forks of the same tone are vibrated about an inch from each ear at the same time. The forks are then moved away from the ears. Normally the tone is heard in each ear from similar distances. If one ear is bad, the tuning fork will not be heard when it is placed close to that ear.

Teal: When a patient says he cannot hear the tuning fork via air conduction, the Rinné test is again performed with the patient blindfolded. On the second trial, a nonvibrating fork is placed against the bone behind the ear and a second, vibrating fork is held a short distance away from that ear. If the patient is really deaf, he will not hear the tone; if he is simulating deafness, he will claim to hear the tone, although he is really hearing the second tuning fork.

When performed: To test hearing function, nerve function, bone conduction; to detect malingering.

Normal values: Each tuning fork test should be felt or heard equally on both sides of the body. Normal, or expected results for each hearing test are described above.

Abnormal values: Whenever the vibrations of a tuning fork are not felt or heard, or where one side of the body perceives the vibrations differently from the other side. Abnormal values for specific hearing tests are described above.

Risk factors: None.

Pain/discomfort: None.

Accuracy and significance: The tests are of major value in helping to identify the part of the body that might have nerve problems. Then too, the combination of all the tuning fork tests is of great significance in arriving at the cause of ear problems. The Teal test is of value in recognizing malingerers.

TYPING AND CROSS-MATCHING (Blood Grouping)

Typing and cross-matching are performed to determine a person's blood type. Blood may be typed according to the common

A, B, AB, and O groups (called the ABO system), the Rh positive and Rh negative groups (called the Rh system, which now has many additional subgroups), the MNS's system, or the Kell system. There are nearly 100 known blood group systems at present. Typing is essentially an **Agglutination** procedure to search for certain antibodies in the blood.

When a transfusion is prescribed by a doctor (usually after severe blood loss or during surgery), knowledge of the type of blood of both the donor and the recipient is not enough. Donor blood may be labeled as the same type as that of the patient, but the two must be specifically cross-matched (mixed) to prevent an incompatible transfusion, which causes hemolysis (destruction of the red blood cells) and can be fatal. Most commonly the donor's red blood cells (which contain the antigens or agglutinating-precipitating factor) are tested for any possible reaction to the patient's serum (which contains the antibodies or response to agglutinating-precipitating factor). At times, the blood may also be tested for sickle cells prior to transfusion. Because of the number and variety of blood type groups and subgroups, the test is one of the first to be performed in **Disputed Parentage** cases.

When performed: The test is performed whenever a blood transfusion is prescribed. A patient about to have surgery will often have his blood typed and cross-matched with potential donors well ahead of time. In **Disputed Parentage** cases.

Normal values: There should be no evidence of agglutination or hemolysis when the blood of the donor and the recipient are mixed.

Abnormal values: Any evidence of agglutination when the two different blood samples are mixed indicates incompatibility.

Risk factors: Negligible (see general risk factors for blood testing).

Pain/discomfort: Minimal (see general pain/discomfort factors for blood testing).

Accuracy and significance: Blood typing is an extremely accurate way to identify blood groups. Its particular significance, in addition to helping identify parentage, is in the matching of blood for transfusion. Every pint of blood used in a transfusion must precisely match the patient's blood. Even though two bloods might have the same ABO system and/or Rh system, they could still be of different subgroups. Imprecise matching of donor and recipient blood can bring on a transfusion reaction, which might prove fatal.

U

ULTRASOUND

Ultrasound is a diagnostic technique that uses sound waves to create a "picture" of certain areas of the body. The technique is similar to an X-ray, but without any of the dangers of radiation exposure (although the absolute safety of ultrasound is also being questioned). High-frequency sound waves (above the range of human hearing) are directed toward a body organ or cavity. The sound echoes back from the selected organ or tissue to form the "picture." The procedure is performed with a transducer (a microphonelike instrument that emits sounds and also detects the echo), which is touched to the body over the area to be studied. Before the transducer is used, a coating of mineral oil is applied to the skin to prevent any air from coming between the body and the instrument. The results may be reproduced in graphic form (resembling an electrocardiograph record) or as shadow illustrations; the latter are especially important for determining the exact location of the fetus during pregnancy (see **Amniocentesis**). The **Echocardiogram** also uses ultrasound as a measuring technique.

At times sound waves that are reflected back from moving objects (such as the heartbeat or blood flow through an artery or vein) show a change in frequency with changes in the speed of movement. This is called the "Doppler effect," and measurement is known as Doppler ultrasonography. Such tests are particularly valuable in discerning the heartbeat of the fetus and in measuring the arterial blood flow to and in the brain as a means of detecting and even preventing stroke. In cases of suspected deep-vein thrombosis (see **Plethysmography**), the tests can sometimes ascertain whether blood is easily flowing through the vein or is blocked by a clot.

With recent developments in ultrasound techniques, the illustrations produced can, in many instances, achieve similar results to **Computerized Tomography** without the hazards of X-ray and at a lower cost. For example, ultrasound scanning can show up a mass in the abdomen (liver, gallbladder, spleen, pancreas, kidney); of even greater value, it can show if the mass is cystic (containing fluid, such as an abscess) or solid (tumor). Lesions only an inch in size can be detected by ultrasonography. An echoencephalogram (brain scan by ultrasound) can show if there are any tumors or other masses (clots or hemorrhages) in the brain. An eye sonogram can reveal pathology inside the eye when there is no other way of seeing inside (see **Fundoscopy**). The thyroid, prostate, and lymph glands may also be tested with ultrasound. An ultrasound scanner is portable and can be brought to the bedside of a patient too ill to move.

When performed: After head or abdominal injury; whenever a mass is suspected in the head or abdomen; whenever there is undiagnosed pain in the abdomen (ultrasound can at times substitute for exploratory surgery); with heart disease when the heartbeat can be observed in its entirety (to test heart valve function); to determine if there is any growth in a body organ; to diagnose prostate disease; to help locate deep-vein thrombosis; to reduce any risks that may accompany amniocentesis by helping to locate the exact position of the fetus and placenta; to detect ectopic (the fetus outside of the uterus) pregnancy.

Normal values: Body organs should appear normal in size and location, and show no evidence of pathology.

Abnormal values: As with several other tests, interpretation depends primarily on the physician's experience rather than on established standards.

Risk factors: None.

Pain/discomfort: None.

Accuracy and significance: Many doctors find ultrasound to be an excellent, safe, noninvasive means of detecting organ pathology. Various studies have shown ultrasound is 80 to 90 percent accurate in detecting internal pathology. The test is extremely valuable in outlining the fetus during pregnancy and helping to detect potential abnormalities.

UREA NITROGEN (Blood Urea Nitrogen, BUN)

Urea is produced primarily in the liver and is the main nitrogen end product of protein metabolism; it is eliminated by the kidneys into the urine. Normally there is very little urea in the blood. When kidney function is impaired by disease, the normal excretion of urea may be decreased and urea nitrogen in the blood (BUN) is therefore increased. Urea nitrogen varies with dietary protein intake. Blood is collected from a vein and the serum is examined. Urea nitrogen may also be measured in the urine.

When performed: When kidney disease is suspected; when there is an indication that urine production is blocked; when the patient displays mental confusion or disorientation; with evidence of increased pituitary activity (acromegaly); with heart failure; after excessive vomiting, diarrhea, or sweating.

Normal values: BUN normally ranges from 10 to 20 mg per 100 ml of blood. Urine urea is measured over a specific period of time and compared with blood urea to determine normal values.

Abnormal values: BUN is increased (over 30 mg per 100 ml) in kidney disease, fever, starvation (increased breakdown of body protein), internal bleeding, and with the taking of a number of drugs, including certain antibiotics, thiazides (diurectics), methyldopa, salicylates, and chloral hydrate. BUN is decreased in liver disease and with increased pituitary activity. At times, urine urea secretion will be low even if BUN is normal; this is an indication of kidney disease.

Risk factors: Negligible (see general risk factors for blood testing).

Pain/discomfort: Minimal (see general pain/discomfort factors for blood testing).

Accuracy and significance: As abnormal values occur in such a variety of conditions, the test serves merely as a rough screening test for kidney disease. It is not considered of enough significance to help in arriving at a specific diagnosis.

URIC ACID

Uric acid is an end product of the body's protein metabolism. The amount varies with certain diseases as well as with ingestion of foods such as sweetbreads, liver, anchovies, and sardines. Blood is collected from a vein and the serum is examined for uric acid levels. A 24-hour urine specimen may be collected for measuring uric acid excretion by the kidneys.

When performed: Primarily when there is suspicion of gout; to aid in the diagnosis of leukemia, toxemia of pregnancy, glycogen storage disease, Lesch-Nyhan syndrome (an inherited form of mental retardation), and other conditions where there is destruction of the body's cells.

Normal values: Normal serum uric acid ranges from 2 to 8 mg per 100 ml. Women and children usually have slightly lower values.

Abnormal values: Higher than normal values are usually found with gout, leukemia, heart disease, toxemia of pregnancy, pneumonia, severe kidney damage (which decreases excretion), glycogen storage disease, and Lesch-Nyhan syndrome. Eating certain foods and taking ascorbic acid, salicylates (such as aspirin), theophylline, or thiazides (diuretics) can also increase values. Lower than normal values are usually found in patients taking coumarin products (anticoagulants) and piperazine (worm medicine).

Risk factors: Negligible (see general risk factors for blood testing).

Pain/discomfort: Minimal (see general pain/discomfort factors for blood testing).

Accuracy and significance: Although this is the basic screening test for gout, it is not significant enough to allow a specific diagnosis of the disease. Furthermore, there are so many foods and drugs that can raise and lower blood uric acid levels that the test is generally repeated several times once the patient is on a special diet and no longer taking the medication that interferes with the test.

URINARY TRACT CALCULUS

When a stone or calculus (plural: calculi) appears anywhere in the urinary tract (from kidney to bladder), it is essential to analyze the stone to identify its composition. If the primary ingredient of a kidney stone can be determined (identification is possible only in about half of all cases), proper treatment can be started much sooner. Stones may come from eating an excessive amount of food high in **Calcium** and **Oxalates,** metabolic problems, dehydration, excessive vitamin D intake, excessive bed rest, **Parathyroid** gland problems and many other conditions. Nephrocalcinosis (stone formation limited to the kidney) is sometimes visualized by X-ray examination, but in most instances diagnosis is made by identification of the type of crystals in the urine.

When performed: When abdominal, back, or groin pain cannot be diagnosed; when there is evidence of blood in the urine; when the amount of urine is decreased.

Normal values: Normally no crystals should be seen in a microscopic examination of freshly passed urine (at times, certain proteins may crystalize when the urine has cooled to room temperature).

Abnormal values: Pathological crystals have uniquely identifiable shapes and colors. Those that can reflect disease include calcium oxalate (the most common), calcium phosphate, uric acid (not always due to gout), cystine (see **Aminoaciduria**), and tyrosine (usually associated with liver disease). The presence of urinary tract stones more often represents a metabolic or inherited disease than kidney pathology.

Risk factors: None.

Pain/discomfort: None.

Accuracy and significance: Analysis of a kidney stone quite accurately reveals the stone's chemical makeup. The test is significant in that once the stone's chemical composition is identified, appropriate therapy can be given and preventive measures undertaken.

URINE EXAMINATION

Many urine tests are described under the names of the blood tests that usually accompany them (see, for example, **Albumin/ Globulin; Glucose; Phenylketonuria**). Urine is one of many waste products that indicate the general health of the body in addition to being a specific measure of kidney function. A routine, or screening urine examination usually consists of tests for specific gravity (concentration of solids), protein (albumin), and sugar (glucose); microscopic examination for bacteria, parasites, chemical crystals, and casts (solid matter made up of bacteria, blood cells, pus, protein, etc.); and examination for acid or alkaline reaction, color, odor, and transparency. Many doctors feel the test for protein in the urine is the best single indicator of kidney disease. A new test is the nitrite test, which can give a rapid indication of bacterial infection anywherc in the urinary tract.

The Addis count is a test of urine sediment to determine the amount of protein and the number of red blood cells, white blood cells, casts, and epithelial cells in a 12-hour urine specimen. The Addis count is elevated in kidney disease.

Approximately 2 ounces (50 ml) of urine is collected, preferably from an early morning specimen, which contains materials excreted by the kidneys during the night and will usually be of less volume (more concentrated, higher in specific gravity). If the patient drinks an excessive amount of fluids, the amount of urine will increase automatically and the specific gravity will be reduced. Today, most urine tests are performed by dipping a multi-chemically-coated paper in the urine, allowing up to ten separate urine examinations to be performed simultaneously.

When performed: As a routine screening test to determine kidney function; when liver disease is suspected; as a measure of any disorder of the urinary, cardiovascular, and metabolic systems.

Normal values: Urine should range in color from yellow to light amber and should be clear or transparent. It is normal for early morning urine to have a spicy odor and to be slightly acid. On microscopic examination an occasional red or white blood cell may be seen; the appearance of a few casts after strenuous exercise is still considered normal. Normal specific gravity ranges from 1.010 to 1.025, with a reading toward the higher limit in an early morning specimen.

Abnormal values: With liver disease, certain anemias, melanoma (a form of skin cancer), and excessive intake of vitamins, the urine may have a greenish or brownish tint. A reddish or brownish tint usually indicates the presence of blood.

Whenever the urine is not clear or transparent, more often than not it contains pus, bacteria, blood and/or chemical crystals. **Gonorrhea** usually causes long, thin, whitish shreds to appear in the urine.

Urine that has an ammonia odor is almost always indicative of some disease condition that causes excessive urine to be retained in the bladder. A sweet or fruity odor is indicative of a dangerous stage of diabetes mellitus.

While the urine normally has a very slight acid reaction, the degree of acidity may increase with kidney disease, heart disease, and diarrhea (from any cause). An alkaline reaction may be seen with certain anemias or various infections and after prolonged vomiting.

Risk factors: None.

Pain/discomfort: None.

Accuracy and significance: Urine examination is one of the simplest and most effective ways to help diagnose a variety of diseases. Even though it is not a diagnostic test for specific diseases, it is probably the most significant medical test for overall health screening.

UROBILINOGEN

Urobilinogen comes from bilirubin (a yellow pigment found in bile and after the normal breakdown of red blood cells). The urine normally contains small amounts of urobilinogen, but in certain disease conditions (anemias, liver damage, certain infections) the urobilinogen level in the urine increases. Maximum excretion of urobilinogen usually occurs between one and three in the afternoon. A 2-hour specimen, or a 24-hour sample, may be required for examination. The test is also performed on feces.

When performed: When there is suspicion of gallbladder or biliary tract obstruction; with blood or liver problems.

Normal values: One Erlich unit per 100 ml is considered normal in a 2-hour collection of urine preferably collected between

1 and 3 P.M. In a 24-hour sample, excretion of 1 to 4 mg is within the normal range.

Abnormal values: Increased amounts of urobilinogen are found with liver damage and hemolytic anemia. Ingestion of salicylates (such as aspirin) will cause the results of the test to be falsely elevated. Decreased urobilinogen is found in obstructive jaundice. Ingestion of antibiotics may cause the results to be falsely lowered.

Risk factors: None.

Pain/discomfort: None.

Accuracy and significance: The test is primarily used as confirmation when particular anemias are suspected. It is also used to help distinguish between obstructive jaundice (gallstone) and non-obstructive jaundice (liver disease). The test is of no great significance.

V

VASOPRESSIN

Vasopressin is a hormone produced in the hypothalamus area of the brain (the part of the brain that translates such stimuli as light, sound, pain, body reactions to the time of day, body positions—especially discomfort—and virtually any emotional excitation into physical, nerve, or hormonal action). It is also known as the antidiuretic hormone (ADH) because it seems to work with the kidney to prevent the body from excreting fluids as urine. In other words, the more vasopressin produced, the more water the body retains, even to the point of edema. When excessive vasopressin is secreted for no reason that can be ascertained, the condition is known as the Syndrome of Inappropriate Antidiuretic

Hormone Secretion (SIADH). On rare occasions certain cancers, injuries, and drugs will increase vasopressin production; more frequently, however, it is emotional upset, apprehension, and anger that cause the increase. In turn the body shows its retention of water through puffiness in the feet and ankles and especially in the face and under the eyes.

Another vasopressin-related disease is diabetes insipidus, in which the patients drink liquids almost incessantly—a condition called polydipsia—while at the same time suffering from polyuria—a condition forcing patients to urinate so constantly they excrete about ten quarts a day. In this case, either there is insufficient vasopressin or the kidneys simply do not react to its presence. With diabetes insipidus, the urine's specific gravity, or amount of solid matter it contains, is very low.

Normally, if a patient takes diuretic drugs, the amount of vasopressin in the body increases as a reaction to the water loss. In addition, the **Osmolality** of the blood helps to control the production of vasopressin. (Generally the osmolality test and vasopressin test are performed concurrently.) Vasopressin is tested from a blood sample, usually obtained from a vein. It should be measured before and after the patient drinks large quantities of fluid for several days; it should also be measured after patients have been deprived of liquids for a prolonged period of time. At times, a patient is given intravenous salt solutions to gauge its effect on vasopressin production.

An interesting observation concerning one form of vasopressin is that when the drug was given to patients, their memories improved markedly and the cognitive benefits lasted for a month following treatment.

When performed: To help diagnose diabetes insipidus; to help diagnose persistent edema; to measure the intensity of certain emotions on the body; to ascertain the diuretic effect of certain drugs, especially lithium; after head injuries; to help diagnose some types of kidney disease.

Normal values: From 1 to 5 pg per ml; when osmolality is measured, the amount of vasopressin should correspond with the osmolality value (e.g., if osmolality is low, vasopressin levels should be about 1 or 2 pg per ml; when osmolality is high—as with water loss—vasopressin levels should be close to 10 pg per ml).

Abnormal values: A vasopressin level that does not accord with the osmolality level (a vasopressin level of 1 to 2 pg per ml when a patient is dehydrated and the osmolality level is high); no evidence of vasopressin with diabetes insipidus; an extremely elevated vasopressin level as a reaction to stress.

Risk factors: Negligible (see general risk factors for blood testing).

Pain/discomfort: Minimal (see general pain/discomfort factors for blood testing).

Accuracy and significance: This is a difficult test to perform. If the blood is not properly collected, stored, and transported to the laboratory, errors are common. In addition, vasopressin secretion is easily influenced by the patient's position (standing, sitting, or lying down), the patient's dietary habits, and, perhaps most importantly, the patient's emotional state at the time of blood collection. All such observations must be noted. In general, this is not a very accurate test; most often its significance is corroborated by other tests.

VENEREAL DISEASES

(This term is no longer used; tests used to aid in the identification of what are now called Sexually Transmitted Diseases include: **Chlamydia Identification; Cytomegalovirus; Gonorrhea; Hepatitis; Herpes; Syphilis;** and the **Torch** group.)

VISUAL ACUITY

Tests of visual acuity (or vision) measure the ability of each eye to perceive the size and shape of an object clearly at standard distances. The tests also measure the ability of both eyes, working together, to discern the distance and depth of objects and their relationship to one another (which object is nearer or further away), called stereopsis or depth perception.

The most common vision test uses the Snellen chart: the patient reads a series of unrelated letters or numbers of various sizes at a distance of 20 feet; for those who cannot read, the letter **E** is used in different sizes and positions (**E**, ш, m). A person with normal vision will easily designate a letter ⅜ inch high from 20 feet away; such visual acuity is recorded as 20/20. The largest letter on the Snellen chart is 3½ inches high; if this is the only letter that a patient can read at a distance of 20 feet, the visual acuity is recorded as 20/200 (reflecting the fact that someone with normal vision could read that letter 200 feet away). The legal definition of blindness is 20/200 vision or worse with the use of the most efficient corrective lens. Normal visual acuity is called emmetropia; a vision defect that can be corrected by the use of lenses is called ametropia.

Myopia, or nearsightedness, is a form of ametropia characterized by difficulty in seeing objects clearly at a distance (usually 20 feet) but being able to read or see objects close up. In hyperopia, sometimes called hypermetropia or farsightedness, patients can see objects clearly at a distance but have difficulty with reading or close work. In presbyopia, usually considered a form of hyperopia as a result of normal aging, the lens of the eye can no longer accommodate (change shape) to focus well on near as well as far objects. With astigmatism, the eye cannot focus properly in certain planes. For example, a person might be able to distinguish all the numbers on a clock except those that are on a line from 11 to 5. Anisometropia is characterized by a difference in visual acuity of the two eyes. This can become a serious problem in children if the eye with the worst vision is not used (amblyopia). Failure to use one eye (sometimes called "lazy eye") can cause **Strabismus,** where the eye no longer focuses on an object and strays outward or inward (cross-eyes). In aphakia, the lens of the eye is absent.

The standard method of vision testing is to have the patient read an eye chart, using trial lenses of different strengths (called refraction) at a distance of 20 feet. Retinoscopy is a much more objective way to test vision, especially with children; it measures the precise way light focuses on the retina in the back of the eye. There are also electronic devices (used mostly by schools, industry, and motor vehicle departments) that can detect most vision problems within minutes. (The Snellen wall chart is best for myopia, but it can easily miss other forms of ametropia.) For more accurate visual acuity testing of patients under 20 years of age whose pupillary muscles are difficult to relax, many doctors use a cyclopegic drug to dilate (relax) those pupillary muscles so that the eye cannot accommodate, or react to light. A simple test for visual acuity involves looking at an object through a pinhole opening. If the object seems much clearer through the pinhole, professional vision testing is indicated.

Measurement of visual acuity is only one of many different ways to test the eyes. For other, more specific tests, see **Color Blindness; Fluorescein Eye Stain; Fundoscopy; Pupillary Reflex; Strabismus; Tonometry; Visual Field.**

When performed: Whenever there is difficulty in seeing clearly;

as a screening test to detect vision problems before they become serious; as a way of following the course of various diseases such as diabetes; as part of testing candidates for certain occupations (flying).

Normal values: Although 20/20 vision (ability to see a standard-sized letter at 20 feet) is considered normal, up to 20/40 vision without the aid of glasses is still considered satisfactory (a driver's license is usually permitted with this vision). Normally an individual who can see clearly at 20 feet also can read tiny print at a distance of 14 inches. When two objects are in line, a patient with normal vision can discern their relative depth (which one is in front and which one is in back).

Abnormal values: Indications of impaired vision include the inability to read at least 20/40 size letters at a distance of 20 feet (some people may be uncomfortable without 20/20 vision), the inability to read small print at a distance of 14 inches or less, and the inability to perceive the relative depth of objects. Poor visual acuity may be inherited or it may be caused by bodily disease, by many drugs and poisons, and, of course, by problems of the eye itself such as glaucoma, cataract, eye muscle weakness, and any trauma to or around the eye.

Risk factors: None.

Pain/discomfort: None.

Accuracy and significance: Most tests for visual acuity, when selected to match the patient's age, are quite accurate and extremely significant when the result is the restoration of a patient's vision to normal.

VISUAL FIELD

Central visual field measurements test the eye's ability to see objects over a wide area (peripheral vision) while looking at a specific point. For example, when an individual looks straight ahead, he should still be aware of any object directly at his side. In most instances, an instrument called a perimeter is used to obtain exact measurements (perimetry) of just how far the eye can distinguish objects above, below, and to the side (called field of vision). Perimetry is usually performed after screening tests indicate a visual field defect.

By charting the visual field for each eye, the physician can diagnose various diseases of the brain, the nerves, and the retina. Blind spots (scotoma) can indicate disease; but the eye also has a normal blind spot (where the optic nerve enters the brain). Locating this specific area can verify the test's accuracy as well as detect patients who are faking vision problems. Hemianopia (inability to see the entire visual field) usually indicates a nerve or brain problem.

The simplest way to test visual field is for the doctor and patient to sit three feet apart and each look at the other's nose while the doctor moves his finger above, below, and to the side; both should see the fingertip at the same places. The physician may also mark the patient's visual margins on a tangent screen (a black felt sheet with circles on it) for a permanent record.

When performed: As a routine screening test in any eye examination; when there is suspicion of a brain lesion or an eye defect that cannot be corrected with glasses (such as glaucoma); when inherited eye disease is suspected; in instances of hysteria.

Normal values: The eye, looking directly ahead at a point, should be able to perceive a small (3 mm) spot (it may be a dot on the end of a stick or a tiny light) at an almost 90° angle to the side (away from the nose, toward the temple area of the head). The field of vision normally extends downward past the top of the cheek to an angle of about 65° and upward to an angle of no more than 45°. When looking straight ahead, the eye should also see anything not blocked by the nose. The normal blind spot (which has no visual receptors) is the point where the eye will not see the test spot when looking straight ahead. The patient's perceptions are recorded on a standard visual field chart.

Abnormal values: Any reduction in visual field is indicative of disease. The reduction may be in one direction only, or it may affect the overall field of vision in equal proportions (as with glaucoma or inherited degenerative retinitis). Most abnormalities of the visual field show specific patterns that aid in the diagnosis of a number of eye and brain lesions. Patients can have a markedly diminished field of vision and still have normal **Visual Acuity.**

Risk factors: None.

Pain/discomfort: None.

Accuracy and significance: The test is extremely accurate in revealing the extent of a patient's peripheral vision. When performed regularly the test allows the doctor to detect glaucoma and nerve and brain disorders at the earliest possible moment.

W

WET MOUNT

This test is considered the most important diagnostic procedure to detect the cause of vaginitis or vaginal discharge, and is often called the saline wet mount test, because it uses a saline (salt) solution. A cotton-tipped stick is dipped in saline and then mixed with a bit of vaginal discharge; it is examined immediately under the microscope for one of the three most common causes of vaginitis: trichomoniasis, a tiny parasite; candidiasis, a fungus; or hemophilus vaginalis, a bacterium that induces certain specific cell shapes. In some instances a woman's sex partner's urine is also examined to make certain that she is not being constantly reinfected (sometimes called a "ping-pong" infection) as a consequence of sexual activity.

When performed: When a woman complains of a vaginal discharge or experiences itching, rash, or swelling in the genital area.

Normal values: No evidence of parasites, fungus, or other than normal bacteria.

Abnormal values: Visible evidence of a specific cause of vaginitis.

Risk factors: None.

Pain/discomfort: None.

Accuracy and significance: The test is extremely accurate when it is properly performed. It is particularly significant when the source of the infection turns out to be the sexual partner, allowing for complete cure.

WHITE BLOOD CELL (Leukocyte, WBC)

The five different types of white blood cells (see **Blood Cell Differential**) are formed and stored in the bone marrow, thymus, lymph glands, and spleen. They are particularly important in fighting infections. The amount of certain kinds of white blood cells usually increases with infection or inflammation in the body, and these blood cells help destroy the causative agents. The white blood cell count is the total of the five kinds of white cells.

A drop of blood from the fingertip, heel, or earlobe (or blood drawn for other tests) is examined. White blood cells are also searched for in spinal fluid, urine, joint fluid, and mucus. The cells may be counted manually under a microscope, but most often they are counted electronically. (With modern equipment, the cells can be viewed on a TV screen and counted automatically.)

The Christmas tree test determines if the white blood cells are performing their function of killing bacteria. A tiny amount of blood is placed on a glass slide stained with a dye. Dead bacteria show up red; live bacteria, green (thus the name Christmas tree). Normally the slide shows very little green color; a lack of red-colored cells indicates the patient's inability to fight infections. The test takes only a few hours (older, similar tests take days).

When performed: When infection is suspected; in toxic reactions to certain drugs (sulfa drugs and other antibiotics, analgesics); in toxic reactions to chemicals or poisons (arsenic); in blood disorders, especially leukemias.

Normal values: There should be 5,000 to 10,000 white blood cells per cubic millimeter (cu mm). Children may have higher values.

Abnormal values: The total white blood cell count increases temporarily with most bacterial infections, blood disorders, emotional stress, hemorrhage, rheumatic fever, and burns. A white blood cell count may be falsely elevated when patients feel tense or embarrassed as a result of undergoing an examination. The white blood cell count decreases following ingestion of certain drugs or chemicals, after X-ray treatments, with malaria, typhoid, brucellosis, certain forms of leukemia, and virus and rickettsial infections. The count also decreases when the body produces autoimmune antibody globulins that stop white blood cell production.

Risk factors: Negligible (see general risk factors for blood testing).

Pain/discomfort: Minimal (see general pain/discomfort factors for blood testing).

Accuracy and significance: The test is a reasonably accurate indication of bacterial infection and such blood disorders as leukemia, providing the many extraneous factors that can affect the white blood cell count are considered. The test assumes a special significance when used to aid in diagnosing those diseases caused by viruses. Although blood cell counting is fairly accurate, recent evidence indicates that when the blood cells are counted by automated machines the results can show false lower-than-normal amounts. Thus, it is important to know when a blood cell count is performed by automated machines.

Z

ZINC

A deficiency of zinc, one of the trace elements (a mineral needed in the body in only minute amounts) has been associated with a number of disease conditions; in fact, in virtually all illnesses, blood zinc levels are usually decreased. Zinc is essential to certain enzyme functioning and the prevention or treatment of certain developmental abnormalities such as hypogonadism and growth retardation. One specific dwarfism condition can be corrected by adding zinc to the diet. On a normal diet, the average adult takes in approximately 10 to 15 mg of zinc per day. Oysters, herring, and whole grains are good dietary sources of zinc. Since zinc is necessary to produce testosterone and the testes are known to contain the largest amount of zinc in the body, the "old wives' tale" of oysters being an excellent treatment for male impotence would seem to have some basis in fact.

Blood serum, plasma, urine, and even hair are examined for zinc levels. For confirmation of a specific zinc deficiency problem, supplementary zinc is prescribed and the patient is clinically observed for reversal of symptoms.

When performed: When symptoms of abnormalities in taste and smell suggest a zinc deficiency; with prostate disease.

Normal values: Normally the level of zinc found in blood serum is 90 to 110 mcg per 100 ml; 0.5 mg per day is excreted in the urine.

Abnormal values: Lower than normal values of zinc are found in alcoholism, during pregnancy, after a heart attack, after surgery when there is poor wound healing, in liver disease, infections, cancers, prostate problems, sickle cell disease, and for a few hours after eating. Certain hormones may also lower zinc levels.

Higher than normal levels of zinc are found in patients who inherit a tendency toward hyperzincemia and also in certain metal workers (usually from breathing zinc fumes); an excess amount of zinc can cause drowsiness, dizziness and muscular incoordination.

Risk factors: Negligible (see general risk factors for blood testing).

Pain/discomfort: Minimal (see general pain/discomfort factors for blood testing).

Accuracy and significance: As little of the body's zinc supply can be measured in the blood or urine, the test is not noted for its precision. It can be of help, however, when other diagnostic tests fail to reveal the cause of illness.

Index of Cross References